Writing at the Margin

Discourse between Anthropology and Medicine

Arthur Kleinman

D0920718

UNIVERSITY OF CALIFORNIA PRESS

Berkeley / Los Angeles / London

GN
296
.K566
1995

h6 13172   PB

University of California Press
Berkeley and Los Angeles, California

University of California Press
London, England

not wd ff

Library of Congress Cataloging-in-Publication Data
Kleinman, Arthur.
    Writing at the margin: discourse between anthropology and
medicine / Arthur Kleinman.
        p.   cm.
    Essays reprinted from various publications.
    Includes bibliographical references (p.   ) and index.
    ISBN 0–520–20099–3 (cl.: alk. paper)
    ISBN 0–520–20965-6
    1. Medical anthropology—Philosophy.   2. Medical
anthropology—Methodology.   I. Title.
GN296.K566   1995
306.4′61′01—dc20   95–35194
                                                            CIP

Printed in the United States of America

    2   3   4   5   6   7   8   9

*For my colleagues in the field of medical anthropology,
so that conversations may continue.*

Man always travels among precipices, and, whether he will or no, his truest obligation is to keep his balance.

José Ortega y Gasset, *Man and People*

Contents

Preface

Without exception, these essays were written in the last five years. Like seed scattered in a strong wind, they have appeared hither and yon in journals, edited volumes, and encyclopedias. I wanted to bring them together in one place, fix them in the scholar's amber. Together the essays attain a critical mass that more adequately than when considered individually represents my efforts to write a cultural critique of biomedicine and to elaborate a social theory of the experience of suffering.

The Introduction, which takes stock of my own intellectual odyssey, and the final chapter, which examines the current state of the field through a long review of the new wave of book-length ethnographies in medical anthropology, were written expressly for this volume. Chapter 8 also has not been published before. Other published essays, to different degrees, have been revised to remove redundant materials and extend and deepen the analyses. Occasionally the rewriting has led me to alter an argument substantially. It has also allowed me to play with style, lightening what had been functional, even heavy prose.

Chapters 2, 3, and 4 have been most extensively rewritten. These three, along with chapters 5 and 6 to a more limited extent, have been enriched with materials from other essays, so much so that chapter 3 is really an amalgam. Chapter 7 has been altered only slightly.

Taken together, these chapters represent the directions my work has taken over the past few years. I have chosen not to include recent work with collaborators on international mental health policy because the major ideas are presented in a recent report, *World Mental Health*, and I have also not included articles with colleagues in which, even when my contribution was substantial, I was not the first author.

The Appendix includes a chronological list of my more relevant publications. Should the intrepid reader feel he or she can tolerate more, if it is not all there, at least what matters is listed—most of it in greatly different publications which reflect the wandering academic life of an interdisciplinary scholar who has written for many different audiences and who has also had the dubious habit of taking on too many responsibilities.

An academic year spent on sabbatical at the Center for Advanced Study in the Behavioral Sciences provided what every scholar would want: time, plenty of it; also the right mix of seriousness and release, and a disciplined yet playful colloquy. Writing nearly full-time in a study nestled close into the fold of a golden hill behind Stanford, among gnarled scrub oak, straight-standing royal palm, spreading cedar and cypress, and clusters of redwoods was everything I had imagined it might be three decades earlier, when, as an undergraduate, I came across the nameplate of the gateway, paused before the long drive that wound toward the crest, and wondered what kind of special place loomed up there in the hills. For the freedom and the re-experience of enchantment I acknowledge with gratitude the support of the Guggenheim Foundation, the MacArthur Foundation, and the Center and its sensitive and sensible staff. I wish also to thank Stanley Holwitz of the University of California Press for his editorial assistance and the two anonymous reviewers who made so many useful comments on the manuscript. All three have strengthened this collection, as has the copy editor, Linda Benefield, and Michelle Nordon, whom I also thank.

Several of the chapters collected below (chapters 5 and 7) were written with my longtime coworker Joan Kleinman, a sinologist, who also happens to be my wife. She has decided for her own reasons not to have her name appear as coauthor of the book. Nonetheless, her ideas, work, and influence in this volume are extensive. This book would not have been put together without her contribution. Chapter 7 was originally written as part of a research collaboration with colleagues in the Institute of Neurosurgical Research and the Ministry of Health in Beijing; while chapter 8 was written with Robert Desjarlais, with whom I have written several other pieces on political violence. I thank each of these collaborators for their contribution. Inasmuch as I have reworked each of these essays for this volume, I alone accept responsibility for their content. I thank Lawrence Yang for his assistance with the bibliography. I also wish to thank my marvelous assistant, Joan Gillespie, who has typed and retyped each of these chapters many times. I suspect she is ready to have me move on to new themes. With this collection, I feel that I have given a fuller form to my work in the context of my several disciplines.

Arthur Kleinman
Cambridge, Massachusetts

1

Introduction

Medical Anthropology
as Intellectual Career

At the Margin

This metaphor figures in the title of this collection in
several senses. It refers to the margin between anthropology and medicine as well as the boundary of Chinese and North American societies, where, since 1968, I have lodged my intellectual project. That is
also the space of my professional career, and it is where I have spent
much of my life. In the strict sense, the usage is accurate, even overcoded. Medical anthropology is at the margin of medicine; it is also at
the margin of anthropology. A medical anthropologist in the field of
China studies is also at the edge of the mainstream disciplines and
professional interests. To write about medicine in 1994, moreover, yet
not locate oneself in the national debate on health insurance in the
United States is surely to make a statement about another kind of
margin, a border that, as the *Oxford English Dictionary* puts it, differs
"in texture from the main body." This collection of essays explores
that difference in medicine's cultural, political, and phenomenological
texture.

The part of the definition of the margin that does not, I hope,
apply is "a condition which closely approximates to the limit below or
beyond which something ceases to be possible or desirable." To write

at the margin is not necessarily to be marginal in that sense of having nearly passed the limit of viability or relevance. It would be bizarre indeed for a professor who heads a large program, has received grant support for his research, and has chaired key committees in health and social science, to claim marginality.

That is not my meaning. Rather I find myself inherently uncomfortable in the center and suspicious of the mainstream, even when that specifies my professional location. A sense of resisting, going against the grain, comes naturally to me. Being at the margin, perhaps at times even at the brink, may, of course, be making a virtue out of necessity, because a quarter century's experience as an intellectual in American society has taught me that I am at the sideline, not in the center of the field of play. Perhaps as a Jew in this century of the Holocaust, I would have felt marginal in any case. Psychiatry, chosen as my clinical specialty after I had begun to study anthropology, is regarded as marginal by the rest of biomedicine, and a cross-cultural and international approach is regarded as marginal by many within psychiatry. Anthropology, as experience has taught me over the years, is in a truly crucial margin between the humanities and social sciences. Thus, for personal, ethnic, and professional reasons, the margin holds superabundant significance for me. But then again, if Anthony Giddens (1991:6–8) is right about the consequences of high modernity, marginalization—in his terminology, "the sequestration of experience"—is everyone's destiny.

Writing about the hidden relationship of autobiography to philosophy, Stanley Cavell (1994) concedes that the pitch or voice we come to arrogate as our scholarly life matures is made out of the special tone of genealogy and the body's remembrance of formative events. Of his own pitch of philosophy, Cavell writes, "I have seemed to myself fated to take what appears as eccentric perspectives, as it were to remain between, to refuse sides" (p. 13). Cavell sees his task as writing against the curious resistance of academic discourse to authorize this kind of self-referential writing. If Cavell is right on this point, and the psychiatrist within my anthropological skepticism intuitively feels he is, then my own fate was to possess what connects yet is utterly separate—sealed as a son who never met his father, a grade school student who bore two utterly separate family names, from two opposed sub-ethnic factions, one in public school, the other in religious school; a scion of a mysterious past about which his Victorian family was silent or whispered inarticulately, so that I had the extra developmental task of figuring out by myself, yet not announcing to others, lest they be hurt, what identified me, which therefore could not be authorized (or denied). My past prepared me to mediate, not through assimilation or accommodation, but by way of existential engagement with different interpretations of constructed differences. I occupy the margin not out of refusal to choose sides, but because I am bound to both, and at the point of their engagement, in order to discover what they are (or are not) and I am, or am not. Hence, the margins I seek are unfinished, even already overstepped, and become something altogether different out of interaction.

While references to neither safety margin nor profit margin (alas) seem apt in my experience, the idea of the liminal—the border as a threshold—does feel right. The margin between social theory and the ethnography of social suffering is a space of vital liminality. It is a threshold to something new, an unoccupied no-man's-land open for exploration. Such a liminal position can animate a critically different reflection on medicine and society, a reflection that need not accept things as they are. And it is in the liminality of illness, poverty, and other forms of human misery that I have found the subject that animates my world, morally as much as professionally. My subject itself, then, is the margin and the marginal.

I might even be willing to accept the idea of "marginal man" as an epithet, if the idea of living in two diverse cultures, two different ways of being-in-the-world—which has been my way of life—is separated from an insistence that it imply an "unstable character." This kind of lived marginality can stabilize; it can even bring a kind of solace.

I would remove the "of" in the cliché "of marginal importance," which derogates something that should be respected: namely, *a small importance.* Scholarship is probably almost always a small importance. Rarely is it an earth-shattering breakthrough. But that does not mean it is of no importance. Scholarship stands for changes and possibilities that widen the intellectual horizon as well as the space of experience. That makes its importance decidedly human. Over time, of course, small though those changes be, they do come to stand for a good deal.

Like scholarship, life itself is a small importance; we live in the margins and at the margin of great events and processes. Children, as the Chinese delight to put it, are little treasures, little happinesses, small importances. So are we all. It is also in the margin of disability that therapeutic change may make a small difference that becomes all the difference in a person's life, a small importance that repairs, rebuilds, reinvigorates, reinvents. Healing usually is transformative at this margin of small yet crucial changes in bodily processes that have social effects. Experience too is about small, local things: including edges and brinks. Unlike depth psychology, the phenomenology of social experience is about surfaces and boundaries, many small importances.

And then, of course, there are marginalia: marginal notes, references, footnotes, figures in illuminated manuscripts which literally step out of the text and come alive in the margin. Scholars spend much of their careers writing in the margin. We write on the sides of manuscripts sent to us for review, in the margin of published volumes, at the bottom of term and examination papers. I like this image because it so thoroughly connects scholarship with intellectual exchange and teaching. In the marginal notation, those three sides of academic experience really are inseparable. Many of the best moments in my scholarly career have come when I could use marginal notes to invite beginning students into a scholarly discourse that was new to them or when there was an occasion to deepen the work of advanced students. I have sometimes felt a moral meaning in the marginalia others have scribbled on my manuscripts, including this one, insisting that the treatment I had given a subject could be different and better. I have tried to bring such a purpose to my own reviews.

It is lamentable that scholarship in medical anthropology, as in anthropology and medicine generally, has thinned out in the current epoch of quick reading and even quicker communication. Authors summarize the contribution of a colleague in a phrase or single sentence, writing a slogan in place of an analysis. I have been treated to this unscholarly strategy more than a few times, and I confess to committing the same delict at least as frequently. While the misprision of the "anxiety of influence," as Harold Bloom put it, is understandable, poor scholarship does violence and should be unacceptable. In chapter 9, I end this book with an old-fashioned review of the literature, allotting enough space for the review of recent ethnographies in medical anthropology to give prominence to the words of the authors and to the intricacies of their interpretive work. I sought to create a review that would do justice to large, complex monographs, and thereby can contribute to the scholarship of the field I have come to inhabit, and that inhabits me. It is no accident that the review is placed last, at this volume's final margin. I could have extended even such a long chapter, and I emphasize that it is unfinished; it points toward the future as a responsibility. We have the responsibility to come to terms with the work of others by deepening disciplinary conversations that grow more substantial and interesting as we engage in their fullness other voices, other visions, and as we come to appreciate the dialogical relationship of our own writings to those of others.

Living and writing at the margin of the wider society, whether it is our destiny or not, can be a statement about what is and what is not at stake. Perhaps it is only at the margin that we can find the space of critical engagement to scrutinize how certain of the cultural processes that work behind our backs come to injure us all, constraining our possibilities, limiting our humanity. And perhaps it is at the margin, not the center, where we can find authorization to work out alternatives that can remake experience, ours and others. In that sense, I suppose, the margin may be near the center of a most important thing: transformation. Change is more likely to begin at the edge, in the borderland between established orders.

However I characterize it, this book of margins, a kind of oblique life of ideas, shares this much with Montaigne's (1992) essays. Like him, I could say, "I have no more made my book than my book has made me—a book consubstantial with its author, concerned with my own self, an integral part of my life" (p. 504).

Rereading My Work: Continuities, Discontinuities, Unexpected Change

My first publications in medical anthropology and in the China field appeared in a cluster in 1973. Reading the titles today—"Medicine's Symbolic Reality"; "Toward a Comparative Study of Medical Systems"; "Some Issues for a Comparative Study of Medical Healing"; "The Background and Development of Public Health in China"—I am lulled into a sense of abiding continuities.[1] The themes run like a deep current through my intellectual career. Yet, when I reread the prose itself, the sense seems not so much false as inadequate: an illusion disperses, yet leaves a residue, an ambiguous trace. For while the thematic consistency is there, the work of interpretation, even the writing, is very different.

The essays assembled in this collection are written two decades later. The involvement with Chinese society, with healing, with the culture of medicine continues. But the commitment to a comparative project has turned away from medical systems—the very idea, with its impression of formal structures and innate divisions, now makes me uncomfortable—toward the lived experience of suffering, toward medical practice as a historicized mode of social being-in-the-world. While I have no desire to deny my roots in symbolic anthropology, an equally long-standing concern with phenomenology has intensified. I also have moved from a preoccupation with symbolic forms and social structures, first toward subjectivity and then on to the intersubjectivity of experience. In my writings, narratives have supplanted models. Medical and psychological categories, which were not mine, have given way to the ethnographic interpretation of intersubjectivity, which feels more authentically like my own way of proceeding. In contrast to what is supposed to happen, and even to my original intention, I started, curiously enough, with comparisons and ended up more and more with particular contexts. All the while, it seems as if I am struggling to find new words and new images to evoke the same recalcitrant *processes* that cross between social space and the body.

In late 1979, the University of California Press published my first book, *Patients and Healers in the Context of Culture*. Widely reviewed and commented upon, the book seemed to take on a life of its own. A generation of graduate students, it seems, was trained in medical anthropology in criticizing its contents. Whereas its contributions perhaps were at first overemphasized, later on it was identified primarily by its shortcomings. Perhaps this is one socio-logic in the career of academic books. Now fifteen years later, new readings of *Patients and Healers* seem to have a more balanced ring.

The book surveyed much of what was then known about medical systems cross-culturally: a difficult but still possible task at the end of the 1970s. In the mid-1990s it seems both less feasible and less desirable. The book took a strong social constructionist position, a position I continue to hold. *Patients and Healers* also was animated by a clinician's gaze. While I was writing the book, I was in active clinical teaching and practice. Because over the past fifteen years I have spent much more time in the anthropology seminar room and much less in the clinic, that orientation is not as pervasive today. In 1980, I found a cognitive orientation useful as a method of relating collective and personal processes. By the mid-1980s, I no longer found that approach congenial, principally because it overcodes one side of experience at the expense of all else and because it fits too neatly into rational choice models that I reject. My emphasis had also shifted from disease categories as an epistemological object of cultural inquiry to the experience of suffering as the object of cultural ontology of everyday practices. And yet, *Patients and Healers* draws from a quarry that I have continued to mine for ideas and materials about patient and practitioner relations, the healing process, and medicine in Chinese society. The quarry itself can support certain mining procedures better than others. Chinese materials made the study of intersubjectivity and sociosomatics unavoidable. (See chapters 5, 7, and 8 below.)

Patients and Healers is motivated by questions large enough to found a career research program.

How can we elaborate an ethnomedical model that can systematically compare different culturally constituted frameworks for construing (and thereby, at least in part, socially constructing) sickness? What would such a model require to be able to provide both accurate phenomenological accounts of the way sickness is experienced in different cultural settings and valid hermeneutic accounts of divergent and perhaps conflicting interpretations of sickness? How would such a model enable us to make cross-cultural comparisons of the way therapeutic responses to the same type of sickness are differentially organized by various lay and practitioner perspectives? And how would an ethnomedical model determine which are the core clinical tasks of healers in different cultures? (p. 18)

This question framework sponsors a set of narrower questions to guide field research:

What are the range of clinical phenomena in a society? How do they relate to systems of cultural meanings and norms on the one hand and institutionalized social patterns of power relations on the other? How and to what extent do cultural conceptions about sickness influence the prevalence, morphology, and course of particular disorders? In what ways do differing cultural views of sickness and treatment affect clinical communication between patient, family, and practitioners? What are the culture-specific and universal characteristics of the healing process? (pp. 18–19)

Today, I am uncomfortable with the style and even the preoccupations of "models," ethnocultural or other, which imply too much formalism, specificity, and authorial certainty, but models were definitely in my mind in the 1970s, a residue of symbolic and structuralist readings. While I have moved away from models, I have continued to hold the notion that to examine the clinical realities constructed in different societies and institutions is no more a form of essentializing or naturalizing research enquiry than is the study of kinship, religion, or economics. Yet, I would not now write so readily about "core clinical functions," both because I am much less certain what they are and because the functionalism of the term rings an alarm. While much new research deepens our understanding of several of the empirical questions, it is impressive how little we still know about cultural constructions of the course of illness or about shared ingredients in the healing process.

In the late 1970s I could write with assurance,

The single most important concept for cross-cultural studies of medicine is a radical appreciation that in all societies health care activities are more or less interrelated. Therefore, they need to be studied in a holistic manner as socially organized responses to disease that constitute a special cultural system: the *health care system*. In the same sense in which we speak of religion or language or kinship as cultural systems, we can view medicine as a cultural system, a system of symbolic meanings anchored in particular arrangements of social institutions and patterns of interpersonal interactions. In every culture, illness, the responses to it, individuals experiencing it and treating it, and the social institutions relating to it are all systematically interconnected. (p. 24)

The idea and cadences are mine, but the blueprint is Clifford Geertz's; it now sounds too complete and deterministic. I, like many others, doubtless including Geertz himself, have become less impressed by systematic connections and more by differences, absences, gaps, contradictions, and uncertainties. Nonetheless, in spite of the postmodernist sensibility, the idea of a symbolic bridge connecting personal and social space has continued to animate my work right through the essays in the second part of this volume.

About "explanatory models" of patients and practitioners, however, I have become much more ambivalent. I introduced the idea as a way to get a rough-and-ready sense of what is at stake for participants in medical dramas. It has proved useful in the clinic, where time prevents even a mini-ethnography, and it continues to be applied in research. But I am extremely uncomfortable when it is misapplied as an entification of medical meanings as "beliefs": things that can be elicited, often outside the vital context of experience, like the reading of the pulse, and coded as a clinical artifact. I meant the explanatory models technique to be a device that would privilege meanings, especially the voices of patients and families, and that would design respect for difference. I intended it to be a *modus operandi* to get at what is at stake in suffering, but also a method that would give anthropologists and clinicians access to the working knowledge of the practitioner as the bearer of the cultural orientation of biomedicine and, therefore, the source of potentially dangerous misrecognitions. I saw explanatory models as a methodology for clinical self-reflexivity, for pressing against biomedical crystallizations, for laying hold of the sources of clinical miscommunication. I wanted to encourage the use of open-ended questions, negotiation, and listening, not the usual mode of clinical interrogation. Clinically the explanatory model approach may continue to be useful, but ethnography has fortunately moved well beyond this early formulation.

Patients and Healers's critique of biomedicine for its ethnocentrism, its reductionism, its essentialism, and its failure to engage the life world of patients recurs throughout my work, as in the next chapter. This I still take to be the deep cultural source of much that is untoward in medical education, research, and practice. Yet my approach to *somatization,* which was one of the sources of that critique, has changed greatly. I now find the earliest formulation too tied to a disease/illness distinction, which becomes less and less tenable, and it is overly psychiatric in its concern with the psychophysiology of depression and the psychodynamics of displacement. Somatization seems normative and often normal; it is not so much a substitution for something more basic as it is a basic way of being-in-the-world. The original formulation also seems to imply a too-simplified cognitive connection between language and the emotions. Since 1986, I have dropped "cognitive coping processes" from my vocabulary, and overall have become less interested in putative psychological universals. Somatic modes of experience now seem to me better understood in a sociosomatic language.

Patients and Healers's studies of family-based treatment, practitioner-patient interactions, and the healing process offer other examples of the continuities and discontinuities in my work. The research on family-based treatment explicitly argued that anthropologists had turned away from mundane everyday responses in the household and neighborhood in favor of more dramatic ritualistic treatments that sometimes provided an aura of exoticism to the study of healing. The study I undertook of the everyday experience and ordinary response to illness is one I still find important and, regrettably, this type of study is still less common than studies of ritual healing. However, the deconstruction of help seeking into distinctive types of resort, together with the diagramming of steps in the process of choosing a caregiver, now seem overly mechanical. Similarly, while the attempt to categorize practitioners with respect to time, space, institutional, and interpersonal aspects of clinical reality remains promising, I no longer am certain that the particular metrics I employed are all that useful. This is an approach I keep coming back to, however; I can't seem to let it alone. It is as if the rich ethnographic detail about clinical encounters itself points to there being something of importance there, but I am uncertain what it is or how best to study it.

Much of what I have to say about efficacy—that it is complex, differentially constructed, even contested in experience, and needs to be examined simultaneously on several levels—I can still stand behind. The question of efficacy hinges on the analysis of cultural processes that continue to be a tantalizing reminder of what medical anthropology might contribute. Yet, the study of a few detailed cases produced a conclusion about the performative bases of efficacy—namely, that cultural healing always must succeed, at least in symbolic terms—that a study I conducted more systematically with a larger sample from 1977 to 1979 contradicted. It is disconcerting that the later study continues to be one of only a few that systematically assess the efficacy of indigenous religious healing (see Kleinman and Gale 1982); it is as if medical anthropologists find it difficult to take on this particularly cherished convention. I too have occasionally misrecognized these findings in settings where alternative healing required defense. (But the review of recent research by Thomas Csordas [1994] and others in chapter 9 suggests important exceptions.)

Montaigne in his classic essay on inconsistency points out that

those who make a practice of comparing human actions are never so perplexed as when they try to see them as a whole and in the same light; for they commonly contradict each other so strongly that it seems impossible that they have come from the same shop. (1992:239)

"We are all patchwork," continues Montaigne. He could very well have said the opposite too. We are all also much of a whole. My own work seems to be both. I went through a sea change, though, shortly after publishing my second book, *Social Origins of Distress and Disease* (1986), which reported on a series of studies carried out to understand the relationship of neurasthenia, depression, and chronic pain to each other and to the Cultural Revolution and other major political and social changes in Chinese society. Before discussing the nature of that change, I should perhaps say something about *Social Origins*.

In writing that book I came to explicitly interpret somatization as an idiom of interpersonal distress, a form of cultural experience rooted as much in political and social structural processes as in clinical ones. Depression, too, I recast as a relationship between person and society. My intention was to deepen the study of "a sociosomatic reticulum (a symbolic bridge) that ties individuals to each other and to the local systems within which they live" (p. 1). I tried to position the analysis so that it centered on this sociosomatic dialectic between symptoms and society, because that is where Chinese cultural processes pointed. The goal was to develop a methodology suitable for anthropological psychiatry and psychiatric anthropology. Like *Patients and Healers,* this book combined narratives and numbers.

At the time *Social Origins* appeared, there were only a few other studies of political trauma, especially during the Cultural Revolution, in the Chinese mainland, a subject that in more recent years has attracted much attention. What started out as a study of the social origins and effects of illness quickly extended to social suffering generally, as it became apparent that neurasthenia was an experiential mode that expressed a variety of different forms of distress. Explicit comparison of neurasthenia, depression, and somatization in Chinese culture and in North American society organizes at least half of the book's chapters. Among the organizing questions were several that aimed at contrasting neurasthenia as cultural representation and neurasthenia as social experience:

- Did the collective behaviors and experiences subsumed by neurasthenia as an illness category decline in the West and greatly increase in China? Or is it a matter of change in the usage of the category?
- Is there something about rapid and disruptive societal transitions—both the long-duration transition of social structures toward modernity and short-duration political and economic transformation—that either place individuals at greater risk for the life problems and bodily dysfunctions mapped by neurasthenia, or that simply encourage the use of this idiom of distress? (p. 35)

This book also signals the beginnings of a shift from treating clinical depression in a disease model to placing it in a much broader array of social suffering. I examined the Western construction of a deep subjectivity in the person as a concomitant to the Western cultural program of rationalization and commented on its global influence. Critiquing psychologization in the West establishes somatization as a different object of enquiry. The body becomes a mediator between individual and collective experience. Affect, then, needs to be examined as the bodily nexus of social relational, moral, and political connections: "to feel is to value or devalue, to connect with or stand apart, to act in resistance to or to be paralyzed by our embodied social circumstance and our socially projected bodily experiences" (p. 177). Rehearsing my founding interest, I pressed an interactionist view, albeit one that now seems to me to make too grandiose a claim of systemization, in which "culture enters into this picture [of depressive emotion] as the *systematized relations* between physiology, feeling, self-concept, body image, interpersonal communication, practical action, ideology, and relationships of power" (p. 179).

Perhaps the book's most salient conceptual point is the idea of a double mediation of distress and disease based in the placement of local worlds as intermediary between the pressure of political movements and other large-scale forces of social change on one side and the resistance or vulnerability of individuals on the other. The second mediation is the body's transformation of that locally refracted force into normal and pathological reactions. How the two processes interconnect became the grounds for linking a social theory of sociosomatics to psychobiological theorizing.

But rather than return to a focus on individual cases, *Social Origins* builds upon the quantitative findings and narratives to discuss their societal implications. The antecedents of the report *World Mental Health* that my colleagues and I have recently prepared emerge from this reconstruction of the object of enquiry:

We now have in hand . . . persuasive findings that mental health problems—suicide, substance abuse, violence, admission rates to mental health facilities, depression and certain other psychiatric disorders, family pathology—also worsen under conditions of social disorder, economic deprivation, unemployment, forced uprooting, and migration. Like health problems in general, mental illnesses and social pathology have their highest prevalence among those in the lowest social statuses in society. . . . There can be little doubt that the health consequences of human misery are most effectively improved by significantly altering the macrosocial sources of misery. But the argument of this book is that local systems mediate the effects of macrosocial forces on groups and individuals, such that in settings of deprivation not all groups and individuals suffer to the same extent. Certain social statuses (the poorest, the least powerful, the stigmatized, those experiencing systematic discrimination) place individuals at greater risk for human misery and its health consequences. (1986:181)

This was my warrant to examine the Cultural Revolution as political violence and to study its traumatic effects on ordinary lives. The survivors' tales I included in the book, though, simply would not sustain too limited a sociosomatic framework. They insisted upon the broadest linkage between the political, the moral, and the bodily as a defining human process, an existential web of continuity and transformation. That conclusion continues to challenge my ideas, as can be seen in each of the chapters in the second part of this book.

I asked Comrade Yu if her major depressive disorder could have resulted from marital incompatibility and strain that only emerged once she and her husband were reunited. She disagreed with this formulation and offered an alternative one—a striking metaphor that I will now paraphrase. Suppose, she said, looking to the ground, you were climbing a mountain and this mountain was very steep and terribly difficult to climb. To the right and left you could see people falling off the mountainside. Holding on to your neck and back were several family members, so that if you fell so would they. For twenty years you climbed this mountain with your eyes fixed on the handholds and footholds. You neither looked back or ahead. Finally you reached the top of the mountain. Perhaps this is the first time you have looked backward and seen how much you had endured, how difficult your life and your family's situation had been, how blighted your hopes. . . . She ended by asking me if this was not a good enough reason to become depressed? (p. 141).

A study that had started as a clinical project had become a project on political violence. Research that began by avoiding the category fallacy—imposition of a classification scheme onto members of societies for whom it holds no validity (Kleinman 1977)—ended by running up against the experience fallacy—imposition of a mode of experience onto members of societies for whom it is not a valid form of life. The epilogue of *Social Origins* tellingly looks in two directions: toward the cultural phenomenology of bodily modes of suffering as collective experience and toward the cultural ontology of the relational self within the historical particularities of Chinese society. Both subjects—the one, cultural bodies; the other, historicized selves—are carried forward in the essays in this book.

The transformation that followed *Social Origins* originated in stories like that of Mrs. Yu which came alive in the margin of the research chapters as a subject larger than the technical one I had fashioned. These accounts stepped outside the pages. The narratives could not be confined by professional classification or clinical purposes; like pictures at an exhibition of the ordinary terror of life in a brutal time, they jarred me profoundly, these narratives whose suffering I could not shake off. They came to reshape the very way I heard patient accounts, the way I thought about my work. What, after all, was it for?

What constrained an overweening anthropological vision of culture so that space was left for the intimate and the intolerable? I followed up the existential turning point with a "popular" book, *The Illness Narratives,* written as much to exorcise these ghosts as for practitioners, patients, and their families. *The Illness Narratives* told stories of sickness much as they had been told to me. I felt a deep compulsion to retell these accounts, most of which came from my clinical experience in North America, not as "clinical histories" but as moral tales of remorse and regret, as social dilemmas, as cultural ironies, as the imperative stuff of myth and tragedy. For me that was a pivotal transformation of what my work was about and what I was for.

At that time, I was only partially interested in the theory of narratology and in the mechanics of narrative analysis, things I learned much more about after I had written *The Illness Narratives.* The book was an existential signifier along the peculiar path I had taken, and, in Michael Jackson's (1989) evocative phrase, that path had led "toward a clearing."

I had more or less found my subject, or it had found me. I worked to control my engagement with the anthropology of suffering in *Rethinking Psychiatry: From Cultural Category to Personal Experience,* where I tried my hand at restating the core questions of psychiatry (What is a diagnosis? Are psychiatric disorders different across cultures? How do cultures and social institutions create a social course of illness? How do they shape the practice of the psychiatrist? What is clinical efficacy?) so that my engagement with suffering did not overwhelm the cultural analysis and cross-cultural content that I needed to privilege to write a psychiatry book. But my preoccupation with the moral and political sides of suffering became so apparent in chapters 4 and 5 of *Rethinking Psychiatry*—the chapters covering the work of the practitioner and the performance of illness—that, at least on my rereading, those chapters overshadow a book that was supposed to have more to do with showing how a cross-cultural perspective alters our understanding of what is a diagnosis, a prognosis, a case, and a treatment.

In an ironic turn that almost became farce, as the second editor of a long-planned collection, *Psychosocial Aspects of Depression,* a carryover from my years at the University of Washington, I bridled at a technical construction of depression. My sensitive though dismayed coeditor, Joseph Becker, one of the great scholars of the subject, allowed me to write what amounted to a separate introduction that dissented from his and from the position of most of the authors whose work appeared in the collection. I could no longer write about suffering as the experience of clinical depression; I needed to write about depression as existential and collective, only one particular form of human misery, and not necessarily the same form in different places.

Essays Written in the Margin

That personal and professional scruple led to the composition of the essays on the experience of suffering in this book, where I, together with my collaborators, have had three goals. First, we seek to redefine suffering as an interpersonal or intersubjective experience: social suffering. The theoretical horizon carried over from the essays in part 1 privileges interactions in the social network, bodily metaphors of societal memory, struggles over the authorization of professional and political representations of suffering, and moral resistance to certain of those authoritative meanings. Out of these cultural processes, my North American and Chinese colleagues and I argue, comes a way of examining human problems that connects anthropological and other humanistic modes of interpretive enquiry with health and medical concerns. We struggle with a way of interpreting interviews, narratives, ethnographic observations, and even survey findings against this intellectual horizon. The materials we work with privilege the experience of recalcitrant human problems over which we have (and can have) only limited methodological grasp. Thus, we come up against the confines (and even the risks) of knowledge. Second, we put in that category of social suffering every different kind of human problem that creates pain, distress, and other trials for people to undergo and endure. We do not, for example, separate illness from political violence or from other forms of misery. Third, we have a go at applying different social theories to better understand the "social course" of suffering and its consequences for social life: for example, how chronic illness possesses not a "natural" but a social history, a moral career. As a corollary, we attempt to balance a therapeutic language with one that privileges normative moral conditions along with societal action.

Our chief concern is neither methodological nor metaphysical. We seek to explore experience—social experience—as a stream of enquiry. Does sustained engagement with the varieties of experience of suffering offer distinctive possibilities for research? Is the framework of social analysis of experience a significant way of doing social theory? Are there potential implications for policy, programs, and practical interventions? Is social suffering a coherent subject? Does our approach to this subject, preliminary as it is, offer novel and interesting insights? The reader can also explore alternative ways of pursuing certain of these, and related, questions that other medical anthropologists have followed, a large and illuminating landscape that I survey in the book's third and final part.

In future, I will explore in more depth the closely related question, What difference does it make—for theory, for research, for policy, and for societal ethics—to change the border between a social and a health problem? Now pulling the edge toward the social side, later on pushing it toward the medical margin—does that disclose a comparative advantage for "medicalization" of human misery under certain conditions, or for "socialization" under others? The moral, the political, and the medical are culturally interrelated, but how do we best interpret that relationship and its implications? This question is partially touched on in this book. I expect it to receive an even broader intellectual horizon in my work in future.

The collection of essays, in sum, follows the three tracks along which my writing has traveled over the past several years. The first (chapters 2–4) is a path of critical engagement with the deep cultural processes that are at work within biomedicine. I extend that cultural critique from biomedicine's peculiar form of rationality and process of knowledge generation to its influence over the development of medical ethics, which originates in the same deep cultural strata. That sovereign cultural frame also shapes the issue of "objectivity" as a central motif in international public health. My concern in each case is not with the obvious strengths that result from this core cultural orientation. That story is overcoded in Western society and now globally. Rather I seek to show how these cultural processes limit biomedicine as a science and form of practice. Ethical deliberation about health care and medical technology is also seriously constrained. And the very way the closely related fields of international medicine and social development go about formulating policy and programs for low-income societies suffers from the same source of limitations.

Perhaps the chief contribution that medical anthropologists can make to these fields is not primarily to assist them to engage different ethnic groups and function more effectively in different social contexts—the

sort of things we are most often asked to do. Instead we need to specify how it is that the very processes that make biomedicine effective as
a technical rationality and strategy of social action so often become,
under particular political and economic regimes, a barrier, at times the
major barrier, to improved health and good-quality health care. A
chief predicament for the professions concerned with human problems
is how they contribute to those problems or, at least, limit the potential for solutions. Cultural critique is anthropology's contribution to
understanding that predicament. Yet there is also a limit to the useful-
ness of this genre of argument. At some point medical anthropologists
must propose alternative ways of responding to human problems. How
I view one of those alternative methods is the subject of the second
half of chapter 3.

The second track (chapters 5–8) is the project on social suffering
that I have just described.

The last track (chapter 9) is an attempt to survey the current phase
of medical anthropology through a close reading of recent ethnographies that represent the varied approaches to the field that attract my
interest. That reading occasionally returns to reconsider the other two
tracks, but more often it covers other grounds. Even if it were feasible,
and it isn't, I would not want to define which are the central questions
in this greatly diverse field, but rather to applaud that diversity, and
to delight in the many reasons why heterogeneous interests and approaches make medical anthropology salient for some of the more significant quandaries in the human sciences in our epoch. This review
can be read as my appreciation of the field.

Thus, the three parts of this book follow the logic of cultural critique, alternative formulations, and fuller exploration of recent ethnographic contributions.

This is not the place to write in detail about my engagement with
things Chinese. I will only say that Chinese culture has absorbed a
large part of my interest and my life for almost three decades. It provides a powerful alternative reality to North American society for thinking about social and health changes. Indeed, Chinese culture has had
a deep influence in my family life and sense of purpose.

Almost all of the chapters in this book give evidence of how broad
that influence runs in my intellectual horizon. From intersubjectivity
to embodied memory of secret history, from moral emotion to political trauma, from Chinese medicine to *shenjing shuairuo* (neurasthenia
as Chinese collective experience) and family responses to epilepsy, the

engagement with things Chinese has pulled me toward certain topics while pressing me away from others. And that is a strength as well as a limitation, not least of all because, while I have had collaborative projects and consultantships elsewhere, my firsthand engagement with social experience is so dictated by the contrast between Chinese and American society that my approach is principally bicultural. That is a condition the reader will need to bear in mind.

And now, to the writing itself—a far better measure of where my work is headed than anything I could conclude here. For I concur with Cavell that "the world calls for words, an intuition that words are, I will say, world-bound, that the world, to be experienced, is to be answered, that this is what words are for" (1994:116).

PART ONE

The Culture of Biomedicine

2

What Is Specific
to Biomedicine?

The Forms of Medicine

Medicine is nothing if not multitudinous. Defined in the broadest sense, as organized health practices and decisive therapeutic choices, medicine is so widespread around the globe that it is surely a universal in human organizations. In the same way that suffering can be said to be a defining quality of the experience of being human, happily not the only one but still one among a rather limited number, so too is medicine, as organized therapeutic practice (the process of care), fundamental to what is deeply human in experience amid the vast diversity of cultural worlds. At this high level of abstraction, it is even possible, if admittedly old-fashioned, by drawing on a large array of sources cross-culturally, to distinguish several general characteristics that would appear to be shared by nearly all social systems of healing, be they forms from small-scale nonliterate societies, low-income peasant societies, or even high-income industrialized states.

These shared characteristics have emerged in comparative studies of medical systems as distinctive as traditional Chinese medicine in Taiwan and China, Ayurvedic medicine in India and Sri Lanka, Bakongo medicine in Zaire, popular healing among laymen and laywomen in Brazil and North America, and professional biomedical practice in Japan, Russia, and Tanzania. They include:

Revised and expanded version of a chapter published in the *Encyclopedia of the History of Medicine,* ed. W. F. Bynum and Roy Porter (London: Routledge, 1993).

22   THE CULTURE OF BIOMEDICINE

- categories by which health is normalized and illness diagnosed
- narrative structures that synthesize complaints into culturally meaningful syndromes
- master metaphors, idioms, and other core rhetorical devices that authorize practical therapeutic actions and the means by which their "efficacy" is evaluated
- healing roles and careers
- interpersonal engagements that constitute a vast variety of therapeutic relationships and modes of clinical interaction
- an immense panoply of therapies, seamlessly combining symbolic and practical operations (a distinction comparative research now shows is no longer tenable), whose intention is to control symptoms or their putative sources [see Kleinman 1980:207–208; 1988b:114–116, for earlier formulations of this list]

Of course, even more impressive is the multitudinousness, the polymorphous differences that distinguish the healing traditions of societies from each other; even the intrasocietal diversity must be for the comparativist disquietingly substantial. Different sociopolitical and cultural-moral contexts contain distinctive, sometimes astonishingly distinctive, forms of medicine. Thus, the gift exchange relationship central to the social structure of Hutu and Tutsi ethnicities in Rwanda shapes therapeutic interactions with native healers that are based upon ongoing, personalized transactions of intersubjective reciprocity (Taylor 1992). This generic mode of social transaction, to be sure, is modified, even nullified, by ethnic conflict and political rearrangements, as the horror of genocide and the forced uprooting of millions in that tragic nation demonstrates. The commodity-based exchanges and institutionalized professionalism in Taiwan constrain the Confucian pattern of paternalistic yet personalized patient-doctor interactions in traditional Chinese medicine, and even in urban shamanism, just as powerfully as they constrain that high-technology society's other bureaucratic practices and commercial activities. As a result, therapeutic relationships get transformed in the direction of an increasingly impersonal consumer archetype. Those relationships are responding as well to the pressure brought by a society-wide democratization movement and the advocacy of groups who support patient rights. That pressure for change marks surgical practice in Taiwan as distinctive from the work of surgeons in China. The movement from authoritarian toward more egalitarian relations in Taiwan, however, is not simply the result of internal changes in its political and moral economy; a powerful global movement is remaking concepts of self and norms of interaction associated with the current stage of late industrial capitalism. The effects of that movement are also intensified by the international politics of democratic rights.

In contrast, the commune and work-unit forms of forced socialist communalism in China, prior to 1980, inflected medical practice like all other professional activities with Maoist priorities—rural, anti-elite, low-technology, yet governed by centralized command and glorifying traditional Chinese medicine's integration with biomedicine while ruthlessly suppressing religious healing—that Taiwan has never experienced. Barefoot doctors, now called rural primary care physicians, and near universal health insurance—alas, now a thing of the past under the surging performance of China's new market economy, the fastest growing on earth—changed attitudes toward doctors and even the actual form of patient-practitioner communication as much as they altered access to biomedical knowledge and technology. Now, under the regime of economic reform, organized rural health care in China has broken down in some areas; it has become less salient in all but prospering rural areas; and the emphasis is all on high-technology practice in urban centers and medicine as a business (World Bank 1992; Henderson 1990). In Taiwan and China at the moment both high-technology biomedicine and folk healing practices are flourishing for a variety of reasons, some shared but some different, owing to those societies' very different recent histories.

There is, then, no essential medicine. No medicine that is independent of historical context. No timeless and place-less quiddity called medicine. Practitioners of Chinese folk religion, *wu-is*, in mainland China and Taiwan may be classified as folk healers, but their attitudes and experiences and those of their patients are distinctive. Malay *bomohs*, Taiwanese *tang-kis*, and Temiar *halaas*, in the same vein, all may be called shamans, yet the concrete ideas they enact and the rituals they conduct are as distinctive as the religious, kinship, and ethnomusicological traditions of their very different societies (Laderman 1991; Kleinman 1980; Roseman 1991). It is simply misleading to relate these types of healers to some idealized notion of the essentials of shamanism. So much variety, indeed, is apparent even within the same society that to talk of "traditional healing," or for that matter "biomedicine," as if the term denotes a homogeneous social reality would be a serious misapprehension of ethnographic descriptions. Bonesetters, herbalists, *bomoh*s, practitioners of traditional Chinese medicine and of Ayurveda, and a wide variety of fortune-tellers and other healers make traditional healing in Malaysia a mélange of immense pluralism. Meredith McGuire (1988) has shown that almost as rich a diversity can be found among indigenous practitioners of "alternative medicine" in suburban America, where experts in various massage and dietary therapy, herbalists, acupuncturists, practitioners of many different Asian traditions of martial arts, Christian Science healers, pentecostal healing ministries, charismatic Catholic healing groups, rabbinical practitioners, astrologers, fortune-tellers, iridologists, chiropractors, homeopaths, naturopathic physicians, spirit mediums, self-styled shamans, hypnotists, together with a bewildering variety of lay psychotherapists compete among themselves and with biomedical practitioners for what must seem to them a dwindling supply of patients. Americans spend billions of dollars on these alternative practitioners (Eisenberg et al. 1993).

Among Bolivians living in the Andean highlands, medical pluralism matches the social pluralism of Catholic mestizos, rural Aymara Indians, and Methodist Aymara town-dwellers. Choice of a particular diagnosis and treatment becomes an idiom for negotiating ethnic and social class position and for claiming access to nonmedical resources, such as land, jobs, urban residence (Crandon-Malamud 1991). Medicine, then, like religion, ethnicity, and other key social institutions, is a medium through which the pluralities of social life are expressed and recreated.

Biomedicine is as plural as primary care practitioners in public clinics, rehabilitation experts in a veterans medical center, heart surgeons in a for-profit hospital chain, nurse practitioners in a rural hospital, psychoanalysts in office practice, social workers on the streets with the homeless mentally ill, and military health planners. The same therapeutic technologies—say, for example, particular pharmaceuticals or surgical equipment—are also perceived and employed in different ways in different worlds. Biomedical practitioners in Thailand and India have been shown to be strongly influenced by local norms (Weisberg and Long 1984). In technologically advanced Japan, the technology of transplantation in surgery is constrained by an unwillingness to accept brain death as the authorization to remove life supports and "harvest" organs for donation (Lock and Honda 1990; Ohnuki-Tierney 1994). Thus, in cross-cultural perspective it is as valid to talk about the cultural processes of *indigenization* of biomedicine as to implicate the *globalization* of local therapeutic traditions.

Nonetheless, for all the heterogeneity, there is something special about biomedicine and its Western roots, something that decisively distinguishes it from most other healing systems cross-culturally such as the great literate systems of traditional Chinese, Hindu, or Islamic medicine and, of course, the vast array of local healing activities described by ethnographers. So that it is appropriate to essay an answer to the question put to me by the editors of the *Encyclopedia of the History of Medicine*: What is specific to Western medicine?

I shall employ the term *biomedicine* in place of "Western medicine," however, because it emphasizes the established institutional structure of the dominant profession of medicine in the West, and today worldwide, while also conjuring the primacy of its epistemological and ontological commitments. These are what is most radically different about this form of medicine (see Lock and Gordon 1988). "Western medicine" is an unsatisfactory appellation for other reasons as well. Biomedicine has long been a global institution. It is no longer only Western, either in its site of practice or even in its locus of knowledge production and technological innovation. "Cosmopolitan medicine," a term fairly widely displayed in anthropological publications (see Leslie 1976; Leslie and Young 1992), also seems less suitable than "biomedicine" because a surgical clinic can be in the distant, parochial periphery or in the cosmopolitan metropole. Moreover, this term doesn't carry the epistemological and ontological resonances that I seek to privilege. "Allopathic medicine," though perhaps widely understood in South Asia, seems to me an unaccustomed term, less well known to readers elsewhere. Intriguingly, if you ask biomedical professionals what word they would use to describe their field, most will say, in a powerfully succinct usage that does capture a sense of the hegemonic self-perception that has become almost a caricature worldwide, "Why not just call it medicine!"

For the purposes of this essay, I will not concern myself with Western religious healing, nor will I deal with other local folk and popular therapeutic practices that are indigenous to the West. The focus on biomedicine will also exclude alternative Western therapeutic professions or heterodox movements among biomedical professionals, such as osteopathy, homeopathy, chiropractic, naturopathy, or most recently "holistic medicine." Furthermore, I will primarily deal with the biomedicine of knowledge creators (researchers, textbook authors, teachers) and of the high-technology tertiary care institutions that dominate medical training and that represent high status in the profession.

I recognize that the working knowledge of the ordinary practitioner treating routine health problems in the community is more complex and open to a wider array of influences. I also know that nurses, technicians, and receptionists perform much of the work of biomedicine, especially through contact with patients and families.

What I seek to emphasize is the scientific paradigm that is at the core of the profession's knowledge-generating and training system (Freidson 1986; Good 1994). Charles Rosenberg, a distinguished historian of American medicine, rightly notes that biomedicine has long contained a holistic, humanly oriented stream that in the nineteenth century prior to the development of microbiology even had very substantial influence (personal communication, 1985). I concur, yet this is not what I take to be the dominant stream in biomedicine today, even though there are impressive examples of patient-centered care and psychosocially sensitive practices in many primary care settings.

Holistic medicine is another problematic term that challenges cultural interpretations of biomedicine that are too simplistically dichotomous. Several decades ago it was widely employed as a code word to juxtapose empathic, psychosocially valued care against medical practices that were viewed by biomedicine's critics (both outside and within the profession) as mechanistic, reductionistic, and inattentive to the human concerns of patients and families. In the 1980s, holistic medicine came to be appropriated by a commercial movement that brought together biomedical practitioners who advocated the use of various nonorthodox interventions (massage, dietary treatments, herbalism, acupuncture, and so forth) and mind-body techniques that had not been widely applied in primary care with a variety of alternative practitioners. Also included in this successfully marketed hotchpotch are New Age spiritual practices. Holistic healers today compete for patients with standard biomedical professionals in primary care practice who themselves have authorized greater use of interviewing and psychotherapeutic treatment skills—a clear example of the influence of a powerful American cultural shift on biomedicine. Anne Harrington (in press), a historian of German science, points to the deeply troubling appropriations by the Nazis in the 1930s of the metaphor of holism to stigmatize reductionistic medical science as "Jewish," and therefore evil, and to tighten ideological connections with the romanticized yearning for organic healing associated with German folkloric traditions.[1] This disturbing irony can serve as a useful caution before I embark on my own cultural critique of "biomedicine." Phenomenologist critics of technological society, such as Martin Heidegger, Arnold Gehlin, and Kitaro Nishida, attacked the inhumanity of the instrumentality of technical rational procedures in the professions, yet they themselves were involved with the Nazis or other fascist movements. This is a sobering reminder of the substantial potential for abuse in the appropriation of criticisms of biomedicine. Holism in the 1930s started out as a movement to reform medicine, but ended up legitimizing political authority and disguising the real sources of oppression. Its salvational ideology came to serve truly dangerous political interests—a serious, destabilizing concern.

Monotheism, Monotypic Order, and Medicine

The historian of Chinese medicine Paul Unschuld (1988) claims that the monotheism of the Western tradition has had a determinative effect on biomedicine, even as it is practiced in non-Western societies, which distinguishes it in a fundamental way from Asian medical systems. The idea of a single god legitimates the idea of a single, underlying, universalizable truth, a unitary paradigm. Tolerance for alternative paradigms is weak or absent. The development of concepts is toward proof of the validity of a single version . . . of the body, of disease, and of treatment. Alternatives may persist in the popular culture or at the professional fringe, but they are execrated as false beliefs by the profession as a whole, not unlike the accusation of heresy in the Western religious tradition. Conversion, ostracism, or sometimes more final solutions result from what William Connolly (1993) has called the Augustinian imperative for complete agreement on what constitutes a universal moral order.[2]

At least, this is the way biomedicine and the Western tradition look from the non-Western world, inasmuch as Chinese and Ayurvedic medical traditions tolerate alternative competing paradigms, seem less troubled by the uncertainty of human experience, and are more pluralistic in their theoretical orientations and therapeutic practices (see Zimmermann 1987; Leslie and Young 1992). Thus, *yin/yang* theory, the macrocosmic-microcosmic correspondence theory of the Five Elemental Phases (*wu xing*), and differing operationalized views of the body in acupuncture and practical herbology exist simultaneously: they are made compatible in the practitioner's practice. Even biomedical concepts and practices are accorded a legitimate place in traditional Asian medical systems. Indeed, in India and Sri Lanka, traditional practitioners of Ayurveda often integrate biomedicine into their practice (Waxler 1984). No viewpoint ever dies out completely; alternatives are never totally discredited (Unschuld 1985).

Drawing from a deep Western cultural source, philosophy in ancient Greece developed a central distinction between reality and appearance. Behind the changing surface of events rests an immutable structure: an immortal soul, an imperishable form of beauty, a universal and objective justice. Rational principle and objective truth can be discovered within the uncertain particularities of changing phenomena. Truth, beauty, and the good are absolute and transcendent (Ames 1991).

"The signal and recurring feature of Western civilization which emerged to dominate the development of its philosophical and religious orthodoxy," according to R. T. Ames,

> was the presumption that there is something permanent, perfect, objective and universal that disciplines the world of change and guarantees natural and moral order—some originative and determinative *arche*, an eternal realm of Platonic *eide* or "idea," the One True God of the Judeo-Christian universe, a transcendental strongbox of invariable principles or laws, a geometric method for discerning clear and distinct ideas. The model of a single-ordered world, where the unchanging source of order stands independent of, sustains, and ultimately provides explanation for the sensible world is a dominant . . . assumption in this tradition. (1991:xv)

Similarly, William Connolly (1993a:176) sees the Augustinian imperative as "the demand that there must be an intrinsic moral order we can pursue and strive to embody in our conduct and politics." The imperative leads to the castigation of anyone who does not accept or fit within this monolithic moral order as an alien Other. The imperative's legacy is easily visible in the justification for stigmatizing and suppressing religious heresies, in the brutal oppression found in colonial movements of conquest, and more prosaically, but equally fraught with dangerous consequences, in the antagonistic absence of respect accorded theories that fall outside the Western canons of philosophy and science. Drawing upon Foucault's late turn to an ethic of "agonistic respect" among plural perspectives in increasingly plural societies, Connolly (1993b) argues for a postmodern moral code that engages with great seriousness alternative and even opposite formulations that broaden the horizon of interpretation, which, in the absence of single truths and universal fundamentals, is all that we can expect. The pressure of alternative medicines is yet another aspect of the pluralism of everyday life that is perceived as threatening by those unwilling to imagine health, illness experiences, and health care as having plural sources, forms, and outcomes.

The entailments of monotheism and monotypic order foster a single-minded approach to illness and care within biomedicine that has the decided advantages of pushing medical ideas to their logical conclusion, uncovering layers of reality to establish with precision what is certain and fundamental, and establishing criteria against which orthodoxy and orthopraxy can be certified. Indeed, from the point of view of Asian medical systems, the uniqueness of biomedicine lies in its method (of controlling existing data within its theory, and the resultant predictions and determinations based on past facts) (Nakayama 1984). While the more fluid complementary paradigms of Asian medical systems appear weak in methodological rigor and not conducive to empirical testing, their categories do represent the active ordering of relationships and have produced many positive practical results. The Chinese approach, for example, is grounded within the phenomenological constraints of time, place, and phase. Though excessive flexibility perhaps limits its function as a science, it presents a serious attempt to codify complex, subtle, interactive views of experience into therapeutic formulations that claim contextual rather than categorical application. Chinese medicine attempts to account for psychological and ecological and even moral as well as corporeal phenomena through the use of dynamic, dialectical, process-oriented methods of clinical appraisal (Nakayama 1984).

Biomedicine differs from these and most other forms of medicine by its extreme insistence on materialism as the grounds of knowledge, and by its discomfort with dialectical modes of thought. Biomedicine also is unique because of its corresponding requirement that single causal chains must be used to specify pathogenesis in a language of structural flaws and mechanisms as the rationale for therapeutic efficacy. And particularly because of its peculiarly powerful commitment to an idea of *nature* that excludes the teleological, biomedicine stands alone. This medical value orientation is, ironically, not nearly as open to competing paradigms or intellectual play of idea as is "hard" natural science, whose ways of approaching problems in cosmology and theoretical physics seem more flexible and tolerant than the anxious strictness of the "youngest science," though ultimately natural science too discloses certain of the same consequences of monotheism.

The "hard" and the "soft," signifiers of a deep cultural logic in North America, figure importantly in biomedicine. Talk and cognitive activities more generally are "soft"; procedures that enter the body (various scopes, surgical operations) are "hard." Psychiatry and the primary care fields (pediatrics, general internal medicine, family medicine) are "soft"; the surgical subspecialties are "hard," as is pathology, which is responsible for autopsies and the interpretation of tissue specimens removed during surgery. The "soft" specialties are the ones that provide the lowest incomes and attract the most women practitioners, whereas the "hard" specialties attract more males and often make them rich. The "soft" specialties increasingly use procedures that make them "harder"; dermatology, which is a specialty of internal medicine, has added surgery to its practice; psychiatry in our time has tried to transform itself, with mixed effects, in a "biological," therefore "harder," direction.

What this cultural logic connotes is a set of deep dualisms between male and female, mind and body, strength and weakness, wealth and poverty, aggressive technological actions and what is popularly held to be more passive styles of intellectual behavior that are metaphors of social structural divisions. Perhaps because biomedicine's rise in status and power took place only since the Second World War, these symbolic markers can be read as residual signs on the road of professional success indicating what succeeds in North America.

In the biomedical definition, *nature* is physical. It is knowable independent of perspective or representation as an "entity" that can be "seen," a structure that can be laid bare in morbid pathology as a pathognomonic "thing." Thus, special place is given to the role of seeing in biomedicine, which continues a powerful influence of ancient Greek culture. Biology is made visible as the ultimate basis of reality which can be viewed, under the microscope if need be, as a more basic *substance* than complaints or narratives of sickness with their psychological and social entailments (Good 1994; see also chapter 9). The psychological, social, and moral are only so many superficial layers of epiphenomenal cover that disguise the bedrock of truth, the ultimately natural substance in pathology and therapy, the real stuff: biology as an architectural structure and its chemical associates. The other orders of reality are by definition questionable (see Gordon 1988).

This radically reductionistic value orientation is ultimately dehumanizing. That which has been so successful a blueprint for a biochemically oriented technology in the treatment of acute pathology places biomedical practitioners in some extremely difficult situations when it comes to the care of patients with chronic illness; situations that, as I review below, offer obdurate resistance to affirmation of the patient's experience of the illness; to understanding the social, psychological, and moral aspects of physiology; and ultimately to the humane practice of medicine. These extreme situations are not created, at least with the same regularity and intensity, by other healing traditions described in the cross-cultural record.

This point is almost certain to be challenged. There is a feeling, not without justification, that anthropologists romanticize traditional healing systems, while at the same time we use that imagery to criticize biomedicine. I myself have raised this concern (Kleinman 1988a). S. X. Li and Michael Phillips (1990), among others, have reported serious abuses by indigenous healers in China. Others have been critical about how effective traditional forms of healing are for serious illnesses. Yet, after reviewing the most recent ethnographies of traditional healers, I am impressed that when these practitioners have been appropriately studied, they seem not to be constrained in the human quality of their care in the same way as are their biomedical colleagues. Rather, the structures of traditional healing—gift exchange relationships, local cosmologies, teleological narratives of suffering, aesthetic codes of performance—center on human experience and its modes of interaction. Less advantaged in technology, they are more advantaged, it seems, in humanity.

Disease sans Suffering/
Treatment sans Healing

Through its insistence on the primacy of definitive materialistic dichotomies—for example, body/mind (or spirit), functional/real diseases, and highly valued specific therapeutic effects/discredited nonspecific placebo effects—biomedicine presses the practitioner to construct *disease,* disordered biological processes, as the object of study and treatment. There is hardly any place in this narrowly focused therapeutic vision for the patient's experience of suffering. The patient's and family's complaints are regarded as *subjective* self-reports, biased accounts of a too-personal somewhere. The physician's task, wherever possible, is to replace these biased observations with *objective* data: the only valid sign of pathological processes, because they are based on verified and verifiable measurements (see Murray and Chen). This is a view from a depersonalized nowhere. Thus, the doctor is expected to decode the untrustworthy story of *illness as experience* for the evidence of that which is considered authentic, *disease as biological pathology*. In the process, the doctor is taught to regard experience—at least the experience of the sick person—as fugitive, fungible, and therefore invalid. Yet by denying the patient's and family's experience, the practitioner of biomedicine is also led to discount the moral reality of suffering—the experience of bearing and enduring pain as a coming to terms with that which is most at stake, that which is of ultimate meaning, in living—while affirming objective bodily indices of morbidity. The result is a huge split between the constructed object of biomedical cure, which is the dehumanized disease process, and the constructed object of most other healing systems, which is the all-too-humanly narrated pathos and pain and meaning-directed perplexity of the experience of suffering (see Jackson 1989; Keyes 1985; Schieffelin 1985; Seremetakis 1991:115, 127, 201).

Thus, biomedicine constructs the object of therapeutic work without legitimating suffering. The physician correspondingly is hedged in in the role of healer. Providing a meaningful explanation for the illness experience is something physicians (and especially those in marginal subdisciplines such as psychiatry and family medicine, which are more oriented to experience) undertake, so to speak, with both hands tied behind the back. They may succeed in using their personality and communicative skills to assist patients; yet they do so, as it were, against the grain, against the consequences of the biomedical orientation for their training and the care they give. Meaning itself is not configured as a central focus or task of medicine. Because it eschews teleology, the very idea of a moral purpose to the illness experience is a biomedical impossibility. That serious illness involves a quest for ultimate meaning is disavowed. Because of distrust of qualitative interpretations and concomitant emphasis on quantitative data, the biomedical framework accords no legitimacy to values. Hence, the practitioner of biomedicine must struggle to practice competent biomedicine, while at the same time searching for some extra-biomedical means to authorize the professional's empathic response to the patient's and family's moral needs to have a witness to the story of suffering, to find support for the experience of illness, and to collaborate with others in the struggle to fashion a meaningful interpretation of what is at stake for them in their local world. It should not be at all surprising then that hospitals and clinics are frequently criticized in the current period of consumer interest in patient-centered care for their dehumanizing ethos. Indeed, it is a tribute to the stubborn humanity of practitioners and to the recalcitrant influence of extra-professional cultural traditions that these institutional settings are not *routinely* experienced as such.

That practitioners of biomedicine are trained in a radically skeptical method that ought to diminish the placebo response in their care is another curious corollary of this peculiar healing tradition, whose many positive aspects also must not go underemphasized. No other healing tradition possesses a significant fraction of the specific therapeutic interventions for serious disorders that biomedicine includes. Nor does any other tradition so distrust and choose not to elaborate nonspecific therapeutic sources of efficacy that are associated with the rhetorical mobilization of the charismatic powers of the healer-patient relationship that persuade patients and families to believe in successful outcomes and thereby enact scenarios of efficacy (Brody 1977; Davis 1992; Frank 1974; see also Lindholm 1990 for a review of the social basis of charismatic power).

And yet, the anti-placebo skepticism of the current phase of biomedicine must also be balanced by its associated antiauthoritarianism, which contrasts strikingly with the paternalism of most traditional forms of healing. Skepticism about charismatic healing power also has protected biomedical professionals from the charges and countercharges of charlatanism that abound in folk healing. Egalitarianism, demystification of medical terminology, informed consent, and concern for patient rights, in cross-cultural perspective, are also rather peculiar to the contemporary Western tradition of biomedicine. The virtues, such as they are, which Max Weber attributed to bureaucratic rationality—namely, generalizability, quantification, prediction, efficiency, quality control—are now ingrained in the professional structure of biomedicine; they have become a central part of industrialized society's processes of risk management (Freudenberg 1993), a protection against institutional recreancy, including medical malpractice. Their absence in folk healing systems makes those practices problematic. The rub, of course, is the iron cage of technical rationality which, as Weber also saw, would come to replace sensibility and sensitivity (Wrong 1976: 247). Sadly, though tellingly, the professionalization of Asian medical systems has not infrequently led in the same direction (see Leslie 1976).

The Progressive Search for Powerful Operations

Biomedicine instantiates the Western tradition's idea of progress. The profession's self-portrait is of a scientific, technological program that is continuously progressing in acquisition of knowledge and especially in deployment of powerful therapeutic operations. Even in spite of limited progress over the past decade in the treatment of the chronic diseases that contribute most significantly to morbidity and mortality indices, biomedicine's self-image emphasizes awesome technological capacity to operate on the patient's organ systems. There is only a poorly articulated notion of an absolute limit to that progress. Organs can be transplanted; limbs can be reimplanted; life-support systems even "prevent" death. It is not surprising, then, that therapeutic hubris is commonplace. Physicians are not educated to feel humble in the face of sources of suffering that cannot be reversed or to place limits on the utilization of powerful technologies.

Indeed, suffering is converted into technical problems that transmogrify its existential roots. Thus, even the approach to ethical issues in the final period of terminal illness, the period when patients are near death on vital support systems, becomes a question not of constructing a good death but of the technical details of "advanced directives." What starts out as an effort to respect the patient's and family's perspectives on a moral crisis, ends up as yet another instance of medicalization—the application of the expert's rational technical rules to deeply human experience. Contrast this social dynamic with the way suffering is valued in rural Greece as moral experience and social commentary (Seremetakis 1991:231).

Whereas in traditional Chinese medicine, as in many other indigenous non-Western healing systems, and earlier within healing professions in the West, the idea of progress is balanced by the idea of regress, and suffering and death are viewed as expected and necessary, biomedicine again represents a radical therapeutic departure. Powerful actions—from the earlier era of heroic medicine with its therapeutic purging and bleeding to our own epoch's stopping and starting the heart, delivering a short sharp shock to brain matter, changing the genes of cells to enhance anti-cancer drugs, or cloning a human embryo—not restraint (still less the appropriate use of inaction, John Keats's negative capability), iconically represent biomedicine's imagery of efficacy. Where Asian medical systems invoke weak treatments as virtuous because they are held to be "natural" and noniatrogenic, biomedicine's therapeutic mandate, for which all pathology is natural, emphasizes decidedly "unnatural" interventions. The historic Western interest in nature's healing powers has passed out of the mainstream of the profession and into homeopathy and the New Age fringe.

The burden on the practitioner of the idea of progress and the expectation of powerful operations is considerable, not least of all through the astonishing claim that ultimately death itself can be "treated," or at least "medically managed." Another aspect of this ideological influence is the euphemization of suffering, which becomes medicalized as a psychiatric condition, thereby transforming an inherently moral category into a technical one. An existential experience of tragedy and loss is reconstructed as a professionally managed experience of major depressive disorder. The consequence is a further transvaluation of therapeutic values (see Bottero n.d.). As a result, practitioners of biomedicine are in a situation unlike that of most other healers: they experience a therapeutic environment in which the traditional moral goals of healing have been replaced by narrow technical and bureaucratic objectives. Psychotherapy, in like fashion, whatever else it is, cannot be construed as a quest for the spirit, though that is what its felt experience is for many (see Shweder 1985; Csordas 1994). That physicians are depicted in the popular culture—for example, in TV soap operas—as inextricably engaged in the moral dilemmas of patients and communities does not disqualify these points. Rather it reflects the still considerable power of the social world to moralize experience, even that biotechnical version which claims independence from parochial passions.

The reader should not misunderstand this criticism. I do not indict the recognition and treatment of a depressive disorder when that psychiatric diagnosis and the antidepressant medications and the psychotherapy it entails can be clinically useful to someone who is in deep distress with a treatable psychiatric condition. But I do call into question the practice through which the suffering that is part of a serious medical disorder is reinterpreted as a depressive disease so that an institutionally efficient technical fix (a drug) can be applied in place of a humanly significant relationship of witnessing, affirming, and engaging the patient's and family's existential experience. That the professional transmogrification of suffering is problematic is seen when virtually all seriously ill medical inpatients can be made to fit the American Psychiatric Association's official diagnostic criteria for major depressive disorder on account of the psychophysiological effects of their heart disease or cancer or their treatment. That is, the suffering of patients has been medicalized, inappropriately, into a psychiatric disease.

One other curious particularity of biomedicine, at least in its present-day form, is its anti-vitalism (see Canguilhem 1989). Traditional Chinese medicine, like many traditional systems of healing, centers on the idea of a vital power—in this instance, *qi* (energy that is associated with movement and breath)—at the core of health and disease. The source of disease is not traced to a particular organ, but to the disharmony of *qi* circulating in the body. Ayurvedic medicine shares a somewhat similar conception of vital breath. Other examples are the *semangat* (spirit of life) and the inner winds (*angin*) of indigenous Malay medicine; *isibo*, the flowing force in the health conceptions and practices of Rwandans; the unbounded souls of the Temiars; *binona*, the vital force that makes the body breathe, among residents of Sabarl Island off of the coast of Papua New Guinea; and, of course, the *pneuma* of ancient Greek medicine (Trawick 1992; Laderman 1991; Taylor 1992; Roseman 1991; Battaglia 1990; Canguilhem 1989).

Vitality, efficacy, power—all capture the idea of a force of life that animates bodies/selves. Biomedical materialism decries a vital essentialism. Things are simply things: mechanisms that can be taken apart and put back together. It is a thoroughly disenchanted worldview. There is no mystery, no quiddity. Therapy does not, cannot work by revitalizing devitalized networks—neuronal or social. There is no magic at the core; no living principle that can be energized or creatively balanced. Thus, though depression feels like soul loss to many persons around the globe, there is no possibility of a lost soul in psychiatry. The devitalized imagery also negates the therapeutic powers within patients, denying efficacy to lay experiences of regaining force and overcoming fatigue. About power, an ordinary human experience, biomedicine is silent.

The attention of biomedicine is also focused on the solitary body of the individual sick person because of Western society's powerful orientation to *individual* experience. That illness infiltrates and deeply affects social relations is a difficult understanding to advance in biomedicine. Population- and community-based public health orientations run counter to the dominant biomedical orientation, which takes for its subject the isolated and isolatable organism. In contrast, African healing systems see illness as part of kinship networks and healing as a kinship or community effort (Janzen 1978; Taylor 1992). The foundation of biomedical psychiatry is also a single self in a single body. The presence of alternative selves or dissociated mental states, measured against this norm, is interpreted as pathology. Trance and possession, which are ubiquitous cross-cultural processes that serve social purposes and can be interpersonally useful, are invariably cast by biomedical nosologies as pathology. In contrast, the sociocentric orientation of various nonbiomedical forms of healing will strike many people as a more adequate appreciation of the experiential phenomenology of suffering cross-culturally.

Bureaucratization, Professionalization, and Medicalization

Because of its long development under the powerful regimen of industrial capitalism, biomedicine is the most institutionalized of the forms of medicine. When, early in this century, the doctor practiced his craft in the living room, kitchen, and bedroom of the patient, or in his own home, the intimate domesticity of suffering with its always concrete implications for treatment loomed much larger in the considerations of the practitioner. Now, at the close of the century, biomedicine is practiced in bureaucracies, whose effect is profound (see Rosenberg 1987; Rothman 1991; Starr 1983; Kleinman 1988b:77–107). The rule of efficiency governs the lived time of the patient-practitioner encounter. Regulations control practice, transforming the doctor into the "provider" of a "product" that is advertised, marketed, and sold. Care is commoditized. Even the lived space of practices is standardized to conform to the institution's blueprint for functionality. The technical rationality of the institution, its priorities and norms, shape biomedicine. The physician is a bureaucrat; the patient is a user, a consumer of the institution's services. The very imagery of care constructs an industrial logic to its delivery and evaluation, reducing the moral space of the career of illness and of the work of doctoring to a minimum.

Equally momentous for biomedicine is its professionalization. Professional "autonomy" conflicts with bureaucratic hierarchy and control. Yet it, too, sets standards that normalize training and practice. If the former, bureaucratization, routinizes efficiency, the latter, professionalization, routinizes the "quality" of care. With these two powerful masters, which concentrate the influence of the state, no wonder the patient's and family's influence on the process of care is weakened. The degree and intensity of specialization is unprecedented. The object of diagnosis, treatment, and prognosis is fragmented into a single organ system. Expert judgment is further legitimated over and against that of the generalist and the layperson. And many other practical consequences make biomedicine different from other systems of healing, even where they are practiced in the same political economy.

Biomedicine is not just any bureaucracy and profession, it is a leading institution of industrialized society's management of social reality. Biomedical constructions of the various forms of human misery as health problems are reinforced by societal regulations that can influence all sectors of experience, from the courts to the workplace to the household. This process of *medicalization* is responsible for certain of biomedicine's most controversial attributes. Biomedicine's sector of influence continues to grow as more and more life problems are brought under its aegis. Alcoholism, other forms of drug abuse, obesity, aging, child abuse, violence—all are presently articulated as health (or mental health) conditions. Medicalization leads us to search for their genetic roots, to assess other individual risk factors, and of course to quest for treatments; yet, while giving the sufferer the sick role, medicalization can stigmatize as well as protect; it can institute a misguided search for magic bullets for complex social problems; and it can obfuscate the political and economic problems that influence these behaviors.

No other therapeutic system can exercise this degree of power, because no other has become so powerful a part of the state's mechanisms of social control. Indeed, in industrialized societies biomedicine along with the mental health, disability, and welfare systems that closely relate to it arguably have become the major form of social control. This may in part reflect the fact that in the current phase of global political economic transformations, so-called disorganized capitalism, the social and behavioral problems listed above seem to be a direct effect of those societal changes that profoundly influence human conditions.

Thus, in the postmodern state, biomedicine has come to serve a major political mission. Its taxonomy holds legal and regulatory significance. Its definitions of what is a problem and how it should be treated carry greater public legitimation than that of most other professions. Its role in the political economy is at the center of the fastest growing sector, which threatens to surpass all other public expenditures. No other healing system is so central to social reality or so wrapped up in the leading political and economic issues of the time. Thereby has biomedicine, at least in the West, outstripped its own professional autonomy and become inseparable from the state.[3]

Another example is the passive acceptance by biomedical practitioners of a patient-doctor relationship that is just another instance of consumer-client interactions characteristic of a market economy. This economistic model represents the diffusion into biomedicine of the most powerful contemporary model of relationships throughout North American society. It runs counter not only to patient-doctor models in other societies' healing traditions but even to the earlier model of a fundamentally moral relationship in medical practice that characterized North American society until several decades ago. It is either another actual instance of the continuing conversion of gift relationships that are based in interpersonal moral meaning to commodity relationships that are based in impersonal market mechanics in the transnational political economy, or an example of the sentimental power of this image of change in social relations to conjure back a world that we are losing and feel the need to mourn.

As a result, the very purposes of biomedicine have been altered from an earlier emphasis on the deeply human grounds of illness and care, shared by other healing traditions, to economic and political priorities, which are the chief influences on research and teaching, organization and delivery of services, and the day-to-day work of the practitioner. Regulation via bureaucratic rationality, state control, and the "market" is remaking biomedicine in North America, for example, into an institution that has more in common with many of the other agencies of government and business bureaucracies than it does with healing systems in other societies or with the biomedicine that existed even a quarter of a century ago.

Much that we have associated with biomedicine at present can also be found in other institutions in technologically advanced societies. To that extent, the sources of these qualities are societal rather than strictly medical. It could be argued, too, that in certain aboriginal Australian societies and other hunter-gatherer/hunter-horticulturalist groups the conceptions of illness and healing are so central to the core religious system that they play as predominant a role in the societal order. These points, however, do not lessen the special significance that biomedical institutions have come to hold in postmodern states.

In this sense, at least, biomedicine is, like other forms of medicine, both the social historical child of a particular world with its shape of experience and an institution that has developed its own unique form and trajectory.

3

Anthropology of Bioethics

The editors of the *Encyclopedia of Bioethics* invited me to write an entry on the anthropology of medicine. They asked that, in a short space, I show readers what the discipline is about and why it might be significant for ethical questions in medicine. I first sent them a contribution that centered on a cultural critique of bioethics. Clearly taken aback by the sharpness of the criticisms I leveled at mainline bioethics, they wrote me that my piece did not sufficiently describe the range of anthropological contributions, nor did they think I was up-to-date on new directions in medical ethics which already met the criticisms I had voiced. I returned to my study to read the more recent articles and books in bioethics that they recommended. That exercise did little to change my interpretation. However, I did take up their suggestion to expand the review of anthropological writings on ethical questions in health and medicine. The corpus is not huge, but it is larger than could be surveyed for a short article. Also, at the editors' request, I made the foolhardy effort to say something in a few paragraphs about medical anthropology more generally. Because it was so thin, that section is deleted from this chapter.

I also have added a response to several recent works by ethicists who have engaged multiculturalism. How could this not become a serious topic, if ethics is to have any pretense of being pertinent to North American as well as global realities. Indeed, I admire the effort

An earlier version of this essay appeared under the title "Anthropology of Medicine" in the *Encyclopedia of Bioethics,* revised edition, edited by Warren T. Reich (New York: Simon & Schuster Macmillan, 1995). It is reprinted here by permission of the Publisher.

of at least those few ethicists who have struggled to treat culture seriously, even if it is a very late trend. Nonetheless, I find the result highly inadequate. Culture, it would seem, is appropriated in ethical discourse largely in an outmoded manner aimed at creating a caricature—cultural relativism—that is meant to act as a foil for continuation of the business of moral philosophy as usual. Not a promising way to engage the multiple cultural realities of everyday life, one would have thought. There is one important exception. Prior to engaging the subject of this essay, I had not encountered feminist writings on moral philosophy. Several recent contributions to this genre I find impressive and consonant with the anthropological argument I advance below.

Admittedly this critique of bioethics as it is usually formulated is strong and fundamental. The reader will rightly wonder, therefore, why I end the essay by outlining an anthropological approach to clinical applications of bioethics. Because I am myself a physician as well as an anthropologist, I share the orientation of many patients and health professionals that the vexing question of human meanings, including contradictory ones, in the face of painful suffering and untimely death, is crucial to health care. If there is to be any approach in bioethics that engages culture, surely it needs to be one that deals with clinical realities, and to do so it must be anthropologically informed. This will not be a panacea; ethnography has its limits. But it is one way to begin engaging the multicultural reality of our times. That is my only defense for first indicting bioethics, and then turning around and offering a glimpse of what an anthropological turn in bioethics might look like.

Anthropological Contributions to Medical Ethics

Because of their concern with meanings and with the practical rationality of everyday decision making, anthropologists have written about the ethical sides of health and health care. For example, Peter Kunstadter (1980) and Morton Beiser (1977), an anthropologically oriented psychiatrist, have discussed the ethical quandaries that development projects, including medical ones, introduce into poor rural Asian and African communities, because the services they provide are temporary and therefore raise expectations that eventually will be frustrated. Mary-Jo Good and colleagues (Good, Hunt et al. 1992) and Margaret Lock and Christina Honda (1990) have examined the moral exigencies of truth telling about cancer and determining death in biomedicine in Japan, respectively. The Japanese may be moving to accept brain death as a formal marker of death and thereby facilitate transplantation, which has been seriously constrained by Buddhist prohibitions, but it is, as Lock (1995) shows, a movement strongly contested by many Japanese who combine religious values about death with the most advanced technological orientation, rendering the distinction between "tradition" and "modernity" meaningless. Emiko Ohnuki-Tierney (1994) has shown that neither in Japan nor in North America can transplantation be modeled as some would suggest as a gift-of-life, since gift exchange relations require reciprocity in sociomoral transactions that is simply lacking in transplantation. Rather the technology of transplantation leads to a series of cultural transgressions of categories of human/nonhuman, rationality/emotion-spirit, self/ other, and life/death that remake what is regarded as "natural" into a new cultural form, a way of being-in-the-world that is unacceptable to many in Japan and which, Ohnuki-Tierney argues, would, if more fully understood in the West as a fundamental alteration of social experience, be unacceptable to many there as well.

Paul Unschuld (1979) analyzed the corpus of Confucian writings and traditional Chinese medicine texts that deal with ethical issues and concluded that professional and cultural values of the literati class colluded to control the medical marketplace. I found that healers in Taiwan in the 1960s and 1970s, regardless of whether they were practitioners of traditional Chinese medicine, shamans, or physicians, were viewed by patients as morally ambiguous: powerful to heal; yet potentially an immoral source of economic gain and even of evil power (dangerous technological procedures or sorcery) (Kleinman 1980: 240, 284, 303–304). This finding of the moral ambivalence central to therapeutic practice would appear to be rather widespread cross-culturally.

Horacio Fabrega (1990), writing explicitly about an ethnomedical approach to medical ethics, sees biomedicine's ethical preoccupations growing out of Greek medicine and from the popular morality of ancient Greece. Following many anthropologists, he asserts that in small-scale, preliterate societies, healing and religion are inseparable; thus, medical mores are tied to ritual and theology in those societies. In larger-scale societies—both peasant and industrialized—the specialized division of labor leads to practitioners who are popularly viewed both as healers and as financially benefiting from the healer's trade. Fabrega argues that all the great non-Western traditions of healers use ethical injunctions to control access to practice and to proscribe certain alternative healers as quacks. He asserts that "bioethics" is a unique version of medical ethics made possible by the development of biomedicine with its knowledge of biology and powerful biological applications. Michel Foucault (1973:199) presses this argument beyond morality. "Bio-power," in the Foucaldian vision, links morality and science and clinical practice through cultural shaping of experience with the deep political processes that are at work in society (Foucault 1980). This line of analysis has been influential among many medical anthropologists.

Writing for a collection of social science treatments of bioethics, Richard Lieban (1990) focuses on anthropological interest in the ethical aspects of controversial local practices such as female circumcision, differential assistance to male children, and the lack of regulation of folk healers as examples of what anthropologists can offer to bioethical issues in international health (see also Grunebaum 1982; Kleinman 1982; Korbin 1981; Scheper-Hughes 1987). Allan Young (1990), in the same volume, demonstrates the value of ethnographic accounts of the hidden moral dimensions of psychiatric practice in a Veterans Administration unit for treating combat-related posttraumatic stress disorder (PTSD) among ex-soldiers who served in the Vietnam War. He argues that what is a psychological crisis or psychiatric disorder in the individual patient for mental health professionals is, for the anthropologist, a crisis or disorder in the politics and ethics of the social body. Vietnam veterans with PTSD are not so much victims of a mental disorder as they are victims of (and victimizers through) the political decisions of their nation's leaders. (See also Young 1993, as well as the review of Young's forthcoming ethnographic monograph in chapter 9 below.)

What characterizes anthropological approaches to ethical issues, in medicine as well as other fields, is an emphasis on questions that emerge out of the grounded experiences of sick persons, families, and healers in concrete contexts. Anthropologists have critiqued universal ethical propositions just as their professional perspective has led them to critique universalist models for economic development. In place of universalist and essentialist propositions—philosophical or political economic—anthropologists, always more the intellectual fox than the hedgehog,[1] have focused upon the interactions of everyday life, the societal hierarchies and inequalities they represent, and the moral issues in which they are clothed. Thereby, anthropologists examine ethics at the intersection of the social logics of symbolic systems, social structures, and historical events (Augé 1984).

In the anthropological imagination, a distinction can be made between the "ethical" and the "moral" (Kleinman and Kleinman in press-a). Whereas ethical discourse is a codified body of abstract knowledge held by experts about "the good" and ways to realize it, moral accounts are the commitments of social participants in a local world about what is at stake in everyday experience. Both are cultural processes, but of a somewhat different kind. As Richard Shweder (1991: 186–240) shows in his research on moral experience in an Indian city, the canonical code becomes part of the moral socialization of children in families. But it is appropriated into settings where many other things are at stake in the local politics of interpersonal relations (Kleinman and Kleinman 1991). While the ethical code informs those relationships, the struggles over differing interests mean that everyday life is inherently a moral process. Moreover, the contexts and process of moral life involve more than individuals. They also are based in collective orientations, social resources, and intersubjective action. The moral is actualized not only in subjective space but in social transactions over what locally matters, often vitally so, such as marriages, family, work, child rearing, education, religious practice, health, death. Conflicts among different priorities create moral dilemmas as social problems that require action.

Thus, Kenneth Read (1955) writing about the Gahuku-Gama of Papua New Guinea, argued that moral issues for this preliterate group were experienced primarily as problems and prospects in social relations. The moral was not viewed as a distinct sphere separate from the rest of life. For the Gahuku-Gama, "moral judgement is largely of a contextual character" (p. 281). They will not judge moral situations in the abstract in which they have not been personally involved. Like the Chinese, the Gahuku-Gama's image of the person is of a relational self, a self in which social interactions, rather than the rationality and free will of the person, are the basis for moral judgment. Not violence in the abstract, but particular violent acts in particular contexts are evaluated morally. For Chinese, morality is also about persons interacting in concrete situations; it is about the subordination of the self to that social relational context of experience, and indeed about the person's use of an interpersonal idiom of what matters—for example, filiality, social favor, "face"—to find and express his or her moral choices (Fei 1992). For the Chinese, social order is more important than self-realization; self-restraint takes precedence over self-expression. But these are not to be understood as different beliefs or values; rather they represent distinctive ways of being-in-the-world, different modes of social experience. As Brad Shore (1990), working in Samoan society, notes, moral decisions are driven not by abstract values but by practical dilemmas, such as whether to respond to a leader's anger toward a kinsman with meek acceptance or violent resistance. Moral decisions, then, represent conflicts between distinctive forms of social action. This is quite a different appreciation of what morality is about than that held by mainstream moral philosophers or theologians in the West.

The remainder of this chapter will adumbrate what anthropological studies tell us about health, illness, and care that is relevant to the practice of bioethics. I start with a cross-cultural critique of leading bioethical orientations and commitments. Thereafter, the more substantial anthropological contributions will be reviewed, followed by a brief discussion of the possibilities and problems with a culturalist orientation. From the anthropological perspective, bioethics shares with biomedicine several inveterate cultural orientations that constrain the standard approach to moral issues in patient care. The anthropological approach, therefore, becomes particularly useful because of the comparative understanding it brings to the analysis of unexamined biases.

The Culture of Bioethics

The *ethnocentrism, psychocentrism,* and *medicocentrism* central to biomedicine are also prominent in the standard bioethical approach (see Lock and Gordon 1988; Weisz 1990). Most philosophically trained bioethicists draw on what Charles Taylor (1990) describes as the orthodox sources of the self in the Western philosophical tradition. The canonical works in that tradition, from those of the Greeks down to the present, assume an individuated self, set off from the collective—single, unchanging, self-defining. Thereby, inter alia, the autonomy of the person is claimed to be a paramount value along with the ideas of justice and beneficence. From a cross-cultural perspective this intellectual commitment, which is reinforced by the deep subjectivism of the Western tradition, is problematic.[2]

Few members of non-Western societies—such as China, India, Japan, or most Southeast Asian or African societies—hold the view that the isolated individual is the locus of responsibility for therapeutic choice, or that therapy should work to maximize the individuation of the sick person, or that personal authenticity is fundamental to health and well-being.[3] Rather, there is usually a paramount sociocentric consensus in which social obligation, family responsibility, and communal loyalty outweigh personal autonomy in the hierarchy of ethical principles. The self, even where it is held to be uniquely individual, is viewed as sociocentrically enmeshed in inextricable social networks, intimate ties that make interpersonal processes the source of vital decisions. More than 80 percent of the planet's population live in cultures outside of North America and Western Europe or are members of minority ethnic groups outside of the Euro-American majority. Among these cultures and ethnic groups, autonomy is often a much less significant value than other, more sociocentric ones. That bioethics is able to avoid serious engagement with these alternative ethical traditions must represent one of the last tenacious holds of ethnocentric mentality. Indeed, there is evidence that bioethicists are commencing such decentering cultural engagements (Jennings 1990; Loewy 1991).

The idea of the primacy of the individual is still, however, the unexamined cultural presumption of Westernization. Spread throughout the globe first by the military successes of colonialism and later by the even deeper forces of postindustrial capitalism, whose commercialism is built so intimately around individual desires, the imagery of individualism has become the international order's central value orientation of "rights." Thus, the very goals by which societies, Western and non-Western, are evaluated turn on the commitments of Westernization. International trade, international peace and security negotiations, international development policies, and international health programs prioritize this value commitment of personal entitlements or consumer preference as fundamental to the enterprise of *globalization*. For this reason, it is not enough to contrast Western and non-Western ethical claims, since the very idea of ethics privileges the Western view of the individual. Globalization brings the deep subjectivism of that ethical design with it, so that that social transformation itself becomes a process of hypertrophic individualization. Simply comparing individualism with sociocentricism, therefore, can never be sufficient. It is essential to make the critique of individualism central to a cross-cultural approach to ethics.

I do not dispute that the international movement on behalf of individual rights frequently has had a laudable effect, especially in highly repressive polities, but I am challenging the cultural assumptions it carries, which too often work to reinforce some of the more negative aspects of Westernization, such as its Orientalism—the construction of cultural difference as an irreducibly alien otherness—and its dissolvent effects on other social modes of experience.

Similarly, from an ethnographic perspective, the use of abstract concepts of justice and beneficence as universal ethical principles in decision making is suspect. This in part restates the cultural critique of individualism. Yet there is also a failure to take into account the local worlds in which patients and practitioners live, worlds that involve unjust distributions of power, entitlements, and resources. It is utopian, and therefore misleading, to apply the remote principles of justice and beneficence to ordinary clinical problems, unless we first take into account the brutal reality of the unjust worlds in which illness is systematically distributed along socioeconomic lines and in which access to and quality of care are cruelly constrained by the political economy. The most desperate and predatory of these contexts would seem, by their very characteristics, to exist somewhere beyond the reach of justice. Beneficent social contracts may make good philosophical theory, but they deny empirical experience in local social worlds. The moral philosopher's "beneficent community" (Loewy 1991), which in ideal terms is supposed to be concerned with minimizing the suffering of its members, is a charming romance; no one lives in such a utopian state. Rather, real communities are sources of suffering at least as much as sources of assistance. They do not contain explicit social contracts, but they are filled with explicitly different interests, status differences, class divisions, ethnic conflicts, and factionalism. Little is gained by installing utopian virtues; in fact, much is lost, since illusion and exaggeration distort the practical realities among which most people on earth live.

Again, this is an instance of the danger of ungrounded analysis of the sources and consequences of ethical choices. On several occasions, I have heard philosophers, who otherwise have made trenchant criticisms of epistemological and ontological positions, intervene in a discussion of medical ethics by adverting to the example, "Suppose a

Martian were to land on earth and were faced with such a problem."
The illustration is probably meant to explode conventional common
sense. Yet it is a telling method to introduce into the discussion of a
particular case, because it so cavalierly steps outside the powerful constraints of real worlds. Happily or unhappily, there are no Martians;
there are unfortunately, many, many humans on our planet who are
faced with desperate choices in situations in which *the concrete details*
of historical circumstances, social structural constraints like limited
education and income, interpersonal pressure, and a calamity in the
household or workplace are at the core of what a dire ethical dilemma
is all about. Thus, there is a deeply troubling question in the philosophical formulation of an ethical problem as rational choice among
abstract principles, because that problem is always the burden of a
man or woman's particular world of pain and possibility. That social
space contains the flows, routines, and everyday practices of moral
experience. Ethnography, biography, social history, literature—all contain methods of entering those local social spaces. They see moral issues from the inside of experience, where those issues appear as they
are so often lived, as fragments, incoherences, things beyond one's
control. Intellectualist perspectives that universalize ethical choice are
flawed, at least for application to serious conflicts in the human experiences of illness and care, because they are, in a fundamental way,
groundless. "Psychocentrism" also installs mind-body dualism, a near
fatal flaw for an approach to the experience of illness and treatment.
But discussion of that intellectual cul-de-sac would overwhelm the
other issues I need to review, and so I set it aside for another occasion.

The third "centrism"—medicocentrism—emerges from comparative
studies as yet another bias of standard bioethical discourse. Like biomedicine, bioethics begins with professional definitions of pathology.
The disease viewed as pathological physiology along with the professionally authorized array of treatment interventions define the clinical
situation (see Canguilhem 1989). The experience of illness is made
over, through the application of ethical abstractions such as those
described above, into a professionally centered construct that is as
divorced from the patient's suffering as is the biomedical construction
of disease pathology. The patient's experience is appropriated by the
rational technical categories of professionals.

The bioethicist, of course, is supposed to take into account the patient's perspective. But by and large the contextually rich, experience-
near illness narrative is not privileged. It is reinterpreted (also thinned

out) from the professional biomedical standpoint in order to focus exclusively on the value conflicts that it is held to instantiate. The categories of patients and indigenous healers are provided with only limited legitimacy; they are after all called "folk," a derogatory label. If they can be restated in the abstract terms of the standard bioethical orthodoxy, they are provided a place in the analysis. But if they cannot, then "folk" categories lose their authoritative imprint to define what is at stake for patients and families. (One extraordinary exception worth applauding is Hoffmaster's [1992] call from within moral philosophy for a more situational, ethnographic turn in medical ethics that is open to the empirical realities that hedge moral questions. See also Davis's [1991] call for thick description in medical ethics.)

Take ideas, for example, of *suffering*—a powerful category in popular cultures worldwide that points to the experiential basis of values. One is surprised to find so many professional ethical volumes in which this word does not even appear as an entry in the index. Indeed, Eric Cassell stands out in both biomedicine and bioethics for writing explicitly about suffering as grounds for research, practice, and theory (Cassell 1982; 1991b). Ethical systems that leave the problem of suffering (and related concepts of tragedy, endurance, and courage) to particular theological or poetical traditions do not adequately engage the human core of illness and care (see Bowker 1970; D. Morris 1991: 261–268). Here perhaps the standard version of bioethics shares yet another biomedical bias, the rejection of teleology (see Emanuel 1991). Biomedicine banishes purpose and ultimate meaning to religion, yet most patients and practitioners struggle to make sense of illness with respect to great cultural codes that offer coherent interpretations of experience (cf. Frye 1982). So important are these codes for patients that efficacy of intervention cannot easily be disentangled from popular conceptions of coherence and significance. Serious suffering is almost always about ultimate meanings, not always theodicy, a decidedly Western issue, but nearly always about what ultimately matters in a particular local world.

A commitment to medicocentrism also leads bioethicists to construct cases that are centered in the professionally approved institutional structures of biomedicine, such as hospitals or clinical research centers, even though most illness episodes, as social studies readily reveal, are experienced, interpreted, and responded to in the context of the family. The family—the mundane, cultural setting of illness and care, where local social processes are so greatly influential—together with the workplace frequently disappear in bioethical discourse, to be replaced by the biomedical staging of more extreme, even exotic value conflicts. Of course, the immense panoply of popular healing settings is even less visible or audible in the bioethical construction of clinical reality.

That professional bioethicists have in the past framed ethical questions in high-price, high-tech, high-drama biomedical settings—neonatal intensive care units, surgical suites, coronary care wards, cancer clinics, emergency rooms—is justifiably arresting. These are after all the same supremely charged arenas that are central to biomedicine's self-image as the cutting edge of the high-technology battlefield where war is waged against death itself. These arenas of soaring technological power are also, of course, the high-status images of the society at large. By placing the most fundamental ethical queries in these settings—the original ethical scene if you will—bioethicists quite obviously, *ipso facto,* have laid claim to that powerful imagery, to those most highly paid health professionals, and to their preeminent status. Not an unreasonable means of fast forwarding the agenda of a relatively new discipline, and yet, in the bargain, something crucial has been lost. Because the biomedical location of ethical issues draws attention away from the mundane worlds of suffering where most illnesses are enacted and most treatments undergone, voice is denied to the vast majority of health problems and outcomes. The extreme is emphasized over the routine. Medical morality is configured as crisis. The primary care clinic, the nursing home, the occupational health unit, the public health nurse's office, places alive with ordinary doctoring and nursing and patienthood, simply are not given the same moral weight as the high-technology settings. Even less are lay settings privileged as the locus of moral choices, yet from an epidemiological standpoint, that is their locus. A patient- and family-centered bioethics oriented to the routinization of suffering is not invisible, but clearly, as in biomedicine, it has been made to count for less.

From the vantage point of social theory the argument might be advanced that bioethics has received authorization to use abstract philosophical terminology that shares a value orientation with biomedicine in order to construct the moral domain in health care so as to assure that professional medical dominance will not be seriously threatened by lay perspectives and everyday life experiences that might generate a deeper critique of that medical-moral domain and the economic interests with which it is inextricably tied. Professional dominance is

maintained, in this view, via the development of a new profession—
bioethics: a handmaiden to the powerful medical bureaucracies and
associations of professionals, which itself gains jobs, prestige, and a degree of influence from this social assignment. An uncharitable social
science observer might even point to the exoticism so characteristic of
the extreme examples bioethicists favor as evidence of mystification,
this profession's unwillingness to challenge the everyday organization
and practice of care.

I would suggest caution in accepting this analysis. Whether as presently constituted it does so or not, bioethics has opened up a legitimated space to examine moral issues of illness and care—a space,
moreover, that is located in the very heart of biomedical institutions
where in principle, if still not in daily practice, the social world of patient, family, and the community can be made a legitimate part of
clinical conversations. Hospital ethics committees, institutional review
boards for medical research, the clinical ethicist on the wards, and the
development of academic programs focused on regulatory and more
broadly societal ethical issues may be, at least at present, unduly influenced by powerful institutional forces, such as the micropolitics of
the "interests" of hospital directors, medical staff committees, and the
barons of biomedical research, yet the very presence of these bioethical activities legitimates alternative perspectives. They hold the very
real potential for importing into the center of biomedical institutions a
sharp cultural critique of the biomedical order and its practices.

Furthermore, I do not subscribe to the vision of biomedicine as a
monolithic force. The medical profession, the hierarchy in a hospital,
the ethical review boards, and the scholars at work developing the discourse in bioethics are greatly heterogeneous. Different interests and
different idioms for communicating about moral problems thrive. The
work of bioethics goes on in local fields of power—societal, institutional—in which contestation is intrinsic and social processes take
unprecedented turns. Indeed, the profession of biomedicine may be
a much smaller player than other interest groups, such as insurance
companies, health maintenance organizations, corporate health plans,
and political coalitions, whose power has grown during the national
struggle over health care financing in the United States. Certainly, in
North America whatever biomedical (and bioethical) hegemony exists
is hedged in by many forces—the state, the corporations, local government, patient interest groups, and professional critics from social
scientists to newspaper columnists. In this contested field of power it

is by no means certain that particular activities in bioethics or groups of bioethicists will support the interests of the profession or of its major institutions: indeed some clearly do not (e.g., Callahan 1987, 1990). Bioethics, like the varieties of clinical practice, could (and sometimes already does) offer internal resistance to the imposition of the interests of the technical biomedical discourse over those of patients, families, and the community. And that, I will assert, is a very good thing.

What an Anthropological Turn in the Practice of Bioethics Might Offer

The portrait of bioethics that I have drawn is all too black and white. I have done so for heuristic purposes in order to draw out the deep difficulties and underline their cultural sources. In the practical flow of events, working bioethicists, like hard-pressed clinicians, struggle to overcome these constraints that limit their engagement with the obdurate particularity and inexpedient uncertainty of their human subjects. And for that very reason the bioethicist will find an ethnographic orientation liberating, even if ultimately she or he is frustrated by its limits too.[4]

In contrast with the bioethicist, the ethnographer begins with the lived flow of interpersonal experience in an intensely particular local world. Not the Western tradition, or North America, nor even New York State, which are too unspecified to provide a positioned *view from somewhere* (Nagel 1986), but rather the Puerto Rican community in the South Bronx, upper-middle-class Scarsdale, a working-class section of Queens, or a network of Russian immigrants in Brooklyn becomes the setting for grounding moral analysis in the concrete historicity, micropolitical economy, and ethnicity of a local world. Even within such a localized flow of experience, perspectives and preferences are further defined by gender, age, and other social categories of persons: for example, the cultural situation of poor women in rural Haiti who are responding to AIDS (Farmer and Kleinman 1989). These indexes of social experience situate groups and their individual members along axes of power such that the force of macrosocial pressures—economic depression, forced uprooting, ethnic conflict, state violence, the organizational control of substance abuse, the social structural sources of chronic illness and disability—is systematically attenuated for some yet amplified for others. Some become successful or at least are protected; others are victims.

Each local world is characterized by what matters for its members. That structure of relevance gives to the meanings of illness and to treatment expectations the sense of something much closer to natural law than a belief or a convention. Families hold the world to be a certain way as an article of fundamental faith in local reality, not as a debatable position in a self-conscious philosophical reflection. In the infrapolitics of family, workplace, and community, which can be described empirically, the processes of strategic negotiation and interpersonal engagement over what is at stake can be properly regarded as those through which a local moral order (i.e., lived reality) is constituted and expressed. Culture, then, is built up out of the everyday routines and rhythms of social life. It is the medium of collective experience, for example, in which chronic pain affects an entire work unit, Alzheimer's disease is shared as an illness reality by a family, and pediatric cancer care is negotiated among parents, child, and professional care providers.

Hospitals, clinics, and disability programs also are grounded in the particularity of localities, as is the bioethicist. The ethnographic task for the practicing bioethicist, then, becomes the discovery of the meanings and relationships in distinctive local worlds, and the interpretation of their actual impact. This process of discovery creates a coherent narrative out of interactions that are ambiguous and changing. This is a type of cultural construction of the moral conflicts and negotiations that take place over plans and practices that make up the flow of everyday living. Unlike the illusion of abstract rational choice, the ethnographer discovers the murky indeterminacy of real lives and the messy uncertainty of real conditions—conditions in which moral dilemmas and contradictions are inherent in the field of transactions, in the flow of social life itself. Though itself a coherent account, the ethnographic narrative must express these incoherencies, this frustratingly nonstop process of social action.

As part of this ethnographic work, bioethicists need to elicit the perspectives of the participants and place them in the contexts of family, workplace, and medical system. To interpret those grounded perspectives, however, they will need to construe the local context in the light of larger societal influences. Thus, by bringing the life world of the patient into biomedical deliberations, bioethicists also bring with that biographical narrative a much larger societal analysis.

The bioethicist's involvement should be to facilitate communication and to help negotiate conflicting orientations. In this work, it is necessary to protect the participants from the dehumanizing imposition of hegemonic principles like autonomy and justice. The focus on the positioned, intersubjective perspectives of participants in a local context—part of what Sen (1994, and see chapter 4 below) means by positioned objectivity—is a radically different vision of how to proceed with the ethical analysis of a case than that which originates in a philosophical quest for an illusory *transpositional objectivity*, a definitive synthesis, an authoritative voice valid for an entire context or for multiple contexts. In the anthropological vision, such a transcendent objectivity is the problem, not the solution.

More specifically, anthropological analysis draws attention to the institutional context of ethical decision making (see Bosk 1979; Fox 1990; Mizrahi 1986; Zussman 1992). Social institutions—a particular type of hospital, a clinic for alternative care, or a religious facility—refigure ethical issues in terms of efficiency and other technical criteria as well as larger social value orientations that make up everyday social routines. Hence, the special characteristics of a Veterans Administration Hospital (VAH), a university-based teaching hospital, a military emergency unit, a for-profit hospital chain, or a highly cost-conscious HMO constrain the day-to-day social processes that create the local moral order. What is at stake for a resident in training in a teaching hospital—generating new knowledge, securing a place in the academic hierarchy, and so on—is noticeably different from what is at stake for a practicing physician at a small community hospital. The difference signals a distinctive institutional context for deciding what level of treatment is "routine," which kinds of issues will be highlighted as "ethical" problems, when and how substantially families will be involved, and so on. Quite obviously, institutional contexts will also be distinctive cross-culturally. In Japan, even in a university teaching hospital, the practice has been not to disclose the diagnosis to patients who are suffering from cancer but to allow key family members to decide if and when "truth" will be told to the patient. In China, as in other non-Western societies, the family members will stay in the hospital with the patient to do the nursing, prepare meals, and make all the major decisions even for the family head when he is seriously ill.

In Zaire and Senegal, members of the kinship-based therapy management group, including perhaps the doctor and the nurse, will decide if the patient is to be part of a research protocol (Beiser 1977;

Janzen 1978). In a Seventh-Day Adventist mission hospital run by American staff in Borneo, the structure for identifying and resolving a moral dilemma will draw on a religious ideology that suffuses the institutional context quite differently than that of nearby medical facilities run by transplanted Javanese Muslims or local Dayak animists. I have compared the responses of North American and Chinese psychiatrists to depressed patients in the United States and in China with respect to their decidedly different institutional contexts for determining what kinds of therapeutic behaviors represent good care and what kinds of moral messages will be given and received in the patient-doctor interaction (Kleinman 1988b:77–108). North American psychiatrists, practicing psychotherapy in outpatient settings where they are paid by patients for each individualized hour-long session, explore pathologies of the self (low self-esteem, narcissism, masochism, "excessive" guilt) with the aim of "helping patients to individuate." Psychotherapists refrain from giving specific advice about concrete decisions lest they usurp the patient's existential responsibilities to the self, including the responsibility to succeed or fail *with authenticity, on one's own*. In the hospital-based practice of psychiatry with its powerful emphasis on the efficiency of getting patients discharged before insurance payments run out and with the outcome objective of getting the patient back to full function (in household and workplace), care is less "permissive" and much more "directed."

The different metaphors are different forms of moral practice. In China, salaried, hospital-based psychiatrists exhort patients with strong messages about what to do or not do, inasmuch as patients are seen as suffering from "autistic" (read, overly individual) desires for which they require disciplined reeducation and resocialization in collective responsibility. Patients perform in group events that range from listening to lectures to singing inspirational, politically authorized songs. Protecting the social order is paramount; patient rights, at least until very recently, have carried little cachet. The development of psychological counseling centers in Chinese urban areas, even if for treatment of only one or two sessions, however, has promoted a kind of treatment that combines aspects of each of the above forms of practice. Thus, institutional values modify and inflect cultural orientations.

Renee Fox and Judith Swazey (1984) have shown how physicians in a Chinese hospital draw on both Confucian views and communist ideology to authorize local patterns of ethical decision making that challenge North American orientations, but that also are changing under the pressure of societal and institutional transformation. Cultural historians disclose how bioethics in North America itself has emerged out of the social problems and responses of a particular era (Rothman 1990). Thus, in the 1960s and early 1970s, informed consent became central to bioethics at a time in which this theme resonated with ethical problems in the political system; just as ethical concern for the limits of treatment and rationing of care, so central to the bioethics of our time, is linked to the political economic crisis in health care (Marshall 1992). Following the Tiananmen Massacre, criticism of China's gulag and its human rights abuses has pressed Chinese psychiatrists to at least make an appearance of addressing patient rights and to dissociate themselves from the highly publicized abuse of dissidents associated in the recent past with East European psychiatrists.

Anthropology (and other interpretive social sciences), then, brings to bioethics a critical approach to the cultural roots of ethical systems and to the cultural process of moral action. The works of moral philosophers who have themselves begun to engage cultural difference indicate why an anthropologically informed understanding of culture that is based in ethnographic study of the lived context of moral experience is essential to such an undertaking. For even such an encompassing yet disciplined moral philosopher as Charles Taylor (1992b) loses his way in the thicket of multiculturalism. Taylor applies a masterly analysis to the contemporary politics of recognition of ethnic difference, in which he seems to move beyond the usual catechisms of individual rights to establish the importance of the right for communities to animate distinctive moral worlds, only to conclude with the rather disappointing cliché that what we need is to show "respect" for other cultures. Coming from one of the major moral thinkers of our era, this surely is not promising.

Another influential moral and political philosopher, Amy Gutmann addresses "the challenge of multiculturalism" by setting up cultural relativism as a "strawman" (Gutmann 1993). First finding fault with a radical version of ethical relativism, in part because, she claims, it fails to register intracultural diversity and change and in part because it fails to recognize that moral reasons can be rationalizations of differences in social power, Gutmann goes on to attack the idea that failure to recognize cultural difference injures ethnic (and self-) identity. Since cultural relativism, she insists, would render justice relative to shared meanings of social goods and since its association of shared meanings and identity is false, cultural relativism's approach to justice is invalid.

In its place she calls for a deliberative universalism that would partly rely on a core set of universal principles of justice which apply to all "modern cultures" and that would also put faith in accountable deliberation to address fundamental conflicts over social justice.

Now, in fact, I shall argue below for an approach to bioethics in clinical settings that is very much like Gutmann's deliberative universalism, though my emphasis is on a method that might be called deliberative relativism. But where Gutmann abandons "culture," under the authorization of a faulty syllogism, I regard it as central to the very process of deliberation, which I will call "cultural engagement." The problem with Gutmann's analysis is her failure to recognize the current understanding of culture within social anthropology. Social anthropologists today define culture not as shared canonical meanings that are distributed equally throughout a community, but rather as lived meanings that are contested because of gender, age cohort, and political difference; meanings that are actualized differently in everyday social transactions so that they exert a partial, uncertain effect are really practices, ways of being-in-the-world. By this definition culture is emergent in particular social interactions. It is neither homogeneous, nor determinative, nor unchanging. And since the misadventures of the culture and personality school in the 1950s, few anthropologists would make a direct one-to-one association of culture with personal identity. A cultureless deliberative universalism may sponsor a useful method for dealing with a particular difference in the theory of ethics. Because it makes no room for culture, however, it begs the question of ethnic and cross-cultural difference, and also, and perhaps most troubling, misrecognizes that the process of ethical deliberation itself is contextualized, emergent, and cultural.

In a more complex argument about culture and ethics, Jorge Garcia (ms.), a moral philosopher and bioethicist, examines several kinds of cultural relativity. He explicitly differentiates a radical relativity ("comprehensive relativity") from "limited relativity." He follows Gutmann in criticizing those who propose "seriously relativist positions" for avoiding the problem of intracultural diversity. He also castigates serious relativists for being capable of bearing only a shallow liberalism, for example, a defense of tolerance—a position he recognizes may be seen as Eurocentric, yet one which he regards as crucial to ethics. Garcia then proceeds with an argument based upon the same inadequate formulation of culture as that held by Gutmann, albeit at least including a place for a stripped-down notion of culture.

Garcia, as he himself recognizes, falls into the problem of ethno-centrism, in this case willfully. But the larger problem is that Garcia misrecognizes moral deliberations. He sees them as deliberations that transcend or avoid culture. He does so by relying, as does Gutmann, on an idea of culture as beliefs, values, and judgments: conventions that can be taken up or put down at will. An idea that leads to simple ethnic stereotypes that are rejected by ethnographers does not offer a promising *modus operandi*. That culture is also a process of action, a mode of collective experience, an emergent in local relationships and situations is not a view Garcia (or Gutmann for that matter) would endorse. If they did, much of their argument against cultural relativ-ism would dissolve.

In a very recent piece, Nancy Jecker, a bioethicist, and clinical col-leagues (1995) propose a set of guidelines for engaging ethical issues in cross-cultural patient care that is quite close to the procedure out-lined in this chapter. The process of negotiation they set out is one that can only improve ethical approaches to patient care. Particularly impressive is their openness to alternative perspectives and their seri-ousness in requiring that genuine patient-provider negotiations over fundamental moral commitments be at the center of bioethical delib-eration. Perhaps because this useful clinical methodology is buttressed by real cases of Navajo patients, we are even more aware of the limita-tions of the conceptual frame that the authors share with Gutmann and Garcia. Values become a surrogate for culture; the description of the local cultural setting is limited to that of the patient's personal his-tory; neither the culture of the clinic, the cultural mode of ethical practice, or financial and bureaucratic interests are brought into the analysis; and the central role assigned to "ethical integrity" is presented as if this mode of behavior were not founded on a very Western set of deeply subjectivist commitments regarding the self, the other, and what is at stake in their relationship. One might well assume that when ethicists finally get around to dealing more adequately with an anthropologically oriented appreciation of culture as moral context, process, and performance that the strategies proposed for clinical prac-tice will be more far-reaching and original. A promising early example is the research program Barbara Koenig and colleagues at Stanford and University of California San Francisco have organized to examine how discussions about terminating care actually proceed among terminal cancer patients, their families, and caregivers across Asian American, African American, and Mexican American groups.

What the philosopher Hans Sluga, in his discussion of Heidegger's mixing of philosophy and politics under the Nazis, writes about the relationship of philosophy and politics (1993) generally will be too strong to transfer verbatim to the relationship of philosophy to ethics. Nonetheless, if in the following excerpt the word "ethics" is substituted for "politics," we are left with a sense of shock that may be worth carrying over into bioethics, not because it describes what exists, but because it cautions against a certain danger while appealing to an impressive strength of what philosophy can do:

> Philosophers, in my view, are not qualified to lay down authoritative standards of political action. Whenever they have tried their hand at this, they have either described useless utopias or given dangerous instructions. It might be more attractive to think of them as playing a critical role. But political critique is productive only if it is tempered by common sense and practical experience. Philosophical critics of politics, on the other hand, proceed all too often from supposedly absolute truths, and what they say then proves generally unhelpful and sometimes even destructive. Insofar as philosophy has any task to perform in politics, it is to map out new possibilities. By confronting actual political conditions with alternatives, it can help to undermine the belief that these conditions are inevitable. If the German philosophers of the 1930s had engaged in such reflection, they would not have surrendered so readily to the false certainties of Nazism. (pp. ix–x)[5]

That it is possible for moral theory, and bioethics in particular, to open a different and more substantial pathway toward culturally salient issues is confirmed by the approach to ethics in a pluralistic society that, as I have already noted, William Connolly draws out of the works of Nietzsche and Foucault for an ethics of agonistic generosity. That continental approach to the diversity of moral meanings encourages empathy for contradiction, contestation, and paradox in a world without an intrinsic moral rule. (James Fernandez [1990] shows how much the same stance emerges from the relativist program in anthropology.) Another promising direction is to be found in the writing of Marion Young (1990) on justice and the politics of difference. Young holds that moral judgment should commence with an understanding of domination and oppression in real social spaces. Her feminist perspective emphasizes that "rights" are more validly conceptualized as relationships and institutionally defined social roles than as things. Because relationships and institutionalized roles take their origin from differences in power, morality must be about those differences in power as found, for example, in cultural imperialism or paternalism.

The focus of ethics should be to empower groups who are the victims of relationships of dominance. For Young, "social justice involving equality among groups who recognize and affirm one another in their specificity can best be realized in our society through large regional governments with mechanisms for representing immediate neighborhoods and towns" (p. 248). Because autonomy at the individual and group level means exclusion of others, she defines justice without privileging ethnic autonomy. Rather her vision is one in which interaction and exchange are the sources of a morality in which difference can flourish among a heterogeneous public. Again this feminist critique possesses much the same thrust as anthropology's relativist interpretations. In both, pluralism and difference are not to be feared; they are affirmed as the source of moral experience, not a threat to moral practice.

Besides cultural critique and comparison, is there a practical contribution anthropology can make to bioethics? The cultural formulation of diagnostic and therapeutic issues clearly should be as significant to the consulting bioethicist as the medical anthropologist can frequently make it for the consulting physician, especially when the patient and family come from cultural and ethnic backgrounds that differ from those of their professional caregivers, or when the setting is outside North America (Kleinman 1982). That formulation involves systematic steps in placing the illness and treatment experience in the culturally grounded context of family, work, and medical/social welfare systems, through the application of a highly focused ethnography—a description and interpretation of how those settings affect, and are affected by, the illness. Cultural formulation identifies lay and professional explanatory models, compares them for evidence of cultural bias or conflict, and sets out a process of negotiation to assure that their inhabitants benefit from studies of cultural sensitivity (see Helman 1992; Kleinman 1988a:227–251; Rogler 1990). These are technical procedures, albeit experience-affirming ones, that can become part of the repertoire of the bioethicist. Ethnographic knowledge of the core ethical orientations and social patterns of different communities will be especially significant in planning and implementing medical research in low-income ethnic and non-Western settings to assure that their members benefit from studies that place them at risk as much as do the wealthy Euro-American groups that sponsor such projects (Christakis 1988).

As this last example suggests, the ethics of the sickroom and the clinical encounter are only one side of medical ethics. Especially important for anthropology are the vexed questions of societal ethics. These questions turn on the control and allocation of resources that underwrite health status and quality of care. They are inseparable from issues of social value, political economy, and history. Societal ethics in North America, for example, needs to be discussed in the political context of the social transformation of North American society and its medical institutions. The ethnographer can examine how these macrosocial changes affect sickness episodes and treatment practices in particular local settings that differ in their rates of unemployment and health risks. That contextual knowledge—for example, of particularly salient local instances of institutional racism and their aftermath in hostility and resistance—is what is missing in medical ethics. The ethnographic method would reshape bioethics's almost single-minded interest in government regulation by emphasizing the dialectical connection between the broad historical processes of change and the local settings in which those changes are exerting an influence on health and illness. Seen in this light, ethnography and social history would seem to be the means by which medical ethicists can obtain culturally valid understanding of the sources and consequences of societal ethics. If we can talk of communities of fate with respect to shared infant mortality rates, job opportunities, and other life chances, then surely we should also be permitted to talk of communities of shared fate with respect to justice; that is how an anthropologically informed ethics should talk. Whether this will be achieved through interdisciplinary collaboration, through the retraining of professionals, or by drawing larger numbers of anthropologists, sociologists, and historians into medical ethics is still an open question.

What are the limits of cultural analysis, cross-cultural comparison, and the sensibility to variation and difference that are the core of the anthropologist's "cultural relativism"? Ethnography can overemphasize the extreme, the exotic case, and not give enough emphasis to the ordinary. The focus for cultural analysis can be so narrow that it encumbers rather than fosters comparisons. In the current era, the privileging of variation and difference can be so automatic and one-sided that there is a partial blindness to the other side of social life: what is shared across human conditions. Ethnographic privileging of interpretive methods may encourage unwarranted rejection of all quantitative approaches and findings. And cultural analysis, when carried to an extreme, can at times reproduce hermeneutic circles that are unhelpful and that discourage the movement from research to practice. Self-reflectivity can also be overdone, as can a reverse ethnocentricism that always privileges the other. But these are correctable faults that the best ethnographies manage to get around. A common and more fundamental critique centers on "cultural relativism."[6]

While epistemological and even ontological relativism—willingness to entertain the idea that there is no single form of knowledge or being in local worlds—will seem defensible to many, ethical relativism of the radical variety, the idea that there are no ethical standards cross-culturally, will not.[7] Critics complain: Are infanticide of female children in South Asia, ritual murder of elderly women accused of being illness-causing witches in East Africa, pharaonic circumcision and infibulation of five-year-old Sudanese girls that leave a pinhole for micturition and, later, menstruation, and rationing of care based on color status under apartheid acceptable because the dominant group says they are the way things should be? Clearly, this would be an unacceptable conclusion. Behind it lurks the terrible transmogrification of medicine under the Nazis, where biomedical ideology and technology, dominated by Nazi values, prepared the way to the death camps (Kleinman 1988b:104–107; Proctor 1988). It is this fear that E. D. Pellegrino (1993), one of the founders of medical ethics, arrogates to dismiss culturalist and postmodernist writings as assaults on the universality of truth, virtue, and the good: in his view the only sure grounds for medical ethics.

The anthropological argument advanced in these pages is for elicitation of and engagement with alternative ethical formulations, a constrained and engaged relativism; it is for affirmation of differences, not automatic authorization of any standard of practice as ethically acceptable because it is held by some people, somewhere (Shweder 1990; Wong 1984). The limit to ethical relativism is that the bioethicist (and the anthropologist) must compare an alternative ethical formulation with those ethical standards she or he holds for the evaluation of a particular problem in a particular context. The outcome of such an evaluation could be acceptance or rejection of the alternative or of the bioethicist's (or anthropologist's) own standard, or negotiation and compromise.

The idea of radical ethical relativism is unacceptable to all but a small group of diehards. It is, in my own view at least, a serious misinterpretation of what ethnography, cultural analysis, and cross-cultural comparison are about: namely, the commitment that before we apply an ethical category we hold to be universal, we had better first understand the context of practice and experience. The job should be to situate a problem in bioethics—clinical or societal—in a deep description of that particular ethos in order to understand what is at stake for the participants, what is contested, and thereby to offer a cultural formulation of conflicting ethical priorities. To do so implies the development of a cultural critique of bioethical discourse in its originating Western context and in its position within the globalization of markets, the media, and professional practice. Those descriptive and self-reflective activities having been done, there are at least three further steps in dealing with societal or clinical ethics. First, we need to systematically compare lay and professional bioethical standards for a particular problem in the contexts of a particular policy's or clinical procedure's social values; second, we need to identify ethical difference and to negotiate that part of the difference on which the various parties deem it ethical to compromise; and third, where a cross-cultural ethical conflict cannot be so resolved, the parties should specify the nature of the problem for further adjudication (Kleinman 1982).

That a cultural question in the ethics of suffering and healing cannot be resolved is not surprising and is not nearly as troubling as failure to engage it as an ethical issue. This ethnographic strategy does not commit the deep error of assuming that "all goods, all virtues, all ideals are compatible, and that what is desirable can alternatively be united into a harmonious whole without loss" (Williams 1981:xvi). Compromise and negotiation may not resolve ethical conflicts, and even where they do, some losses must occur. By definition ethical dilemmas leave a sense of remorse and regret. The quest is not for agreement on a transcendent (transpositionally objective) universal but for positioned pluralism. Indeed, identifying the deep sources of local ethical conflict may be more important for authorizing the process of cultural engagement in general than for handling a particular case.

Where possible, it is the obligation of the anthropologically informed bioethicist not only to respect the specific views of others and to affirm the validity of the process of formulating moral alternatives but also to develop deep knowledge about those positioned Weltanschauung in order to engage with alternative categories and practices as a potential way to resolve ethical conflict. This ethnographic approach emphasizes the process of engagement and negotiation with the engaged moral orientations of others; it attempts to minimize the

application of bioethical categories that derive from the Western philosophical tradition to settings for which they lack coherence and validity. It attempts to prevent a commitment to that ethical tradition
from becoming a kind of partisanship that "knows the answers to the
questions it asks" (Sluga 1993:5). The ethnographic approach is not
averse to leaving questions undecided.[8] The ethnographic vision recognizes the limits of our knowledge. Social experience always exceeds
our grasp; description can never be complete. A large residue of human
experience resists or exceeds understanding. This perspective also attempts to introduce sensitivity to the way ethical positions are contested locally as well as recognition that what may seem to an outside
expert to be an ethical conflict may in fact represent a conflict over local resources or a form of resistance to state and professional control.

In other areas of cross-cultural research and practice, sensitivity to
cultural difference and professional bias is established procedure. This
approach also protects the responsibility of the professional consultant
not to accept value decisions that contravene human rights and other
pan-national moral conventions. But it makes that universalist responsibility the final stage in a lengthy process of cultural translation that
gives priority, initially at least, to the social reality of alternative worlds
of experience interpreted in their own terms.[9]

In this respect, an anthropological approach to medical ethics would
have much in common with William Connolly's (1993b) version of an
ethic of agonistic generosity. If ethical and political positions are always contingent so that there is no fundamental, intrinsic ethical and
political ground, but each belongs to a historical epoch and cultural
context, then what is required, Connolly avers, is that each position be
presented strongly but that the presenters must also accord contesting
views affirmation as alternatives that have to be taken seriously, that
have to be brought into a process of critical moral and political engagement. Recognition of and respect for alternatives (not patroniz-
ing attitudes, but genuine expression of the worth of difference) are
central to a process that moves from empathic affirmation through
critical assessment toward encouragement of contestation and ultimately to constructive integration or resolution of another sort. (See
Kekes 1993 on value incommensurability and the unavoidability of
conflicts, as well as the place of conflict resolution, in a pluralist version of ethics.)

A number of these sensibilities are brought together in Joan Tronto's

(1993) notion of an ethics and politics of care. Drawing upon various sources in feminist studies, Tronto describes care as a practice of reciprocation involving "caring-receiving." The process of care embraces attentiveness, responsibility, competence, responsiveness. It requires moral engagement as a political form of life, a way of acting that simultaneously engages the power of context and the context of power. Tronto seeks to establish caring as an alternative language for policy as much as for ordinary human interactions. John Caputo (1993), in *Against Ethics,* a curious combination of substantive thought and egregious exuberance, makes a complementary argument for understanding obligation in the face of social exigency as the grounds of moral experience, a "language game" that challenges the Western canon's discourse on ethics. For Caputo the social sources of obligation create a subject who suffers the powerful constraints of social history (p. 11) as much as she or he is active as an agent of choice (pp. 95–97). The process of events, especially disastrous ones (p. 29)—occurring, blowing up, resolving—creates a field of obligation and response, which *inter alia,* lends to powerlessness its power (p. 5) and to moral life its undecidability and its passion.

Such interpositional engagement is very much in the ethnographic mode. It also echoes Emmanuel Levinas's (1988:156–167) idea that morality is a process of interaction that results from a person's empathy for the suffering of "the Other." That empathic interaction creates the ethical as an "inter-human" experience of "suffering for the suffering of someone else." Or put differently, only in the engagement with the Other (and with what is at stake for that person, family, or community)—in a cross-personal interaction modeled on the lines of a cross-cultural one—does ethics emerge as a process of moral enactment that is sustainable in a multicultural world.

Of course there is no anthropological consensus for doing medical ethics. Complementary to, yet still different than, the anthropological way I have fashioned would be a Gramscian emphasis on the creation of "strategies of interference." By applying such strategies, practitioners would assist patients and families in disrupting or otherwise resisting the dominant institutional discourse with its tendency to commodify and to prescribe uniform, one-size-fits-all, practices. Although such a vision is too easily romanticized, when in fact its limits and potentially dangerous side effects are apparent, there is something to be recommended for bioethicists, only in carefully defined contexts of course, in considering obstructing the institutional efficiency of routinizing guidelines that they believe undermine care on behalf of the poetics of the experience of illness and the humanity of the clinical encounter. This is likely to be controversial; in fact, clinical consultants of many kinds, in my experience, silently apply something like this strategy on occasion in the hospital when they have identified the institution itself as the chief obstacle to good care. The tension that already exists in bioethics between the theoretical and the applied would likely be intensified by this way of proceeding, but that might be salubrious, both for the field and for its audiences (cf. Hoffmaster 1992; Pellegrino 1993).

The cardinal contribution of the anthropologist of medicine to bioethics, then, is to deeply humanize the *process* of formulating an ethical problem by allowing variation and pluralism and the constraints of social positions to emerge and receive their due, so that ethical standards are not imposed in an alien and authoritarian way but, rather, are actualized as the outcome of reciprocal participatory engagement across different worlds of experience. This would be a way of doing the work of ethics that is parallel to what the distinguished moral theorist Martha Nussbaum (1990:141) has pointed to in the work of Henry James as a narrative ethic that authorizes the moral sensibility of the ethicist. She writes,

Human deliberation is constantly an *adventure* of the personality, undertaken against terrific odds and among frightening mysteries, *and* . . . this is, in fact, the source of much of its beauty and richness, that texts written in a traditional philosophical style have the most insuperable difficulty conveying to us. If our moral lives are "stories" in which mystery and risk play a central and a valuable role, then it may well seem that the "intelligent report" of those lives requires the abilities and techniques of the teller of stories. (p. 142)

Ethnographic stories and literary stories are not the same, yet both genres draw upon a sensibility to context, the confounding connective tissue of intersubjectivity, and the ambiguous figures in the multiplicity of experience that would seem an essential tool also for bioethicists, if they are to avoid constructing an artifact of rational choice that inevitably will homogenize and therefore possibly dehumanize sufferers.

4

A Critique of Objectivity
in International Health

This material was originally prepared as a response to two chapters written for a book on social science contributions to international health of which I am an editor (Chen, Kleinman, and Ware 1994). In that volume, a section was organized to review conceptual and methodological problems in the measurement of mortality and morbidity in low-income societies. The chapters included a review by Christopher Murray and Lincoln Chen, two international public health researchers, which essayed the chief difficulties in the measurement of morbidity and their implications for health research and policy, titled "Understanding Morbidity Change" (chap. 4), and a more theoretical piece by Amartya Sen, an economist and philosopher who has written extensively on famine and female mortality in Africa and Asia, titled "Objectivity and Position: Assessment of Health and Well-being" (chap. 5). My commentary tried to balance the section with a contrasting cultural critique of "objectivity": a core concern for these authors. I have further reworked the material in order to include several related themes with a different audience in mind.

Economists and public health experts (Murray, Chen, and Sen included) have traditionally worked with mortality rates. These they have aggregated for countries and regions in order to correlate them with large-scale economic and social changes that also are measured by aggregate statistics. There is increasing awareness even in these disci-

Revised and expanded version of a paper published in *Health and Social Change: An International Perspective,* ed. L. C. Chen, A. Kleinman, and N. Ware (Cambridge: Harvard School of Public Health and Harvard University Press, 1994); pp. 129–138.

plines, however, that mortality rates are social fabrications that are based upon often seriously inadequate sets of data of questionable accuracy. They serve bureaucratic purposes of the state and the international community, certain of which come to distort their significance and uses. In spite of this by now well-recognized problem, economists and public health experts are not deterred from working up aggregated quantitative data in elaborate statistical programs that create the illusion, at least, that certain parameters of the knowledge base are well supported and their policy implications clear. (Sometimes they are, though more frequently they are not.)

Chen, Murray, and Sen are sensitive to this problem; indeed each has made important contributions to the understanding of how serious a problem it is and what can be done to control it. Moreover, they recognize that as suspect as mortality statistics are, they do not raise the degree of uncertainty that data on morbidity—the experience of sickness and its disabling effects—do. These authors, though quantitative researchers, wish to see measures of morbidity (and of well-being) added to international health statistics so that those statistics more accurately reflect the serious problems of chronic illnesses in aging populations which produce substantial distress and disability while not usually taking the life of the sufferer until many years later, if at all. That information, they argue persuasively, is needed to more effectively plan for health care and preventive programs. It is for this reason that the question of measurement looms especially large for them. Yet, they have even greater difficulty with anthropological sources of information, because they are largely qualitative and local, recalcitrant to aggregation at national or global levels.

All three authors felt that my commentary painted them into positions that were overdrawn and not sensitive enough to the subtleties of their arguments. Hence I should warn readers that they must read the chapters by Murray and Chen and Sen before they assume that what I have written is fair to these scholars. Nonetheless, I feel the general points I discuss hold for the field of international health and development in the main, and for that reason I have extended the original argument in a final section added expressly for this collection in order to touch upon other points that deserve to be brought into the compass of the critique.

The reader of *Health and Social Change* might rightly ask why a volume of social science and international health studies should include several chapters on theoretical questions concerning the measurement of health status. The reason, as the chapters by Murray and Chen and Sen should make clear, is that the measurement of morbidity necessitates assessment of subjective complaints and recognition of the situated knowledge of health indexes. Subjectivity and the positioning of knowledge intensify the challenge to a positivist approach to measurement which is already strained nearly to its limits by problems in the measurement of mortality. While both chapters indicate the need and even necessity for taking into account patient reports and practitioner interpretations, they come down on the side of the requirement for some form of objective measures that can be used to make more reliable intrasocietal and intersocietal comparisons. Those measurements in turn can be used to test claims about changes in health and their relationship to social change. Ultimately, these authors argue, there must be a determination of the legitimacy of claims about ill health so that resources can be allocated fairly and justly to those who are in the greatest need.

This is an understandable and salient goal. It is a goal, moreover, whose theoretical grounds and entailments are all too often taken for granted by epidemiologists, public health experts, and many social scientists. One group of social scientists among whom this aim is not taken for granted is anthropologists. Indeed, critiques of the way positivism and objectivism function in the health sciences are central to the intellectual program of medical anthropology. And it is from the vantage point of this intellectual program that I join the debate that the chapters by Murray and Chen and Sen seek to advance. Because Sen offers a philosophically elaborated discussion that seems both generally compelling and particularly challenging to a culturalist analysis of "health transitions," I offer my comments on the objectivist position as Sen so carefully articulates it. Nevertheless, these comments can be extended to the position set out by Murray and Chen, a position that I think accurately represents the dominant orientation in international health and social development studies. (See also Dasgupta 1993.) The critique I offer does not attempt to represent all relevant culturalist responses to this challenge, but simply those that emerge from my own work over two and a half decades as a medical anthropologist who, in the course of doing cross-cultural research on illness and care that is mostly qualitative, even when it mixes stories and statistics, routinely comes up against the demand by public health experts for objectivity.

Amartya Sen's "Objectivity and Position":
Assessment of Health and Well-being

Sen (1994) argues that "objectivity requires explicit acceptance and extensive use of variability of observations with the position of the observer." For Sen such "positionality" is an intrinsic feature of objectivity that needs to be distinguished from subjectivity. Sen distinguishes between "positional objectivity," a statement about the objectivity of observations from a certain position, and "transpositional objectivity," which builds on the former but goes beyond it. Subjectivity, in contrast, pertains to the inward-looking nature of subjective judgments and to interpersonal variance.

Observational claims, in Sen's way of putting it, are a specific form of objectivity that is prior to the objectivity of generalized presumptive claims. Although observation and conceptualization influence each other, and observations are dependent on a person's positionality, there is also "some *invariance* vis-à-vis the subject" (p. 116). Drawing on Thomas Nagel's *The View from Nowhere* (1986), Sen reasons that some observations or claims based in observations are more objective than others because they are more accessible to a range of subjective capacities, and because some positioned observations have priority over others. To move from "positional" to "transpositional" objectivity "calls for rules of assessment—of 'priority'—that have to go beyond what is needed in examining the demands of objectivity of observations from an amply *specified position*" (p. 118). Transpositionality can be built up out of congruence of "*all* the relevant positional views," or out of a particularly decisive positional view (p. 120). Moreover, even if there is a fair amount of subjective influence, a positional observation can be specified. Indeed, such specifiability may help to control subjective influence. But Sen holds that much of what goes by the name of subjectivity in the domain of health is really a matter of positions that have not been specified. Specify the economic, institutional, professional, and ideological positions of practitioner and patient and you will so constrain the clinical construction of reality that there will be positional objectivity even if there is "non-objectivity in a transpositional sense" (p. 123).

Morbidity can be assessed from the positional objectivity of the patient's point of view. But this is a slippery slope because perception may be variable due to interpersonal and intertemporal differences, and owing to systematic social influences. Once we start specifying the positionality of illness perception, where do we stop? Because Sen is concerned with morbidity in settings of deep deprivation where there are few or no formal health services, as in the poorest regions of India, he is especially concerned that systematic experience in the use of health services in more resource-rich settings may both reduce morbidity and increase self-perception/reporting of symptoms. That would render comparisons across regions which are based on questionnaires invalid. Hence the need to view self-perception of health status as positional. It is objective only where its positional qualifiers are specified, and it is of less priority than other positional observations (perhaps the doctor's) which can be made more accessible and specifiable.

Sen is most convincing when he suggests how gender inequality in India creates positional observations that systematically underreport illness because of deprivation in education and also "acceptance of greater discomfort and illness as part of the prevailing mode of living" (p. 125). Those local observations, though capable of being constrained as a kind of positional objectivity, "would not readily translate into transpositional objectivity of women's relative deprivation, nor into positional objectivity from the general position of being an Indian rural woman" (p. 126). Yet, they might well, Sen qualifies, have local "explanatory and predictive relevance."

This brief summary cannot do justice to the precision, balance, and subtlety of Sen's argument. There is much in that argument that I find persuasive and can agree with. But I wish to draw out a tension between Sen's cautious commitment to objectivity, which for all its complexity and qualifications is still a positivist orientation, and the orientation of many social anthropologists who conduct ethnography.

The Primacy of Categories to Observations: Reliability versus Validity

Sen emphasizes the observational basis of verification, though he qualifies the classical example of the mirror held up to nature by addressing the relativity of perspective. All perspectives are positioned. What we observe depends upon where we are. Therefore, we need to control our observations to assure their accuracy. In research parlance, we refer to the verification of observations as reliability. A finding is considered reliable when it is verified with a high degree of confirmation. For example, different raters may observe whether or not a patient demonstrates weakness in the performance of a task, or exhibits unsteady gait when asked to walk in a straight line, or reports feeling sad. Their degree of agreement after observing the same patient sample is frequently quantified as a correlation coefficient of the reliability of their assessment of a particular feature of morbidity.

But observations, as Sen also notes, involve conceptual assumptions about what is being observed. If you are going to measure ischemic heart disease, you need to begin with a concept of the condition and its operationalized criteria (chest pain, narrowed coronary arteries, stress-induced, or other causes of, insufficiency in oxygenation of heart muscle). The concept—be it a professional or lay category—precedes and guides the observation. Thus, both symptoms (complaints) and signs (observable indications) of disease are in fact *interpretations.* Conceptual categories shape our interpretation of observed states, be those observations subjective or objective. (And these are categories and interpretations from which one can die: biological processes may be understood through cultural construction and shaped by those constructs, but they and their prepotent effects are real nonetheless.) Put differently, *validity*—which is the verification of the conceptual categories that organize our observations—is both different from and a more fundamental aspect of verification (i.e., measurement) than *reliability.*

Elsewhere I have given an example from psychiatric categories that applies equally to any other conceptualization of health (Kleinman 1988b:10–14). Suppose ten trained observers are asked to interview the same ten adult American Indian informants who have experienced the death of a spouse, parent, or child in the previous month. The interviewers will determine with a high degree of agreement that the same informants report the experience of hearing and/or seeing the recently deceased family member beckoning them to the afterworld. This experience is very common among adult American Indians. Yet it is distinctly uncommon among other adult North Americans. Now if the observers agree nine out of ten times that the same eight American Indian informants have had this experience, they will have achieved a high degree of reliability indicating an observation about which we can be highly confident. But if they describe this observation as a "hallucination," that is, a pathological percept indicative of mental illness, which it might be for adult non-Indian Americans, they would have an empirical finding that was reliable but not valid. Validity would require the qualifying interpretation that this percept is not pathological—in fact it is both normative and normal for American Indians since it is neither culturally inappropriate nor a predictor or sign of disease—and therefore it could not be labeled as a hallucination. Rather it would require some other categorization, for example, a pseudo-hallucination or a culturally appropriate and personally normal percept, in order for the observation to be both reliable and valid.

When measuring morbidity of any sort, reliability is necessary but insufficient to verify the condition and its effects. Take chronic fatigue syndrome as an example. Are we talking about the same thing when we observe the fatigue noted by an otherwise healthy long-distance runner with a postviral syndrome; a middle-class single father in a North American suburb with chronic fatigue syndrome associated with grieving for a dead wife; a desperately poor mother of six malnourished children living in a hovel in a *favela* in northeastern Brazil who has experienced chronic starvation; or an elderly man who has struggled with the disabling lifetime effects of childhood polio, to which his body is now giving in? If assessments lack validity, then morbidity has not been adequately measured. The problem with findings that have reliability in the absence of validity is by no means limited to mental, culture-bound, or new conditions; it is a serious, generic problem in cross-cultural assessment of patient complaints as symptoms and signs of illness.

Hilary Putnam (1993:151–152), a distinguished philosopher, drawing on a decade of publications, puts the issue in more general terms that go much deeper and further into the limits of objectivity.

First, I contend that there is not *one* notion of an "object" but an open class of possible uses of the word "object"—even of the technical logical notion of an object (value of a variable of quantification). The idea that reality itself fixes the use of the word "object" (or the use of the word "correspondence") is a hangover from pre-scientific metaphysics (Putnam 1987). Secondly, the idea of the world "singling out" a correspondence between objects and our words is incoherent. As a matter of model-theoretic fact, we know that even if we somehow fix the intended truth-values of our sentences, not just in the actual world but in all possible worlds, this does *not* determine a unique correspondence between words and items in the universe of discourse (Putnam 1981). Thirdly, even if we require that words not merely "correspond" to items in the universe of discourse but be causally connected to them in some way, the required notion of "causal connection" is deeply *intentional*. When we say that a word and its referent must stand in a "causal connection of the appropriate kind," then, even in cases where this is true, the notion of causal connection being appealed to is fundamentally the notion of *explanation*. And explanation is a notion that lies in the same circle as reference and truth (Putnam 1989).

Context, Interpretation, and the Experience of Suffering

For anthropologists conducting studies in international health, the focus of research, unlike that of epidemiologists and economists, is on individuals and small groups in local worlds: a village, a group of villages, an urban neighborhood, a social network. (For public health researchers, it may seem like the study of a single, "uncontrolled" case, even though the case is a community rather than an individual.) The research (ethnography with or without quantitative surveys is what I have in mind) usually involves relatively long periods—often months, sometimes a year or more—living with informants, engaging in participant observation of daily activities, and interviewing and reinterviewing a relatively small group of key informants. Over time the ethnographer gets to know the local setting well, establishes relationships of trust, and comes to understand the long-term tensions, supports, and negotiations that underwrite daily happenings. Such research seeks to describe informants' indigenous categories of the body, the self, health, illness, and healing, but not as abstract responses to questions cut off from social life. Rather the ethnographer interprets the effects of these meanings in the sociopolitical context on the way the group experiences suffering and responds to illness. Or the ethnographer focuses on some other daily life engagements in which these categories are part of social action. Conversely, the ethnographer also describes the way that illness alters social relations, disrupts patterns of interaction with key institutions, and transforms personal behavior; again, within the exigencies and uncertainties of real social contexts. (See chapter 9 below for examples.)

Those descriptions are understood, in current cultural theory (Bourdieu 1990:10–27; Kleinman 1988b:5–17; Kleinman 1992; Shweder 1991:27–72), as positioned interpretations of positioned interpretations.[1] In other words, the ethnographer establishes his own position as a usually nonindigenous field-worker of a particular age, gender, and cultural background and with particular social commitments, who possesses a certain conceptual orientation and focused problem framework from which he or she encounters members of the community who are themselves positioned (on account of gender, class, caste, etc.) participants in local worlds. The empirical result of this utterly human—because contextualized and uncertain—though professionally disciplined engagement is positioned knowledge; that is, a view from somewhere. Context and interpersonal dialogue are understood to shape the knowledge so that it is always particular to a local world. The ethnographer, if honest, is also compelled by the nature of the experience to be aware of the limits of her or his grasp of uncertain and changing human conditions.

From the perspective advanced by Sen, as I have qualified it, the ethnographer's account carries a positioned validity. Often its reliability is untested. But even its validity is not regarded by the ethnographer as "objective," because it is never a transpositional "view from nowhere" (Nagel 1986), nor can it be verified straightforwardly as a positional observation or series of observations. That is to say, it can be neither fully specified (because it is always more than observation) nor made broadly accessible. Rather the ethnographer constructs a professional category based on the interpretation of local popular or expert categories, which are themselves held by native actors engaged in parochial actions vis-à-vis others. The ethnographer interprets a field of interpersonal experience as he or she narratizes (forms a story of) the felt flow of that interpersonal world, a world that is encountered as stories told to the ethnographer (a positioned witness), stories of illness, disability, and therapy.[2] That interpretation is a creation as much as an observation; it is a constrained yet storied observation that is made for a professional discourse and into a genre.

The knowledge the ethnographer produces is never impersonal; it represents not only the public, focused account of informants but also the subsidiary, tacit knowledge that is part of their (and the ethnographer's) practical life activities (Polanyi and Prosch 1975:22–45), what Pierre Bourdieu (1990:66–69) calls a feel for the game, or sense of the field. Thus, the anthropologist's ethnography cannot be, in any strict sense, objective, even when it concerns social "objects" (people, institutions, exchanges, power), because it is embedded in the subtleties and complexities of subjective and interpersonal understandings. The ethnography is constructed from those particular interpersonal engagements in such a way that two ethnographers working in the same community would (and, in fact do) construct distinctive ethnographies.[3]

Anthropologists strive for interpositional knowledge of a local world by comparing understandings of positioned participants. They also struggle to place their findings in a transpositional professional discourse of academic writings, one that is external both to the local world of their informants and to their own institutional and cultural settings. What anthropologists seek to achieve, however, is not objectivity of observation, but a multisided interpretation. Only because it includes multiple, situated interpretations can it be considered "transpositional." Translation of findings into what is more accurately called an interpositional discourse, furthermore, should be a final stage in anthropologists' work, not a precommitment or initial move.[4] Hence, even though their goal sounds much like Sen's, their way of going about achieving it seems rather different, and that difference in practice makes for a difference in outcome. The ethnography reads more like a work of social history or biography than a publication in economics or the health sciences.[5]

Anthropologists in international health credit the knowledge of local informants concerning everyday health practices, illness episodes, and therapeutic actions. Are they mistaken in doing so? Both Murray and Chen (1994) and Sen (1994) offer reasons for regarding this practice as epistemologically unsound. After all, patients do not have privileged access to objective "knowledge" about their underlying conditions that can be measurably verified with a high degree of probability. The patient's "subjective knowledge" is less reliable than the medical researcher's "objective knowledge." Doubt is cast on the informant's (and the ethnographer's) constructions.

Two comments need to be made here. First, the researcher's knowledge—that of the epidemiologist, the economist, the public health physician as much as the ethnographer and clinician—is a construction not so very different in kind, though often quite different in degree of systemization and control, from that of the informant. (I believe Sen's analysis also supports this point.) The histologist interpreting a surgical pathology slide or autopsy specimen of tissue presumed to be cancerous constructs the object of his or her inquiry (see Canguilhem 1989). The histologist works with a historically derived, changing set of categories that defines malignancy, that distinguishes, for example, premalignant or borderline cases, that stages invasiveness and spread in different systems of classification, and that relies on his or her focal and tacit knowledge to diagnose. Anyone who has ever looked under a high resolution microscope—say at cells, certain of which are malignant melanoma cells and others of which are dysplastic ones—knows that one has to be taught the categorization with its operationalized diagnostic criteria to distinguish the two, and even then it takes "experience" to "feel" confident one is making an objective assessment. The same can be said of "reading" a chest X-ray or interpreting a CT scan of the skull, listening to abnormal heart sounds, examining a rash, and conducting an epidemiological survey based on such interpretations. Categories construct experience, and in turn socially constructed experience validates the working knowledge and practices through which those categories are interpreted as "objective." Peter Berger and Thomas Luckmann (1967), in their classic statement of the social construction of reality, regard the internalization of cultural categories, through socialization, into personal experience as involving incorporation followed by objectivization. Thus, in their view, objectivity is, at least in part, a projection of internalized but socially derived categories onto the external world, where they are then "felt" to be "objective" structures of reality, because personal experience, through a grand tautology, does indeed match public definition.

Second, informants at times actually can be shown to possess privileged knowledge of the body that predicts at least certain health outcomes. That is to say, "subjective" knowledge may sometimes be more valid and useful than "objective" knowledge. For example, Richard Lazarus and Raymond Launier (1978) have demonstrated that individuals' "self-appraisal" of stressful events can predict what will be experienced as stressful. More impressively, Ellen Idler (1992) and colleagues (1990) have found that "subjective" self-assessment by the elderly of their health condition is a better predictor of their own mortality than are "objective" biomedical measures. In a similar vein, Edward Yelin and colleagues (1980) demonstrated that self-assessment was a better predictor of return to work among disabled chronic pain patients than more objective clinical or radiological tests. Working with informants in Mexico who believe they suffer or are believed by others to suffer from a "culture-bound condition," *susto* (soul loss), Arthur Rubel and colleagues (1984) determined that even though biomedical measures could not diagnose the condition or determine the pathology, sufferers had higher mortality rates than matched community control subjects. This indicated to them that subjective complaints and lay interpretations were sensitive to disease processes that biomedical methods could not measure. Finally, the ethnographer's use of positioned subjective accounts is an interpretation based upon multiple accounts so that there is the potential for cross-checking and for consensual validation, for example, of illness narratives from different members of the social network.

The chapters by Sen and by Murray and Chen refer to surveys in which better-educated populations living in higher socioeconomic settings who utilize health care services more frequently, and therefore are presumed to be healthier, report more symptoms than poorer, less-educated populations, who utilize services less frequently and who live in settings with poorer indexes of general health. Thus, Sen reviews survey data showing that people in Kerala, the state that has the best health status in India, report more symptoms than populations in certain of India's poorest states, who would also be expected to be in poorer health, while in international comparisons the self-reported illnesses of Americans in surveys are of greater magnitude than those of Indians, who again would be expected by objective standards to be in poorer health. This finding—which needs to be qualified by surveys in the United States that show the opposite, namely that African Americans, low-income persons, and the elderly do in fact rate their health status lower than do whites or higher-income and "younger" persons in keeping with objective measures (Barker et al. 1991; Idler 1990)—should not diminish interest in the pertinence of personal complaints. It is well known in the social survey literature that perception of the relative significance of a problem in a person's life or in the experience of a group is highly dependent on the context and increases with rising expectations. It is also well known that members of disadvantaged groups will tend to suppress complaints of misery, especially when they are interviewed by members of dominant groups, if they feel there is little that can be done or that their complaints may cause trouble (Guarnaccia et al. 1990; Scott 1990).[6] In fact, I take this to be Sen's point.

The positioned place of patient and family reports of symptoms, then, does not make those interpretations erroneous; it only qualifies that local knowledge. Some patients with peptic ulcer craters in their stomachs may not complain of pain; other individuals with the "classical" abdominal pain associated with peptic ulcer disease may have no gastrointestinal pathology. That does not mean that such patients are not conveying valid information about their experience of bodily processes; it only demonstrates a gap between experience and biology. Social expectation, cultural priority, and personal response fill that gap. Why should the materialistic determination of pathology and its projection into prognostic predictions about the future be considered as more authentic or real than the culturally and personally positioned human expression of suffering in the exigency of the here-and-now? I think Sen would agree on philosophical grounds, but Murray and Chen probably would not, because this distinction is, in fact, an operating tenet in international public health studies.

The tacit health knowledge of informants is used to inform health-relevant choices and actions, such as whether to smoke, wear a condom, wash one's hands, draw upon a social tie for strategic assistance in gaining access to health services, and so on. It contributes thereby to health outcomes. The sufferer's interpretation of suffering needs to be taken into account in the assessment of pain, distress, or dysfunction in order for such assessments to have validity in the experience of real people in real worlds.

Suffering is, moreover, not only a "subjective" phenomenon but also an interpersonal one. The distress of an Alzheimer's patient is part of a micro-context of serious trouble in which the family becomes a locus of the suffering and indeed even of the illness experience. We do not dwell in worlds where dichotomies between real/unreal disease, objective/subjective health problems, valid versus reliable diagnoses, or mind/body are part of everyday experience. These are professional constructions that are imposed on local worlds. Many chronic pain patients, for example, experience serious, disabling pain in the back or the head with objective evidence of only very modest, if any, "real" pathology on the CT scan or MRI. Pain for them is certainty, whereas for their health professionals it is doubt (Scarry 1985). A chronic back pain patient who is told not to worry because there is no evidence of "real" disease may be furious because that disaffirms his or her bodily experience. This is the logical outcome of the overvaluing of the biomedical understanding of objective measures and the devaluing of subjective or interpersonal ones—a characteristic of high-technology biomedicine. It has been shown repeatedly to have a dangerous effect on care (see Good, Brodwin et al. 1992). By delegitimating the interpersonal experience of suffering, this approach manages to be simultaneously inhumane and invalid.

Veena Das (1994), writing in the same volume in which this debate first appeared, criticizes the response of health professionals to the plight of the victims of the chemical poisoning at Bhopal. Her criticism turns on the insistence by those physicians that objective measures, not in Sen's sophisticated and qualified sense but in commonsense biomedical terms, replace self-report and family experience to determine the consequence of exposure. Thus, for the health experts, the complaints of many victims—impoverished adults and children who dwelt in a slum near the Union Carbide plant, and, therefore, whose health status was likely to have been poor before the disaster—were suspect because no "objective" evidence from "before" documented the "baseline" level of respiratory functioning and other physiological performance so that current status could be verified and any change that was documented could be attributed beyond any doubt to the disaster and not some other cause. For these professionals, the absence of objective baseline evidence meant that evidence gathered after the accident could never be objective enough to determine the cause. Thus, the victim was medicalized into a suspect who might be making unjustified or even illegal claims on welfare and disability funds—a profoundly disturbing transformation.

When objective indexes are used, they measure biological change as if it were fungible, separable from the experience of distress and the bearing of suffering. Indeed, "objectivity" in medicine is formulated so as to require such an artifactual, context-independent metric. Yet, can such an objective health index validly measure the consequence of industrial poisoning on the person, and on the experiential processes that integrate the affective, interpersonal, and neurobiological changes that together constitute the human quiddity of that person's suffering?

In one sense, ethnography comes closer than other methodologies to being "transpositional," because it requires specification and analysis of multiple (including self-) perspectives. Yet in Sen's analytic schema, ethnography may not qualify as providing transpositionally objective knowledge at all, inasmuch as the knowledge it constitutes remains positioned, or at best interpositional, experiential even if the ethnographer seeks a transpositional framework. Sen's carefully worded analysis clearly does not require that objectivity leave out human experience. Yet that may well be the unintended result when the quest for transpositional objectivity involves a leap from interpositional to extrapositional grounds and from intersubjective to objective claims. In this sense, an illusive ideal in measurement may become the enemy of a practical *modus operandi* for international health objectives: too rigorous a requirement for transpositional objectivity may lead the researcher to reject positioned knowledge. When this happens, say through the sole use of HIV sero-status and AIDS fatality rates to measure the AIDS pandemic, something fundamental to the human experience of suffering may be lost: namely, its grounding in greatly different local worlds and local lives (Farmer and Kleinman 1990). One impetus for the Chen, Kleinman, and Ware volume (1994) is disquiet among at least some international health researchers over too narrow an indexing of human suffering. This occurs, for example, when infant mortality rates obscure other measures of child "health." If child survival is accurately assessed but made into an "objective" sign of a community's positive health status, yet is followed by malnutrition, disability, and mental health problems among those same survivors—findings that clearly point in a more negative direction—then this measure is "objective" yet invalid. Perhaps the goal for international health studies should be to combine just that degree of transpositionally objective reliability which can be achieved while still making feasible a high degree of interpositional, experiential validity.

As the chapters in the section "Conceptual and Methodological Issues" in *Health and Social Change* clarify, classical metrics of mortality and morbidity are necessary but not sufficient to describe health transitions. They need to be supplemented by measures of disability and behavioral and social pathologies, and by humanly grounded descriptions of suffering. Narrative-based evaluations of the latter will differ in a fundamental way from numerical measures of the former. The same degrees of reliability and validity should not be required. Or, if they are, different kinds of measures (surveys enriched by stories of sickness) should be employed reciprocally to assure that both features of illness are assessed.

If these strictures are pertinent to the measurement of health changes, they are even more significant for the assessment of social change and the mediating processes that lead from particular social processes to health outcomes. To understand what urbanization in a low-income African society such as Kenya is about and to assess its effects on health, it is insufficient to treat urbanization as a unified variable that can be objectively operationalized, inquired about, and assigned a quantitative value for any population. Rather, urbanization as a concept needs to be unpacked—separated into subprocesses and understood in the historical context of particular settings of rural migration and urban resettlement.

This social change can be greatly different for a marginalized woman who migrates with her children from a community undergoing serious breakdown into a big city slum without support from husband or kin, as compared with a woman and her children who migrate from a vital rural community to which they retain effective social ties into a market town where husband and maternal kin have occupied a compound in a neighborhood of fellow villagers and are engaged in a thriving business. The characteristics of the rural-urban migrants (their ethnicity, age, gender, class, employment, education, and health status), the community from which they come, their resources, the type of uprooting (voluntary, forced), the forms of migration, the situation into which they migrate—all contribute to qualify the variable, urbanization, as does the history of migration in that society and the large-scale political and economic forces that push and pull the displaced. To measure the mediators that transform social processes into health outcomes, the way to proceed would be to parse urbanization as a social category into those components that are locally valid. No social change could be validly assessed without evaluation of its contextual meaning for those who experience it. That meaning will mediate between the larger social world, the microprocesses of family and neighborhood, and the person's psychobiological processes; indeed, as a result of that mediation between the social, the biological, and the psychological those body and self processes are transformed into sociosomatic ones. Meaning will itself be a changing mix of cultural code, what is at stake in social negotiations over resources, personal experience, and conversations with positioned others, including the ethnographer. Measurement will need to canvass meaning in context, social process, and historical event, and their relationship to health indexes. Such relational measures will require both "objective" and "subjective" information.

Clearly, the requirements for this type of research cannot be met unless we move beyond the objectivist/subjectivist dichotomy, even with transpositional and positional qualifications. That movement either can be toward interdisciplinary forms of assessment that integrate quantitative and qualitative evaluations, or toward studies that encompass the separate contributions of narratives and numbers. Our terminology may be different, yet I interpret Amartya Sen's analysis as a complementary call for widening the space of measurement to make room for what is interpersonally at stake for human beings.

Objectivity and the Basic Values of International Health

The search for solid assurances of objectivity, as important as it is for international public health, is by no means an end in itself. If you ask experts in international health to explain just why objectivity is so important, they do not offer a basic scientist's defense of the scientific process. Nor do they launch into a discussion of epistemology and ontology. Quite to the contrary, they insist theirs is an applied field. And it is for a thoroughly applied reason that objective surveys are said to be crucial to their mission. International health professionals like to tell down-to-earth stories about desperately poor people dwelling in miserable urban slums or in villages on the dangerous margin of survival whose family members are suffering from sometimes fatal, yet potentially preventable, disorders—diarrheal diseases, measles, malaria—while the governmental agencies of those societies are expending the funds that should support progressive programs to control these serious problems on other, less essential, sometimes downright inappropriate services, too often ones that benefit those with power and wealth.

The moral of these paradigmatic tales is that "objective" measurement of the magnitude, distribution, and cost of health problems is essential if advocates of the health needs of the poor and powerless are to be able to effectively persuade the representatives of health and finance ministries to expend the resources necessary to control (or eradicate) preventable diseases. A second lesson these professional tales offer is that only objective measurements can establish, equitably and justly, who are the truly deserving and which problems are most serious and would benefit most from specific public health interventions. Hence, objectivity is ultimately necessary to authorize action, and action, based upon rational technical guidelines, is the moral mandate of this profession. (See Dasgupta 1993 for a similar argument within development economics.)

A child of Enlightenment thinking if ever there was one, international health, which is one of the pivotal fields of social development, sponsors a rational technical discourse that regards health as the progressive achievement of societies that modernize. Among the many things that modernization denotes is movement through a transition that separates underdevelopment from development; high fertility from low; poverty and ignorance and passivity and superstition from a modernity based upon education and rational choice; and high infant mortality rates, high infectious disease rates, and compromised longevity from the improved health indexes of industrialized societies (see, for example, Caldwell et al. 1990).

This transition—variously called the demographic, epidemiological, or simply the health transition—is held to be one of the major milestones on the path of progress. The movement along this path is described in the objective measures of improving health and social indices: fertility, mortality, education, gross national product, and so on. Progress should be continuous along axes of increasing industrialization, technology transfer, democratization, professional expertise, individual autonomy and empowerment, and, of course, health. Action is needed to remove obstacles, advance the pace of change, and control or eradicate disease. Thus, the idea that objectivity underwrites practical applications is linked, "objectively" as it were, to the idea of progress. Together they constitute the moral basis of the profession of international public health.

From the perspectives of anthropology and social history this positivist value orientation is obviously more than a little problematic. To begin with, the ideas of progress and development assume a universal standard against which the experiences of different societies can be compared as evidence of greater or lesser success. The particularities of social change in a region or series of local contexts must be ironed out to fit the universal metric. The process of "ironing out" is one of aggregating data at ever higher levels, ultimately ending up in a comparison of the "developed" and the "developing" societies, or the nonindustrialized, the industrializing, and the industrialized, a dual or tripartite categorization into which all societies are made to fit. Aggregated data are also "cleaned" so that what is peculiar to a context is removed from what is shared and therefore generalizable. Cross-cultural ethnographic comparisons, much like social histories, tell a very different story, of course. Here there are few instances of progressive advance toward health, or universal principles guiding the aggregation of greatly different societies and regions. In their place, there are detailed stories of the local history of particular places and peoples undergoing many kinds of social change with all sorts of antecedents and consequences.[7]

Nancy Scheper-Hughes (1992; and see chapter 9 below) describes a *favela* in a small Brazilian city in the impoverished northeast in which misery is endemic and health problems multiple and seemingly incorrigible, even as the region and the rest of the city "progress" economically through the production of sugar and as certain health problems are improved. The infant mortality rate may be reduced through earlier access to more effective treatment of diarrheal disease with associated life-threatening dehydration, but malnutrition, other infectious disorders, and mental health problems are widespread. Is this an indubitable instance of success? Few would regard it as such since the poverty and violence and suffering of everyday life are so extensive; yet for public health purposes, the improvement in outcome of severe diarrheal disease will be depicted as a story of success. Here medicalizing social problems, focusing upon an individual disorder in a field of interrelated problems, and applying the positivist metrics of objective measurement woefully mislead.

China in 1994 offers another example of the complexities of development. The coastal edge, where perhaps 200 million people reside, possesses the world's fastest growing economy (a 13 percent growth rate). Urbanites and rural villagers enjoy a greatly improved standard of living. But China has also an interior where 750 to 800 million people, mostly very poor peasants, are experiencing "development" at a very different pace. Whereas the coast from Guangdong to Jilin has transformed China into the world's third largest economy (according to Purchasing Power Parity), after the United States and Japan, the huge interior is closer in living conditions to India than it is to Singapore, Hong Kong, or Taiwan. In the southwest and northwest provinces, yet another 200 million Chinese live in conditions of often extreme poverty. Here infant mortality rates can be five times higher than the rate in Shanghai; the poorest peasants rarely eat meat and often get inadequate amounts of vegetables. Some can't afford rice on a regular basis. Housing is also inadequate, and there are not enough clothes to go around. Whereas peasants in the coastal periphery can afford a fairly high level of fee-for-service health care, in the most impoverished interior, they cannot. And as a result they suffer without biomedical care, inasmuch as the rural health care system and its insurance schemes, in impoverished areas, have broken down under the pressure of decollectivization and privatization. Some claim that the situation of the poorest peasants is no different than under the Qing Dynasty. This third sector of the Chinese economy and polity contains most of China's minority groups, whose standard of living is far below that of Han Chinese.[8] Tens of millions of internal economic migrants who are encamped in China's cities come from this "other" China. Economic and health conditions of this "floating population" vary greatly, but many are destitute, their shantytowns sites of violence and sickness.

In many areas of China, crime, prostitution, drug abuse, and sexually transmitted disease have returned to the high rates that prevailed under the Nationalists, after forty years during which they were effectively contained by the diffused political control of the communist state, which simultaneously created political violence and human rights abuses on an immense scale. New problems have arisen related to appalling levels of industrial hygiene, inadequate environmental safeguards, man-made catastrophes such as explosions at munition manufacturers' plants, and the early onset of an AIDS epidemic. Success and failure are systematically related, as in the case of cigarette smoking, which places tens of millions of Chinese at risk for lung cancer, emphysema, heart disease, and stroke, yet also fills the coffers of the state's tobacco monopoly and thereby contributes to economic success.

How are these predicaments of health to be assessed within the paradigm of "development"? There is evidence of economic and health successes, economic and health failures, the dark side of rapid economic reform, and continued underdevelopment. Intrasocietal diversity, and indeed fragmentation, is so extensive as to defeat a single index of socioeconomic and health change. Does it even seem sensible anymore to use aggregate statistics to describe China as a single social unit? Do such statistics describe an "objective" entity? Is aggregation across regions valid? Can there be a "transpositional objectivity" when there are so very many "realities" that stand for China's economic and social conditions? Will a single narrative of health and social change in China do?

What interests are served by the quest for objective data? Clearly, first served are those interests of the professionals whose technical construction of a public problem can then become the basis for developing and evaluating intervention programs (see Gusfield 1981).

Doubtless at times those professional interests will correspond with the needs of the public. The eradication of smallpox is an outstanding example. Yet, frequently the acquisition of technical data is self-serving and does not contribute in a significant way to the health of the community. By privileging questions of the objectivity of observation, public health surveys routinely avoid questions of the "interests" that stand behind and direct the search for objective findings. Therefore, the political and economic interests of the state or of dominant factions are ultimately served.

This need not be the case. Professional formulation of the health components of societal problems can articulate (and occasionally have done so) interrelated problems of powerlessness, poverty, and suffering as a broader social policy horizon requiring political and economic transformation. Indeed, historical, anthropological, and sociological studies regularly do so, as do, less frequently, epidemiological surveys. The question, then, becomes one of discovering how professional public health interests have been subordinated to dominant political economic interests. While students of this topic have examined the politics of health policy and the sociology of the professions (see, for example, Justice 1985; Freidson 1986), I think it is equally important to examine the relationship of scientific epistemology and public health practice to cultural orientations that are closely linked with political economic interests and institutions.

The entire field of social development, involving the academy, the foundations, governmental agencies, nongovernmental agencies, and international institutions such as the World Bank, is oriented around what is called "science-based" development. But what kind of science? In the main, not that kind of science which emphasizes critical engagement with the purposes and concepts of social change and its relationship to health, or which points to the variety and diversity of changes and outcomes. Rather, science-based development all too often builds upon economic, epidemiological, and policy analyses that privilege the transpositionally objective measurement of narrowly articulated professional categories—the view from nowhere (Nagel 1986)—over the anthropology, history, and sociology of the view from a particular somewhere by a particular somebody with some special interest at stake.

In this way, the social development field connects with the idea of a value-free, objective domain of health and human development.

Here progress and flourishing are "natural" and social and health difficulties are professionally articulated as "human problems," obstacles to progress that require technical remedies. Thereby, poverty is constructed as a risk factor, unclean water and uncontrolled sewage are precipitating causes, and microorganisms are the agents of ill health for which technical fixes can be arranged. Their systematic relationship to one another and to political and economic structures, however, goes unaddressed.

This approach is not without its utility for the solution of narrowly conceived, though still important, problems such as water and sewage control, a utility which no one could argue against. Yet the emphasis on science-based development, I would suggest, is also at times what is wrong with international development and public health. The sources of human misery are based in the dynamic effects of large-scale political and economic forces working within local worlds. Those causal effects are mediated by cultural and historical processes that place certain categories of persons under great pressure while protecting others, that provide resources for some while blocking access to resources among others. It is not that these forces, processes, and effects cannot be objectively measured, but rather that the narrow technical pursuit of objectivity, as currently constructed by the international health professions, gets in the way of the larger conceptual and methodological task of reconstructing and reinterpreting those social sources of human misery so that their powerful interconnections can be targeted for interventions.

Thus, what at first glance seems to be a fairly recondite question of the epistemology and ontology of objectivity points to deep values in international public health that are themselves a major barrier to understanding the sources of ill health and studying ways to effectively address them. Anthropology and social history offer a needed complement because they critique the deep-grained assumptions that need to be recast. Only through the concrete understanding of particular worlds of suffering and the way they are shaped by political economy and cultural change can we possibly come to terms with the complex human experiences that underwrite health.

And yet, the quest for objectivity also offers certain strengths that cannot be waved away (and indeed are not) by most historians of medicine and anthropologists of health. These strengths complement and go beyond interpretive approaches and suggest that an adequate study of international health problems requires both narratives and numbers. To more adequately formulate and assess leading international health issues such as AIDS, drug abuse and related violence, forced uprooting and migration, and malaria and tuberculosis, the appropriate goal should be to work out *modi operandi* that reciprocally use quantitative and qualitative measures, that insist on validity together with reliability, and that balance history with epidemiology and ethnography with policy analysis. That reciprocal engagement is also the way to test the significance and practicality of conceptual as well as methodological practices.

There is, of course, a huge barrier to the integration of anthropological and international public health approaches. Although some anthropologists have learned to work effectively with international health experts with impressive achievement—say, in assisting public health programs to proceed in culturally appropriate ways in local communities (Nichter 1989; Kendall 1988; Nichter and Kendall 1991)—they have usually (and, given their goal, appropriately) not challenged the fundamental orientation of public health. Yet, taken to an extreme, the critique of the cult of objectivity does lead to an almost insurmountable divide, an epistemological and, one wants to say, ideological disjunction between the two professions that I for one find uncomfortable, unnecessary, and unhelpful. To explore the divide at the most extreme point, let's examine a position set out by Nancy Scheper-Hughes (1992:171–172), a medical anthropologist who has employed ethnography to provocatively challenge policy directions and criticize the alleged abuses of medicine.

Explicitly following in the well-trod footsteps of the European tradition of critical theory, she notes that "commonsense reality may be false, illusory, and oppressive" (p. 171). The goal of the critical medical anthropologist is to search out buried truths in order to "'speak truth' to power and domination" (p. 171). This means exposing the role of "traditional" intellectuals and experts who are "bourgeois agents of the social consensus" that maintains "hegemonic ideas and practices" (p. 171). Doctors are such experts, and therefore serve a crucial social function by misidentifying the hidden indignation of the oppressed poor who are sick and its sources in the sociopolitical order. Anthropologists who fail to speak this class truth occupy the same role as doctors (p. 172). The medicalization of folk complaints—that is, the doctor's diagnosis and treatment of folk idioms of complaint—is a kind of appropriation that may treat the symptoms but simultaneously camouflages their social cause. Therefore medical treatment is "bad faith," "an oblique but powerful defense strategy of the state" (pp. 169–170).

This analytic line is not hyperbolic for its own sake. It is obviously meant to draw a dividing line between critical theorists and others, including international public health professionals and anthropologists who do not accept the idea that they are collaborating in "bad faith" with hegemonic projects of the state and transnational corporate capitalism to boot. The critical theorists claim moral superiority and accuse others of immoral behavior; that is, other professionals in the health field are implicated as working with bad faith or false consciousness, mystifying the political reality via medical applications.

So unqualified a revolutionary claim will strike many—especially given the current vicissitudes of revolutions—as mischievously overdrawn. This margin is untenable. After all, has not even Henri Lefebvre (1991:25), one of Europe's leading Marxist theoreticians, pronounced: "Critical theory, after being driven into practical opposition—and even into the most radical form of it—has had its day." Fortunately, relatively few medical anthropologists, including perhaps even Scheper-Hughes in her more generously collaborative style, would go along with this extreme position, based upon which any useful collaboration with health professionals short of revolutionary change would seem almost impossible. (Indeed, the purpose of the extremist position may be to make interdisciplinary collaboration much more difficult.)

And yet, I also think many medical anthropologists will properly regard a critical perspective (including the important findings in Scheper-Hughes's ambitious ethnography of everyday violence in the lives of the chronically poor and hungry) to be an important *modus operandi* in their work. I certainly do. A critical cultural analysis is needed to unpack international health's value commitment to the objective measurement of change in health status based upon the cultural idea of progress. Cultural critique is also necessary because of our epoch's construction of the great issues in health largely (and sometimes solely) as questions of economic costs and their control. The historical relationship between cultural practices, politics, and economics in the latest phase of capitalism should be at the heart of ethnographic studies, be they in Africa or America. Anthropology's project in international health (not the only one but surely an important one) should be to sponsor critical studies at several levels and also to encourage research that balances or complements objectivity with criticism. That means that besides collaborating with international health professionals in programs that are organized within a public health framework, anthropologists need to organize alternative frameworks for international health studies that conceptualize health, health conditions, and health care in social theoretical ways that can use ethnography and cross-cultural comparison as chief methodologies.

Although useful efforts to do so are under way, it is not at all surprising, given the early stage of research and the difficulty of securing core research funding, that these efforts have not yet created a substantial body of work that is comparable to economic, policy analytic, and epidemiological contributions.[9] Because questions of the objectivity of methodology and findings have dominated the latter approaches to international health research, the conceptual basis of international health has remained remarkably underdeveloped. Hence there is a special opportunity for critically informed social theory, though of a somewhat more circumscribed variety, to define and fill in the conceptual space of international health. It is for this reason that an analysis of objectivity, as remote as it may seem at first from the exigent social problems of human conditions, is an occasion to critique what has been done so far and offers an opening to suggest what could be done in future. It is a rebuke to frustration over established strategies (see Desjarlais et al. 1995).

Hilary Putnam suggests that with respect to objectivity we might as well

accept the position we are fated to occupy in any case, the position of beings who cannot have a view of the world that does not reflect our interests and values, but who are, for all that, committed to regarding some views of the world—and, for that matter, some interests and values—as better than others. This may be giving up a certain metaphysical picture of objectivity, but it is not giving up the idea that there are what Dewey called "objective resolutions of problematic situations"—objective resolutions to problems which are *situated*, that is, in a place, at a time, as opposed to an "absolute" answer to "perspective-independent" questions. And that is objectivity enough. (1993:156)

Amen!

PART TWO

Suffering as Social Experience

5

Suffering and Its Professional Transformation

Toward an Ethnography of Interpersonal Experience

Interpretation and Experience

An effective strategy in medical anthropology is to demonstrate how a patient's illness complaints and convictions reproduce a particular moral domain. Via visible social archetypes and invisible social processes, pain and lay modes of help seeking are shown to replicate a cultural world, one, moreover, that the anthropologist can validly interpret. The theory may come from Durkheim, Weber, Marx, Freud, or Foucault, and the style of ethnographic writing may be no-nonsense naturalism or vexed postmodernism, yet the accomplishment is to show that illness is a socially constructed reality to which the ethnographer has privileged access.

This interpretative strategy is often followed by a second analytic feat in which the anthropologist reveals how the clinician reworks the patient's perspective into disease diagnoses and treatments that reproduce the health profession and its political-economic sources. The

This chapter is a revised and expanded version of an article written with Joan Kleinman which was originally published in *Culture, Medicine and Psychiatry* (15[3]:275–301) in 1991. The expansion draws upon materials from Arthur Kleinman and Joan Kleinman, "How Bodies Remember" (*New Literary History* 25 [summer 1994]:707–723).

semiotic iteration of the suffering of lay men and women into the tax-
onomies of healing professionals is then shown to distort the moral
world of patient and community.

Thus, when a psychiatrist transforms the misery that results from
political calamity—say, the horror of the Cambodian genocide or the
numbing routinization of poverty in urban ghettos—into major depressive disorder, posttraumatic stress, or sociopathic personality disorder, the anthropologist claims that, notwithstanding technical and
ethical intentions to the contrary, psychiatry ends up delegitimating
the patient's suffering as moral commentary and political performance.
At least by implication, psychiatrists are held to trivialize the experience of their subjects, and even perhaps render them more difficult to
work through. The anthropological accounts, then, claim to make a
fundamental critique of the psychiatric transformation of that irreduc-
ible existential quality of illness. That professional transformation, it is
claimed, sometimes with more than a little suggestion of moral superiority, re-creates human suffering as inhuman disease (J. Cassell 1991).

The anthropologists' *interpretive dilemma* is that they participate in
the same process of professional transformation. The interpretation of
some person's or group's suffering as the reproduction of oppressive
relationships of production, the symbolization of dynamic conflicts in
the interior of the self, or as resistance to authority, is a transformation
of everyday experience of the same order as those pathologizing re-
constructions within biomedicine. Nor is it morally superior to an-
thropologize distress, rather than to medicalize it. What is lost in biomedical renditions—the complexity, uncertainty, and ordinariness of
some man or woman's world of experience—is also missing when illness is reinterpreted as social role, social strategy, or social symbol . . .
as anything but human experience.

Please do not misinterpret our intention. We are not positing an anthropological oxymoron like suffering as experience taken neat, without its cultural meanings and historical changes. There can be no such
acultural, ahistorical human phenomenon. But we are suggesting that
anthropological analyses (of pain and passion and power), when they
are experience-distant, are at risk of delegitimating their subject matter's human conditions. The anthropologist thereby constitutes a false
subject; she or he can engage in a professional discourse every bit as
dehumanizing as that of colleagues who unreflectively draw upon the
tropes of biomedicine or behaviorism to create their subject matter.

Ethnography does participate in this professional transformation of an experience-rich and -near human subject into a dehumanized object, a caricature of experience. That it occasionally resists such transformation seems to have more to do with the constraints imposed by participant observation as an empirical practice—by its very nature a way of knowing difficult to isolate from the messiness and hurly-burly of daily living—than with anthropological theorizing about experience and its modes.

Categories for the Ethnography of Experience

What categories might an ethnography of experience, in particular one concerned with the study of illness and other forms of suffering, draw upon to resist the tendency toward dehumanizing professional deconstruction, or simply to become more self-consciously reflective about the human core of human experience? It is our opinion that a contextual focus on experience-near categories for ethnography should begin with the defining characteristic of *overbearing practical relevance* in the processes and forms of experience. That is to say, *something is at stake* for all of us in the daily round of happenings and transactions.[1]

Experience may, on theoretical grounds, be thought of as the intersubjective medium of social transactions in local moral worlds. It is the outcome of cultural categories and social structures interacting with psychophysiological processes such that a mediating world is constituted. Experience is the felt flow of that intersubjective medium. In Pierre Bourdieu's (1989) terms it is the social matrix out of which habitus is structured and where shared mental/bodily states in turn structure social interactions. Yet, in practical terms, that mediating world is defined by what is vitally at stake for groups and individuals. While preservation of life, aspiration, prestige, and the like may be shared structures of relevance for *human conditions* across societies, that which is at stake in daily situations differs (often dramatically) owing to cultural elaboration, personal idiosyncrasy, historical particularities, and the specifics of the situation.[2] What is at stake in life settings, then, is usually contested and indeterminate (Kleinman 1992).

Ethnographers enter the stream of social experience at a particular time and place, so that their description will be both a cross-sectional slice through the complexity of ongoing priorities and a part of the temporal flow of changing structures of relevance. That such structures are contested, indeterminate, novel, and changing means that the ethnographer's descriptions are always about a local moral world that can only be known incompletely, and for which the relative validity of observations must be regularly recalibrated. Moreover, what the ethnographer experiences matches how individuals encounter the flow of experience (Dewey 1957:269). They do not dominate it, or invent it, but rather are born or thrown into the stream of lived interactions. (See Jackson 1989:1–15 for a review of phenomenological sources for this existential appreciation of experience.)

A central concern in ethnography should be the interpretation of what is at stake for particular participants in particular situations.[3] That orientation will lead the ethnographer to collective (both local and societal) and individual (both public and intimate) levels of analysis of experience-near interests that, we hold, offer a more valid initial understanding of what are social-psychological characteristics of forms of life in local worlds than either professional sociological categories (roles, sets, status) or psychological terminology (affect, cognition, defense, behavior).[4]

The focus on what is at stake encourages the ethnographer to build up an ethnopsychological inventory of key indigenous conceptions, but not to stop the analysis at that point. The level of indigenous categories qua categories can quickly become artificial—as the misadventures of ethnoscience clearly disclose—because it leaves out precisely what orients those categories to practical experience. Moreover, a list of ethnopsychological categories in itself can only partially provide the grounds for understanding what is shared in human conditions and what social psychological processes mediate experience. The former, the conditions of being human, refers to the existence of certain defining rhythms and limits to experience: birth, life cycle change, moral development, death, and bereavement. Human conditions—for example, the subject of this chapter, suffering—constrain lived experience. They offer a resistance in the flow of life to the elaboration of life plans.[5] The dialectical dance between these shared resistances and the culturally elaborated yet simultaneously idiosyncratic structures of relevance creates the "bewildering inexpediency" of human experience (Manning 1981). It also shapes the character of danger, the scope and possibilities of transcendence, and the other existential quiddities that taken together represent whatever is meant by the expression *human nature.* That is to say, the flow of experience is not the product of a human nature (personality, instinct, etc.) but the condition for its emergence as both shared and culturally particular, and therefore far from the determinative agency that has been claimed by psychoanalysts, cognitive behaviorists, or most other psychological theorists.[6]

The upshot of this phenomenological vision is that viewed from close up, the density of personal awareness (the actors' and the observers') of the richness of human experiences is difficult to express and uncertain owing to its repleteness, subtlety, and complexity. Yet when viewed from afar the historical shape of experience is apparent as are cross-culturally shared elements and rhythms. The ethnographer's focus moves back and forth. The task is to interpret patterns of meaning within situations understood in experience-near categories; yet, ethnographers also bring with them a liberating distance that comes from their own experience-near categories and their existential appreciation of shared human conditions. That means that ethnography, like history and biography and psychotherapy, holds the possibility of a way of knowing more valid to the dialectical structure and contingent flow of lived experience than reductionistic forms of knowing that by definition distort the existential conditions of life. This perspective also suggests why understanding ethnopsychological categories, though essential, is insufficient: we know much more than we can say or understand; we are awash in the meanings of experience; the historical flow and cultural elaboration of experience lead us to organize figures out of grounds that are greatly relevant to particular occasions. (Our informants and our audiences are also trained in varying levels of irony, as Geertz [1988] puts it.) Getting at mediating psychological processes requires that eventually we shift to the view from afar—we cannot otherwise abstract universalizing processes from the particularizing content of ethnopsychological meanings—but to understand actual situations we must use both lenses.

In sum, then, what is at stake for particular men and women in their local worlds offers an example of the type of category we regard as crucial for advancing an ethnography of experience.[7] In discussing this category, we have all too quickly touched upon other aspects of experience—for example, the existential pressure for coherence and unity (see Oakeshott 1985), the immediacy of its felt quality (Cassirer 1962:78; Merleau-Ponty 1962), the confusing multiplicity and indeterminancy of its flow (à la Bergson [1889] and William James [1981:

279–379]), the notion that it is emergent, achieved, and contested, not preformed (as in Dewey 1957:269), the character of brute resistance to life plan that must be transcended and that expresses the finitude of experience (Jackson 1989:1–15), the existential responsibility to come to terms with its teleology (Sartre 1956:553–556; Frankl 1967: 84–93), and so on. These recognizable aspects of experience suggest other categories that must inform our ethnographies. For the purposes of this chapter, however, a single category will be all that we can handle, though we shall return to certain others later in the chapter.

Human Suffering

We will examine the suffering that is a concomitant of illness and its social sources as an illustration of the ethnography of experience. Biomedical interpretations of illness have properly been criticized for leaving the experience of suffering out of assessment of the disease. In order to depict suffering, anthropological accounts disclose how the idiosyncrasies and divided interests and cross-purposes of personal life lived under the strenuous constraint of disease processes are actually culturally patterned into recognizably shared forms: for example, the desperate withdrawal and isolation of seriously ill Gnau patients near the Sepik River in New Guinea (Lewis 1975), the neurasthenia of Chinese with major depression in Beijing or Taipei (Kleinman 1986), the *nervios* of Puerto Rican immigrants to inner city ghettos on the East Coast of the United States (Guarnaccia 1989) and so on. To accomplish this analytic feat the illness experience is frozen at a certain moment as if the illness narrative had reached completion or the illness course had terminated at a final stop. Of course, in the actual flow of illness experience, there is no final stop. Even death is followed by bereavement and the further and influential trajectory of the remembered past (for the family and the practitioners). The anthropologist creates the illusion of finality and continuity and coherent meaning, when in fact even the simplest illness episode has more complex resonances than can be accounted for by the analytic models that are available to us. The abstraction of a definitive cultural form out of the inchoate transitoriness and recalcitrant uncertainties of the everyday experience of illness does violence to the personally idiosyncratic and the situationally particular, to the "blooming buzzing" confusion of the stream of living. As shown in *The Illness Narratives* (Kleinman 1988a), cultural representation is only one of at least several discrete kinds of illness meanings—the others include the personal and interpersonal meanings in a local setting—yet in numerous medical anthropological accounts it is all that readers learn about an illness. The authors hold that the anthropological tendency to create cultural archetypes out of the always messy and uncertain details of a personal account of illness—an approach to which we too have contributed—is as invalid an interpretation of the human core of suffering as is the biomedical tendency to create a purely biological metaphor for pain. Both render the peculiarly human quality of suffering—that which is most at stake for the participants—fungible. By alienating the illness from what is at stake for particular individuals in particular situations, cultural analysis creates an inhuman reality every bit as artifactual as the pathologist's disease entity. If there is no purely "natural" course of disease, there also can be no purely "cultural" symptomatology.

Suffering can be defined from the historical and cross-cultural record as a universal aspect of human experience in which individuals and groups have to undergo or bear certain burdens, troubles, and serious wounds to the body and the spirit that can be grouped into a variety of forms. There are *contingent misfortunes* such as serious acute illness. There are *routinized forms of suffering* that are either shared aspects of human conditions—chronic illness or death—or experiences of deprivation and exploitation and degradation and oppression that certain categories of individuals (the poor, the vulnerable, the defeated) are specially exposed to and others relatively protected from. There also is *suffering resulting from extreme conditions,* such as survivorship of the Holocaust or the atom bomb or the Cambodian genocide or China's Cultural Revolution. The cultural meanings of suffering (e.g., as punishment or salvation) may be elaborated in different ways for current-day Sri Lankan Buddhists or medieval Christians, but the intersubjective experience of suffering, we contend, is itself a defining characteristic of human conditions in all societies.

To illustrate this point in order to draw out its significance for understanding human suffering as the focus of an ethnography of experience, we will turn to a case of the bodily mode of experiencing personal and political distress—that is, somatization—in Chinese culture.

Case Illustration

Huang Zhenyi is a worker from a rural county town in his late twenties with depression.[8] He attributes his chronic headaches and dizziness to a traumatic childhood experience during the Cultural Revolution, about which he can talk only to his wife. During winter vacation from school, when he was twelve, Huang Zhenyi returned to the schoolyard. Someone had tacked up a piece of paper with "Throw down Chairman Mao!" written in bold characters across it. Not knowing what to do about this anti-Mao slogan, he ran to see his close friend, who told him to quickly inform their commune leaders. This he did, and those cadres responded by calling in the public security (police) agents. Three of them interviewed Huang Zhenyi at his school. They asked him who wrote the poster, and when he could not respond they accused him. The policemen threatened that if he didn't confess they would not let him return home. Frightened after being interrogated for several hours in a small room at the school, from which he was not allowed to go to the toilet in spite of a painful urge to urinate, he told the police that he had found the slogan but was not the one who wrote it. He was angry at his friend for not supporting his story by telling what had actually happened. Eventually, late at night, his interrogators allowed Huang to return home. There he found his mother distraught over his absence. He explained the problem to her and assured her he was not at fault.

The next morning the three agents came to Huang Zhenyi's home and took him to the public security building. Brutally, they assured Huang Zhenyi that this time he would never leave the small interrogation room until he confessed. Terrified that he would not be allowed to eat, relieve himself, or see his mother again, Huang Zhenyi signed the confession, accepting sole responsibility for writing the poster.

When he returned home he told his mother that he had written the poster, fearing that if he told her the truth it would only create greater trouble for her and for him. Huang Zhenyi still recalls with obvious pain his mother crying and cursing him, "If I knew before you'd end up like this, I wouldn't have wanted you." He remembers breaking down in tears, but he found himself unable to tell his mother the truth. "I felt like a coward. I couldn't tell her."

This experience recalled for him an earlier one. At age eight he had gone with several classmates to fish in a nearby pond, instead of walking to school. They were very late getting to class. The teacher punished them by locking the boys in a small mud-walled room. They escaped by knocking a hole in the wall and hid in a nearby cotton field. Their teacher, who was known for being a strict disciplinarian, ran after them and caught Huang Zhenyi's two friends but not him. "I was so frightened I froze in my place. I could not move." Later in the evening he returned home, and the next day went back to school. The teacher, greatly angered by Huang's behavior, ordered him to do menial work around the school rather than study. Huang Zhenyi refused to do the hard labor, and this led his teacher to criticize him severely in front of other teachers. After this experience, Huang Zhenyi reported "my liver became small, and I became frightened, cowardly." From this time onward he felt "paralyzed" whenever he had to "stand up" for himself before adults.

Because of his confession, the twelve-year-old Huang Zhenyi—who again felt "paralyzed," unable to break his silence before his adult accusers—was marched through the local county town wearing a dunce cap, carrying a sign around his neck on which he had written a self-criticism for the "terrible act," surrounded by thousands of local peasants and cadres, who cursed him, spat at him, and threw dirt and pebbles at him. The next day he was sent to work as a peasant at a local production team. He was expected to do the work of an adult. No one would talk with him at first. The heavy labor was so exhausting that Huang Zhenyi thought he would not survive. Each day he had to undergo self-criticism, while local groups of children jeered at him. In a mass criticism session he felt himself go numb, as if paralyzed. He wanted to yell out the truth but couldn't get himself to do it, to break his silence. No one would believe him, Huang Zhenyi reasoned. He had been patient so far, he would endure the unendurable, since there was no way out. Finally, after a year of hard labor, a year during which he several times thought he could no longer stand the work and the isolation, his fellow peasants praised him for doing the work of an adult and enduring his punishment in silence. They pleaded on his behalf with the local authorities that he be allowed to return to school, which he did.

Eventually Huang left this commune and moved to a county town in another province, where he finished high school and where his past was unknown. He became a key worker and joined the Communist Party. He was able to do the latter since the local party officials, owing to the chaos of the time, knew nothing about his past and because of his highly regarded poor peasant background. He never told his mother his version of what had happened. When she was dying he thought of confessing to her the full story but decided against it. "I was too frightened to speak out and didn't think it would do any good." Huang's mother died not knowing of her son's innocence, a point he returns to again and again as a palpable reason for his current feelings of desperate shame and self-hatred.

Now, looking back, he feels depressed, hopeless, desperate. He retains great anger at the three policemen and at his classmate, who would not admit to the interrogators that Huang Zhenyi had told him he had found, not written, the anti-Maoist poster. He feels a searing sense of injustice, a feeling that he associates with a burning sensation in the head, dizziness, and exhaustion. He is fearful that someone in the party will learn of his past and expel him on account of it.

Huang believes he will never recover from this event. "It has affected my character. I am withdrawn; I don't like to be too friendly with others. I am a coward. I cannot trust others." He sees his only hope as writing a novel about his experience that would fictionalize it to protect his anonymity and generalize it so that it comes to represent the "losses and defeat" his generation has experienced. "Like me, we are a lost generation that has suffered so much." But Huang Zhenyi doubts he will accomplish this goal. He has no formal training or natural skill to write fiction. He actively fears the consequences of others learning about his past. He feels trapped. Each time he takes up a pen to write the story, he is overcome by a self-defeating lassitude, dizziness, and sense of his inefficacy. Hence Huang's physical complaints are amplified (perhaps created) by the literal embodiment of chronic frustration, inability to act—if we use his word, "paralysis," but of will, not muscle—and the unbearable inner hurt of shameful "injustice" that he can neither publicly articulate (save through the personally unavailing neurasthenic pain) nor privately expiate.

Huang Zhenyi's own statement that his losses during the Cultural Revolution represent those of his generation signifies a collective awareness in China that the Cultural Revolution deeply affected the lives of entire cohorts of Chinese, in this case adolescents. Unlike others I have interviewed to understand the relationship of neurasthenia to political oppression, his losses during these terrible times were not the physical loss of close family members (his mother died after the Cultural Revolution). Instead Huang is talking about the loss of self-esteem, self-confidence, the normal developmental period of becoming an adult, the normal relationships with family members, and also of hope in his future and that of his society.

Doubtless there are parallels in pre-Communist China and in other societies, the United States included. We are not trying to suggest that what happened to Chinese in the Cultural Revolution is without precedent or cannot be compared to social sources of misery in other societies. But it is also the case that we mean to implicate an entire generation in Huang's distress. His demoralization and anguish may be (and probably are) greater than that of others, owing to his personal vulnerability and the magnitude of the crisis he experienced. He developed a disorder, most others did not. Yet it is precisely because Huang's disorder exposes the inner hurt the Cultural Revolution caused that we may suspect this type of psychological wound is fairly widespread among the members of his generation. To our minds, it represents the personal effects of a society-wide delegitimation crisis; a loss of engagement with the dominant moral order (see chapter 6). For most members of that generation the psychological effects of the Cultural Revolution are unlikely to have led to the despair that Huang experiences. We do not know with what intensity and quality of distress it has afflicted them. We can be sure it has left its mark, however, and that that mark is more like a wound than a blemish. China's leadership seems to have written this "lost generation" off, concentrating instead on the new generation of students, who are expected to be better prepared, educationally and psychologically, to take maximum advantage of the new emphasis on technological and economic growth.

The story of Huang Zhenyi, including the interpretive paragraphs, was published in 1986. By September of 1989, it was eerie to read the closing words about hopes for the new generation. In the Tiananmen Massacre and its repressive aftermath, the Chinese government has gone on, it would seem, to create a second "lost generation." There is a popular cultural delegitimation of the party and the state every bit as widespread and deeply felt as at the end of the Cultural Revolution. One can only wonder what has happened to the man to whom I gave the pseudonym Huang Zhenyi, or how many other Huang Zhenyis will arise out of the ashes of the latest democracy movement? In the face of such ongoing oppression is it surprising that bodily idioms of distress are commonplace, that neurasthenia again seems on the rise?

A student of Chinese culture will experience little difficulty interpreting even this brief illness narrative in light of core Chinese cultural configurations. One of Huang Zhenyi's chief complaints, dizziness or imbalance, *tou yun*, resonates with a central metaphor in traditional Chinese medicine, balance or harmony between macrocosm and microcosm, between the constituents of the body/self and the social world. Huang Zhenyi's disharmony is in the circulation and amount and forms of his *qi* (vital energy), and in his past experiences; they in turn disharmonize his emotions and create illness. To be dizzy—a common though usually unmarked symptom of neurasthenia in the past and of chronic fatigue syndrome at present in the West—is to be unbalanced, to experience malaise, to be dis-eased. Dizziness was understood by our informants to be the embodiment of alienation. The broken moral order was quite literally dizzying. To experience dizziness was to live and relive the memory of trauma. It was as close as many could come to expressing political opposition and cultural criticism, at a time when overt expression of such hidden viewpoints could lead to dangerous political outcomes: public violence, humiliation, demotion or job loss, forced self-criticism, exile, imprisonment. Dizziness also expressed for some the felt experience of falling (or fear of falling) from a higher to lower social position. The topsy-turvy cycles of the Cultural Revolution spread this experience across all social positions. One group ascended via struggle, was in turn struggled against, and then was passed by, as another group grasped for higher position, only to fall in turn.

Huang Zhenyi's exhaustion and pain can be analyzed in the same way. Exhaustion from sleeplessness, and the paralyzing fatigability and weakness associated with it, recalled shared traumatic events. Months of working frenetically in political campaigns, often at contradictory purposes, convinced sufferers that they and perhaps the nation had reached the end of revolution. Vital resources were exhausted. Personal and collective efficacy had been drained. Fatigue and weakness in traditional Chinese medical theory express loss or blockage in the flow of *qi* (vital energy). Devitalization is understood to affect the body-self and the network of connections, the microcosmic local context and the macrocosmic society.

Pain—headaches, backaches—also recreated the effects of the Cultural Revolution's turmoil on human lives. This lived metaphor, like the others, was easily extended from personal anatomy to the social body, from the anatomical network of muscles, bones, nerves, and blood to the social network of interpersonal experience in conflicted work and family settings. Pain, inner resentment, collective suffering, and social resentment merged. Each complaint, elaborated in the context of a story that integrated social and bodily suffering, extended the metaphoric reach of the pain, exhaustion, and dizziness as moral commentary, first, about the self and its local life world, ultimately, about the society. That is to say, somatic complaints expressed what was at stake in the flow of experience. There is not one source of symptoms; different social experiences engage the same culturally prepared bodily processes (Kleinman and Kleinman 1994).

A student of Chinese culture could follow this line of emic analysis to interpret Huang Zhenyi's physical complaints as a somatopsychic idiom of distress that expresses the psychosocial effects of political problems in a politically acceptable and culturally sanctioned collective rhetoric of complaint. Indeed, one could write an entire book on the relationship of neurasthenia to depression in China and its mediation through culturally shaped bodily experience among patients whose complaints are similar to Huang Zhenyi's (in fact, Kleinman 1986 is one such book).

Yet Huang Zhenyi's tale has so very much more in it than the cultural semiotics of symptoms and disease that violence would be done to the account—we would suppress its echoing misery—if we stopped at this level of analysis. If we left off at that point, we would turn Huang Zhenyi into a passive object, a caricature unworthy of the tragic tale he had told us and the moral significance it held for him that he wanted us to take away from the encounter to transmit abroad. The same inauthenticity would occur if we interpreted this story solely in psychodynamic terms or even as a political tract. Those implications are also present, but they, like the illness experience, are only facets of a complex narrative of suffering, the human veracity of which is its concentration of multiple divergent meanings. What is most at stake for Huang Zhenyi—the historical injustice, the obdurate sense of shame, the frustrated desire to express his grievance and right a terrible wrong, and the practical need to protect himself from the machinery of oppression—was only in part at stake for the Chinese psychiatrists who listened to his story, and was not at all relevant for us. Yet understanding what was at stake in this encounter, we are now convinced, tells us something more valid about Huang Zhenyi's actual experience of suffering than separate cultural, political, or psychodynamic interpretations.

Suffering in Chinese Culture:
The Limitations of Cultural Analysis

Take a recent piece in *Ethos,* the *Journal of the Society for Psychological Anthropology,* by Sulamith Heins Potter (1988), a Berkeley anthropologist who has conducted field research in China. In that anthropological article, Potter contributes to a growing literature that seeks to distinguish non-Western cultures from North American and Western European cultures by emphasizing the point that whereas Western societies are individual-centered, non-Western societies are sociocentric. This dichotomy seems to be one of the basic orientations of contemporary psychological anthropology.

Potter's argument asserts, based on her rural field research, that Chinese regard emotions as irrelevant idiosyncrasies lacking in serious implications for social relationships. The Chinese, she tells us, do not locate significance in the connection between the emotions, the self, and the social order. For them, emotions are "a natural phenomenon" without important symbolic meaning for the maintenance and perpetuation of society. Emotional experience and expression of feeling have no formal social consequences. Suffering, she avers, is not understood by the Chinese as inner personal experience. Nor would the personal experience or expression of suffering, by extension of her argument, hold social significance in Chinese society. Rather a Chinese person's anguish, resentment, ominous feeling of menace, bitter demoralization, hopeless despair, or raging alienation are of no intrinsic importance to the social order. Feelings are never the legitimating rationale for any socially significant action undertaken by Chinese, insists Potter. Americans, of course, are described as the absolute obverse of this caricature. For us, emotions are everything. They are the "legitimating basis that establishes a relationship between a person and a social context." Social action for us is spurred by feelings; the form and meaning of our lives derive directly from our emotions.

Thus, we have Edward Said's (1978) *Orientalism* equation, albeit with a reversal in the values, now favoring the formerly colonized. The cultural other is the alien opposite of what we hold ourselves to be. What is flawed in our world is perfected in theirs. But to accomplish this interpretive feat, what evidence is adduced must (1) portray homogeneous, unidimensional stereotypes, not real people; (2) discount examples of the opposite, which of course abound in Chinese (and also in American) culture; and (3) above all, leave out any shared human qualities that suggest there is an obdurately panhuman grain to human conditions. The upshot of Potter's transformation comes dangerously close to what Said accused the orientalists of accomplishing: narrowing the humanity of the other and thereby of ourselves.

To make such comparisons, one tends not to, one *must not,* emphasize actual experiences of suffering or narratives of personal misery; they are too powerfully human; their concrete details—always original and affecting and usually plural and ambiguous enough to contest—disintegrate abstract dichotomies; they smudge the cold prose of social analysis with the bitter tears of moral sentiment. It is not that Huang Zhenyi after all is not more sociocentric than his North American counterpart but that that very sociocentric orientation to the world is the medium in which his individuality is expressed. Or rather, as Nan Lin (1988) has pointed out in a powerful recent essay on the Chinese family, Chinese, like Huang Zhenyi, are both sociocentric members of family groups and rugged individualists. Different patterns of transmission from generation to generation of moral authority and material property, argues Lin, foster a divided orientation of the self. (See also Ellen Oxfeld [1992] on divergent constructions of the self among Chinese.)

Any culturally valid theory of psychosocial dynamics for Chinese society would have to transcend the simplistic sociocentric/egocentric dichotomy and also, to our mind, would find inadequate and distorting a number of standard psychoanalytic presumptions. Rather we should begin with a historical reconstruction of Chinese cultural categories of personal experience and interpersonal engagement. Emotion (*qing* or *zhih*) is not presented as an independent phenomenon, separable from the rest of experience. The Su Wen section of the pre-Chin *Huang-di nei jing* (*The Yellow Emperor's Classic of Internal Medicine*) sets out an indigenous theory of the emotions as they relate to health and illness. Suicidal grief, immobilizing sadness, manic passion, and other extreme emotional states are held by the dominant Chinese medical tradition of systematic correspondences up to the present to be etiological factors that cause organic pathology; they are also signs of social pathology. They are *pathogens,* internal etiologic factors (*nei yin*) that create organic dysfunction. In traditional Chinese medicine (TCM) emotion is not a general phenomenological descriptor. Instead, there are seven specifically named entities, the *qiqing,* seven kinds of situationally embedded emotional reactions, namely joy (*xi*), anger (*nu*), melancholy (*you*; also translated as anxiety/depression), worry (*si*), grief (*bei*), fear (*kong*), and fright (*jing*). These, if excessive, may become pathologic factors. These factors are said to influence the normal circulation of *qi* and the blood in the internal organs, thereby causing morbid conditions. In this view, the human body as well as its pathological changes are in a continuous state of adapting to the variations of the "natural environment." This is the concept of *tian ren xiangying*—nature and man adapt to each other—and here "nature" includes the four seasons, the physical and social environment, and the physical structure and physiological processes of each person. Thus, emotional pathology may become both sign and cause of social pathology, and balancing the emotions means harmonizing social relations and vice versa. Dizziness or imbalance is a sign of illness. Suffering simultaneously affects and is affected by the relational balance between body-self and the natural world. (In a vast civilizational culture like China's, plural traditions abound, and we could find a few exceptions to support another interpretation of the emotions. But this we take to be the paramount view.)

From at least Zhang Jiebin's (1710) *Qing Yue's Medical Text* right up to the most recent writings of China's leading theorists of psychopathology, the prototypical Chinese view of emotions and emotional disorders has recognized various sources and consequences of depression and anxiety states, while holding a somatopsychic view within which the causal line from environment to person is held to be mediated by the body. The body is also regarded as the main idiom or medium through which psychological, social, and psychosomatic problems are expressed.

Francis Hsu (1985) points out that *affect* in Chinese culture is understood as *specific* feelings: love, hate, loyalty, sympathy, betrayal, aspiration, despair, and so on. It is further understood to be inseparable from the performance of particular tasks in specific situations that are part of one's social role, says Hsu.

In Taiwan today there is a major movement by academic psychologists to sinicize psychological theory and methodology. A leading figure in the sinicization movement is K. K. Hwang, professor of psychology at the National Taiwan University, who offers, to our mind, the most conceptually satisfactory interpretation of emotion among Chinese. Hwang (1987) defines *renqing* (the emotional response of an individual who confronts various concrete situations in daily life) as the essential meaning of emotion. *Renqing* is happiness, anger, fear, love, hate, and desire.[9] If a person understands other persons' emotional responses to various circumstances in life and can respond empathetically to their reactions, then that person is said to "know *renqing*." Emotions need not be expressed openly. A sensitive person "knows the tone" (*zhih yin*). For example, close friends are "those who know me" (*zhih jizhe*).

Thus, emotion means a contextualized response, a response one feels or senses in experiencing the concrete particularity of lived situations. The person who knows *renqing* reads his and others' responses to the situation through all the senses: sight, smell, sound, and other sensations, including an inner resonance. *Renqing* is also a *resource* that is part of social exchanges. Affection, like goods or services, is exchanged. But unlike money, it is difficult to calculate. Indeed, it is said that "one is never able to pay off debts of *renqing* to others." And that is why social relations involving establishment of networks of influence so central to Chinese daily life transactions turn on whether *renqing* is withheld or given as gift. Thus, "reading," "exchanging," and "repaying" *renqing* (here understood as favor) constitute what is at stake in relationships. Finally, Hwang argues, *renqing* is also a set of social norms by which one has to abide in order to get on well with others in Chinese communities. Hwang relates *renqing* to *mianzi* (face) and to *la guanxi* (creating networks of relationships or connections) and *bao da* (repayment or reciprocity) as the central Chinese models of experience. *Renqing* is both social and deeply personal; it captures the dialectical quality of experience; it is individual and interpersonal. It represents the moral core of experience. Sociocentricity alone is an inadequate category to interpret what the Chinese mean by emotion; this term points to something that is simultaneously sociocentric and individualistic in experience.

The methodological question is how to elicit both sides of the dialectic. And here there is a major problem. For as the leader in the movement to sinicize psychology, Yang Kuo-shu (1987), also a professor at the National Taiwan University, has shown, research must confront the tripartite division of all social relations among Chinese. The nearest compartment is occupied by family and close friends. Here trust is unconditional, and certain private feelings can be revealed. The second compartment contains distant family and friends. Here trust is conditional, and feelings will only occasionally be expressed, and always with great caution. The most distant compartment contains relations with strangers, including researchers (i.e., professional strangers). Here there is an absolute lack of trust, and inner experience is not to be expressed lest it is used against one's family and social network. Such a worldview is likely to lead the researcher toward certain conclusions (i.e., the Chinese are sociocentric) and away from others (i.e., the Chinese are also strongly individualistic).[10]

Other key indigenous sources that create a more valid understanding of experience, and therefore of the experience of suffering, include the third-century text *Renwu zhi* (On human personality, chapter 2), by Liu Shao, who presents a political and transactional view of the self. The ideal person is to be *bland;* one is to blend with others and situations "like salt, that by itself is not salty. One is clear, but not sharp; substantial, but not overbearing; attractive, but not obvious . . . decisive and cautious, there is no knowing all one is capable of. With this one can regulate and control." Balancing emotion and situation is essential to master social relations with others. Demonstrating strong feelings, including the menaced and aggrieved affects of suffering, is dangerous, because it gives others power over relationships and restricts one's flexibility to respond effectively. Ultimately, uncontrolled emotional displays threaten one's position in a world of power. Balance, blandness, control provide greater access to power and protect one from the feared effects of power: loss of resources or status or life.

As for Potter's deconstruction of emotion among Chinese, one has only to point to a few classical sources to challenge her conclusion that emotions in Chinese society are irrelevant to the legitimation of the social order.[11] Qu Yuan (332–295 B.C.), hero of the *Li Sao* (Encountering sorrow) has traditionally exemplified the delegitimation of an unjust social order.[12] His tale of sorrow is that of the wanderings of an upright official outcast from a corrupt court, a lonely individualist. The poem is a deeply moving meditation on his grief. The poetry's haunting sadness becomes the idiom of moral accusation. Qu Yuan's suicide is the ultimate act of delegitimation of the social order; a paradigmatic moral exemplar for Chinese remembered each year at the time of the Dragon Boat Festival (the fifth day of the fifth moon), and embodied in the eating of *zonqzi* (glutinous rice wrapped in leaves), both by participants in the festival and, after they are thrown in the water, by Qu Yuan's spirit. (Perhaps Huang Zhenyi, who came from Qu Yuan's homeland, even had Qu's lament in mind as a model for his own dirge of personal suffering and political injustice?)

From pre-Chin times the songs or odes of the land, defined as *shi yan zhi* ("verbalized emotion") were gathered together to record, somewhat like an ancient Gallup poll, how well the realm was governed. These songs were thought of as not just the upwelling and outpouring of personal sentiments but as deriving from the social ethos. Joy, sadness, and disgruntlement, as conveyed in the odes, were believed to express the tangible conditions in the political order and to comment on the moral climate of the times. Confucius indicates this quite clearly in the Great Preface to the Book of Odes, the *She King* (*Shi Jing*).

> . . . in an age of good order [the odes are] quiet, going to be joyful;—the government is then a harmony.

> . . . in an age of disorder [the odes are] resentful, going on to the expression of anger;—the government is then a discord.

> . . . when a State is going to ruin, [the odes are] mournful, with the expression of [retrospective] thought;—the people are then in distress. Legge 1960

Classically, Chinese poetry explored concentrated life experiences, like the endurance of suffering, for their echoing emotional quality and universal significance. Writing such poetry was itself a way of witnessing and also of protesting one's times. Here is Arthur Waley's translation of Zuo Si's (Tso Ssu) third-century classic, *The Scholar in the Narrow Street*, a scholar-official's criticism, through the portrayal of suffering, of himself and his era. (The moral sentiment is as appropriate for intellectuals in present-day China as for those in past periods.)[13]

> Flap, flap, the captive bird in the cage
> Beating its wings against the four corners.
> Depressed, depressed the scholar in the narrow street:
> Clasping a shadow, he dwells in an empty house.
> When he goes out, there is nowhere for him to go:
> Branches and brambles block up his path.
> He composes a memorial, but it is rejected and unread,
> He is left stranded, like a fish in a dry pond.
> Without—he has not a single farthing of salary:
> Within—there is not a peck of grain in his larder.
> His relations upbraid him for his lack of success:
> His friends and callers daily decrease in number.
> Su Ch'in used to go preaching in the North,
> And Li Ssu sent a memorandum to the West.
> I once hoped to pluck the fruits of life:
> But now also, they are all withered and dry.

Though one drinks a river, one cannot drink more than a bellyful;
Enough is good, but there is no use in satiety.
The bird in a forest can perch but on one bough,
And this should be the wise man's pattern.

(1940:75)

The tradition of using the emotional response of readers or an audience to indict the system of political power extends right down to modern times through the writings of Lu Hsun, Lao She, Ba Jin, and many other Chinese authors. Shame, menace, loss, grief, and other emotional expressions of suffering are master symbols of China's revolutionary literature. For Lu Hsun (1963), the most influential of all Chinese writers in this century, the suffering of common people, as depicted in the social roots of their sorrow and desolation, represented the moral delegitimation of cultural as well as political authority. In the revolutionary theater put on for villagers by local representatives of the Chinese Communist Party (CCP) during the years of civil war, their emotional response to memories of suffering under cruel landlords was used to sanction land reform and the destruction of their class enemy. The campaigns of the Great Leap Forward, Anti-Rightists, and Cultural Revolution reenacted this bitterness of experience as the transformation from "eating bitterness" (i.e., suppressing resentment and grievance) to expressing it publicly, often in the most extreme forms, against those designated at the time as the enemies of the people. The killing of landlords, the ritual degradation of intellectuals, the expulsion of party leaders, the erasure of alternate political memories—all were sanctioned through the conjuring of intense emotional reaction to the experience of suffering. The literature of the wounded following the Cultural Revolution, to which Huang Zhenyi's story belongs, is another example of the political uses of public sentiment; here it is used to delegitimate the Cultural Revolution.

Social Origins of Distress and Disease (Kleinman 1986) describes the case histories of individuals whose distress and disease resulted from the excesses of the Cultural Revolution. The stories of suffering they told were meant in large measure to articulate pain and despair as a moral commentary on the sources of their tragedy. Their idea was the classical one described in this chapter: ruinous social policies ultimately ruin personal lives, the felt experience of whose haunting tragedy becomes the most telling political commentary on the times; precisely because that account is lived and powerfully felt, it has moral authority. Those stories were told as a moral witnessing of the Cultural Revolution: personal bitterness and defeat passed a sentence of condemnation.

To interpret such problems, because of the bodily idioms that frequently accompany them, solely as illness is to medicalize (and thereby trivialize and distort) their significance. The idea of *posttraumatic stress disorder* in North American psychiatry, which is increasingly being applied to victims of political trauma such as Cambodian and Salvadoran refugees, is the latest example of this invalid transformation of moral into medical meanings of suffering (see Young 1990 and chapter 8 below). For here the intimate physiological consequences of political violence are converted into an anonymous medical euphemism. In so doing, their moral significance is weakened or even denied entirely.

Think of what "stress" means for an elderly Chinese as opposed to a similarly aged North American. The former has lived through the breakdown of social order in the 1920s and 1930s, when epidemics and other consequences of a disintegrating social order dominated personal experience. What would be the equivalent in North America of the "stress" of the Anti-Japanese War when 20 million people died and 180 million were uprooted? During the first eight years of the People's Republic, Mao Zedong admitted that eight hundred thousand counterrevolutionaries were killed. The aftermath to the 1989 Democracy Movement has taught us what counterrevolutionary means! From 1959 to 1961, following the disastrous policy of the Great Leap Forward, China experienced perhaps the most deadly man-made famine in history: perhaps as many as 30 million died of starvation. And so on. The very idea of posttraumatic stress as a disorder invalidates the moral and political meaning of suffering. After all, in both traditional Chinese and Western cultures, the idea of suffering turned on the idea of having to endure or bear great hardship. The idea of suffering carried the moral significance of endurance, and in its Buddhist and Christian senses, there is the idea of transcendence. Those teleological connotations are lost when suffering is configured as a stress with which we cope (either adaptively or ineffectively) or a disease that can be "cured." Foucault's analysis of the practice of the professions in modern society emphasized that the responses of experts to stress and disease—experts, that is, who define *rationality* as a self-designation of what they think and who regard suffering as having no teleological significance but rather as an opportunity for technical intervention—become a very powerful, perhaps the most powerful, source of social control for just this reason.

One need only read Susan Sontag's (1989) recent cultural analysis, *AIDS and Its Metaphors,* to see that for the other side of our comparison—suffering in the United States—we would need to fashion an equally rich and complex indigenous analytic framework to get at the cultural elaboration of personal experience in North America, a society by the way where to bear or endure hardship for most of its members seems to run counter to the now-dominant secular text of a world without pain or suffering.[14] The ideas of personal responsibility for suffering, hidden contagion silently transforming genetic codes into cancer or AIDS and thereby threatening at the very core our society's myth of technological control and our penchant to view as predictable and therefore insurable risks the quiddity of human tribulations, the banishment of death from our response to AIDS, and even Sontag's utterly American wish to remove the meanings AIDS inflicts on sufferers—all are examples of the significance of suffering among North Americans that we can only mention in passing. They show obvious differences but also a few surprising similarities with our Chinese materials (see Kleinman 1988a:100–120,146–157).[15]

And then? Having in hand different analytic frameworks and different accounts of suffering, then what do we do? If we stick to the texts, we might be tempted to throw up our hands over radical untranslatability. But we will not do this, we the authors of this chapter believe, if we stay close to the ethnographic context of experience.[16] For there is, we hold, something panhuman in the experience of distress of the person, in the bearing of wounds, in the constraints to the human spirit, in the choke and sting of deep loss, in the embodied endurance of great burdens, in the search for coherence and transcendence. There is something definitively human at the core of the experience, which to be sure is elaborated in greatly different ways in different cultural settings, but something that would emerge as universal from cross-cultural translation in the final stage in cultural analysis, if ethnographers focused their descriptions more self-consciously on experience and its modes. That is, translation must be not the first but the last step in cultural analysis, as Stanley Tambiah (1990) has put it. Not the first, as it all too often is in psychiatry and psychology, because then ethnographers lose the valid cultural grounding of experience. But at the last it must be carried out—because if we fail to compare, we are not merely left with cultural solipsism, but with inhumanity: something less than the moral grounds of human experience.

Conclusion

Thus, just as biomedicine delegitimates the suffering in somatization by entifying it as *disease,* so too do the other professions and institutions of postmodern society (including all too frequently medical and psychological anthropology) transform somatization into something other than human experience. Michael Taussig's (1987) writings are to our mind among the more troubling examples of doing violence to the authenticity of the flow of lived experience—they undermine the status of suffering as a legitimate moral domain—but he is not alone.[17] We, each of us, injure the humanity of our fellow sufferers each time we fail to privilege their voices, their experiences. Accounts of the responses of poverty stricken mothers in the *favelas* of Northeastern Brazil to the high rates of death among their children (Nations and Rebhun 1988) and of the experiences of survivors of interethnic violence and of the Bhopal disaster (Das 1994) are exemplary contributions to the anthropology of suffering precisely because they privilege the experience of sufferers to such an extent that it simply is no longer possible to disregard or disguise their grief, or to deny its implications for understanding the experience of the moral orders behind the distancing categories of public health or anthropology.

The professionalization of human problems as psychiatric disorders, undeciphered anthropological codes, or class warfare causes sufferers (and their communities) to lose a world, the local context that organizes experience through the moral reverberation and reinforcement of popular cultural categories about what life means and what is at stake in living. Experts are far along in this process of inauthenticating social worlds, of making illegitimate the defeats and victories, the desperation and aspiration of individuals and groups that could perhaps be more humanly rendered, not as representation of some other reality (one that we as experts possess special power over), but rather as evocation of close experience that stands for itself.[18]

We human beings live in the flow of daily experience: we are intersubjective forms of memory and action. Our experiences are so completely integrated—narratized moments, transforming narratives—that the self is constituted out of visceral processes as much as expressed through them. Because the order of that flow is historical and cultural, what we feel, and see and recall, is a symbolizing physiology. Because of the social construction of the flow of experience, psychosomatic processes are transmitters and receivers of cultural codes. Because of the psychophysiological grounding of experience, cultural codes cannot make of each of us precisely what they will. There is also a panhuman constraint on the continuities and transformations that represent our lives and our networks which derives from the limited number of social ways of being human. Because of the political economy of experience, that panhuman constraint is itself twisted and turned by the local contexts of pressure that encourage or oppress our aspirations, that defeat us, that defend us, that are us.

Can there be a society without sadness? Can there be a culture without menace? Can the flow of experience, no matter how fantastically different is its cultural elaboration of loss or how serene, optimistic, or trivial its historical configuration of that which must be endured, escape suffering?

This essay is not saying that anthropology or psychiatry provides invalid knowledge. Far from it. We believe these two fields have greatly enriched our understanding of the social and psychological origins and consequences of illness, and of the powerful influences of social context and psychological orientation on the forms and processes of care. Even when it comes to the experience of suffering, both fields have opened up important directions for investigation. And yet, the materials required to understand suffering are of such a different order that we believe research approaches to it must deal directly with an experiential domain that heretofore, perhaps with the exception of the work of phenomenologists (which has its own problems), has been the grounds of art.[19] How social and behavioral science is to transform that realm into a suitable subject matter is not entirely clear to us. We feel certain, though, that this must happen if human suffering qua experience is to be part of the problem framework of our disciplines. Inasmuch as outstanding works of ethnography, biography, and history aspire to engage the phenomenon of experience, we feel comforted that the challenge, though a great one, can be met. That challenge, however, is not to create a universal science of human suffering, which would be archly ironic.[20]

We also most definitely are not insisting that the topic covered in this chapter is the most central or important topic for psychological or medical anthropology. The study of experience is simultaneously both another subject and a way of examining several of these fields' concerns. It deserves a place in medical and psychological anthropology.

Finally, we are not saying that suffering defies understanding or that it cannot be defined. We are not implying an irrational or mystical quality to suffering. Human beings find their plans and actions resisted by forms of resistance in the life course, in social relations, in biophysical processes. Out of these forms of resistance emerge what is shared in our human condition: loss, deprivation, oppression, pain. Human conditions are shaped as well by our responses to those forms of resistance: grief, rage, fear, humiliation, but also by what Max Scheler (1971:46) called transcendent responses: endurance, aspiration, humor, irony. Yet these are so greatly elaborated by systems of meaning and individual idiosyncrasy that human conditions must always contain great divergence too. Suffering is constituted out of these shared forms of resistance and by our greatly different ways of reacting to inevitable misfortune. Suffering and transcendence are among the things most at stake in the practical forms of daily experience. For that reason they deserve to be the self-conscious subject matter of ethnography and cross-cultural comparisons.[21]

6

Pain and Resistance

The Delegitimation and
Relegitimation of Local Worlds

Chronic pain's uncertain etiology and even more uncertain treatment, its inseparability from the local worlds of sufferers' lived experience, its changing forms and significance in different social contexts, perhaps above all its intractable opposition to interpretation—all make it a particularly rich subject for anthropology. Chronic pain challenges the simplifying Cartesian dichotomies that still are so influential in biomedicine and also in North American culture: for example, the complaints of chronic pain patients regularly defeat easy definition as based upon "objective" or "subjective" evidence. The condition most perplexes those family members, clinicians, and researchers who have not liberated their thinking from "real" (i.e., physical) versus "functional" (i.e., psychological, therefore imaginary) categories.

Bioethicists, who regard personal autonomy as the only solid ground of ethical choice in the hospital, do not know what to make of chronic pain. They do not want to hold cancer patients accountable for their pain, yet the bodies of most other chronic pain patients reveal either no biomedically ascertainable pathology or only such modest pathology that it seems grossly incommensurate with complaints and the cost

This chapter was originally published in *Pain as Human Experience: An Anthropological Perspective,* ed. M.-J. DelVecchio Good, Paul E. Brodwin, Byron J. Good, and Arthur Kleinman (Berkeley, Los Angeles, Oxford: University of California Press, 1991). It has been expanded and revised, including material from Kleinman and Kleinman 1994.

of care. Are these millions of sufferers responsible for their conditions? Should their care be rationed because it is not "really" necessary? Are they malingerers? Because most workers disabled by chronic pain earn considerably less from disability support than from their job, because many have taken years to grudgingly receive even the limited, stigmatized compensation they do win, and because many are seriously depressed by their disabled condition, it is hard to accept the standard claim of political conservatives that rewards for illness behavior directly encourage malingering (Osterweis, Kleinman, and Mechanic, eds. 1987). Psychodynamic, behavioral, and most social psychological conceptualizations, though they may at times help in the care of a particular patient or even a special group of patients, also appear seriously inadequate when applied to the broad, multiform class of chronic pain patients.

Social science research on chronic pain syndromes has in the past emphasized the obvious economic costs of these conditions—costs to the health care and disability systems and to industry and the economy generally. The professional discourse of economists and political scientists—both constructing the terms for political debate over disability compensation—dominate policy analyses of chronic pain (ibid.). Sociologists who have studied the institutional settings where pain is treated, such as hospitals, clinics, and rehabilitation units, have drawn attention to the negative consequences of the medicalization of pain: professional misuse and abuse of dangerous and expensive tests and treatments, patient experiences of enforced dependency and alienation, and the transformation of human experience into a bureaucratized object and even standardized commodity: the pain patient, for whom countless drugs and all sorts of standard and off-beat interventions are marketed as pain *relievers* (Kotarba 1983; Strauss 1970). Studies have repeatedly documented that pain patients feel biomedical practitioners routinely delegitimize the experience of their illness, pressing them to believe that it is not real or, at least, not as serious as they fear it to be (Hilbert 1984). Their subjective reports of distress are challenged and disconfirmed. They feel violated by practitioners, betrayed by biomedicine. And that enervating and deeply angering sensibility carries over into their family and work settings (Corbett 1986; Kleinman 1988a: 56–99).

The questions for anthropologists, then, are perforce diverse. They overlap with the topics that other social scientists have seized upon, yet reflect abiding interests in medical anthropology: the influence of the political economy on social construction of illness categories; the cultural patterning of the course of illness as a form of experience; the biocultural interactions between family, work, and the psychophysiology of the person in pain; the micropolitical use of symptoms as idiom of distress and rhetoric for conducting interpersonal negotiations; the ethnography of differing reactions to care across gender, ethnic, and class lines. The chapters in *Pain as Human Experience* (Good et al., eds. 1992) attest to this diversity of interests, exemplifying how even members of the same anthropological research group construct the subject of anthropological enquiry into chronic pain in rather different ways. Pain's sheer inexhaustibility as a subject for conceptualization and empirical study is a statement about how deeply its roots tap the sources and express the forms of human conditions. Pain eludes the discipline's organized explanatory systems as much as it escapes the diagnostic net of biomedical categories.

Against this background, I choose to address two sides of chronic pain: (1) how different intersubjective experiences of suffering get constructed, and particularly, in the case of pain in North America and China, how that construction turns on experiences of delegitimation and relegitimation; and (2) how one particular cultural interpretation—conceptualizing the experience of chronic pain as the embodiment of *resistance*—can represent the possibilities but also the limitations of anthropological interpretation of suffering.

I will draw on the illness experiences told to me by several of the patients in the Harvard study of chronic pain patients in urban North America to illustrate these aspects of chronic pain. Elsewhere (Kleinman 1988a), I have written extended illness narratives of three of the patients I interviewed in order to understand the varieties of suffering as moral experience. Here I sketch the outlines of several exemplary narratives in order to demonstrate how pain emerges in the micropolitics of social relations that have come under larger, menacing societal pressures as *resistance* to the flow of interpersonal experience. To further develop this line of analysis, I draw a comparison with chronic pain patients I interviewed in China (Kleinman 1986).

Local Moral Worlds and the Intersubjectivity of Experience

In his evocative, if enigmatic, thesis *The Normal and the Pathological*, Georges Canguilhem (1989), the middle link in the intellectual chain of remarkably influential French philosophers of science from Gaston Bachelard to Michel Foucault, argued that the central task for a cultural analysis of science is to disclose how a particular scientific practice constructs the object of its enquiry. Canguilhem reasoned that for biomedicine, at best only a partial science, this construction must begin with the determination of the normal from the pathological. In his formulation, this determination had to reflect two conditions: the *norms* that the dominant social group establishes to evaluate and, therefore, control behavior, and also the vital condition of *abnormality* in the biological processes that participate in experience. Thus, for Canguilhem, the question of disease/illness is simultaneously a violation of the *normative* (the moral structure of society) as well as of the *normal* (the enfolding of that sociomoral structure into the body of the individual—its *embodiment*). The dialectical processes mediating the socially normative and the biologically normal are, for Canguilhem, the epistemological *and* ontological grounds for understanding health and disease.

I wish to rephrase this position to bring it in line with an emerging anthropological theory of human suffering, its sources, and its consequences (Kleinman and Kleinman 1991). What distinguishes the anthropological theory from Canguilhem's approach, and also from that of phenomenologists such as Helmut Plessner (1970) and Maurice Merleau-Ponty (1962), who have addressed a similar question, and from Bourdieu (1977, 1989), who has explicitly called for a dialectical resolution to opposing subjectivist and objectivist accounts of social reality, is its emphasis on the central importance of the microcontexts of daily life. This anthropological approach to the study of human suffering also emphasizes the crucial work of ethnography to describe how microcontexts mediate the relationship between societal and personal processes.[1]

In the ethnographic perspective, those contexts of belief and behavior are *moral worlds*, where, *inter alia*, the experience of illness is constructed (Kleinman 1980, 1986, 1988a). Be they an East African village (a classical ethnographic context), an inner-city neighborhood in Istanbul, or a social network in North America's universe of plural life settings—these micromoral settings are *particular, intersubjective*, and *constitutive* of the lived flow of experience. They are not simply reflections of macro-level socioeconomic and political forces, though they are strongly influenced by such forces. The micro-level politics of social relationships, in the setting of limited resources and life chances, underwrite processes of contesting and negotiating actions. Yet microcontents are *not* for the most part so greatly fragmented or disorganized as to be lacking distinctive forms or coherence. What unifies

divergent statuses and conflicting interests are the symbolic apparatuses of language, aesthetic preference, kinship and religious orientation, rhetoric of emotions, and commonsense reasoning, which, to be
sure, derive from societal-level cultural traditions, yet are reworked to
varying degrees in local contexts (Cassirer 1953–1957). These symbolic forms work through individual and collective involvement in community activities to construct the flow of experience. Hence, universal types of loss and menace—death, disease, disaffection—are made
over into particular forms of bereavement, pain, and other experiences
of suffering. For example, in a sensitive ethnography of the Kaluli of
New Guinea, Steven Feld (1982) describes the construction of bereavement out of the memory associations of deceased persons with
local places, the cosmology with its charter for teleology, the psychophysiological resonance of culturally marked sounds with similarly
shaped sentiments.[2] The outcome is a world of bereavement that is
experientially greatly distinctive, yet is not so completely foreign as to
lose all resemblance to what is shared in human conditions.

I emphasize the moral processes in these worlds because it is the
construction of what is most at stake for persons and families which
assembles from contested preferences and differing priorities a sociosomatic linkage between symbol systems and the body, between ethos
and the person. This linkage allows cultural meanings to provide structure for attention, memory, affect, their neurobiological correlates, and
ultimately experience.[3] Experience, seen in this structured way, is only
in part subjective. A developing child in her or his cultural context is
part of an ongoing flow of intersubjective feelings and meanings; in a
sense, the child awakens cognitively and affectively within that flow.
How to orient him- or herself, what to orient to, the child's sense of
what is most relevant result from the development of moral sensibility
to this social space. Ethnic as well as personal identity emerge in this
process of entering into and finding a structured place within the flow
of experience. Social status, gender, and the micropolitical ecology will
inflect those identifications, as will personal temperament. We will become ourselves as well as participants at home in the world. And this
plurality of influence is the basis of the novelty and indeterminacy of
experience. But learning to live within and through the vital medium
that emerges when symbolic forms interact with psychobiology places
our lives squarely in the flow of things, bound to others and to the
moral meanings that define a world of exigency and expediency.

And here, where persons encounter *pain,* is where we need to center the study of its sources and consequences. Thus, studying chronic pain patients means that each must be situated in a world. That world must be described, and the description must include an account of the experience of pain in the wider context of experience in family, workplace, and community. To understand what chronic pain signifies, what its experience is like, ethnographers must work out a background understanding of local knowledge and daily practices concerning the body and the self, and misfortune, suffering, and aspiration generally. And they must relate this background understanding to episodes of pain, courses of pain, and other aspects of the world of patients, families, and practitioners who are responding to the constraints of pain. They must also interpret pain in the trajectory of a unique life course as it is told to them in a narrative of suffering that emerges from their positioned engagement with a person in pain. And therefore they must include in the analytic focus pain both as a culturally constituted (biological) object for researchers as well as a biological heritage that constrains cultural meanings. This agenda, though daunting, should sensitize the researcher to the generative matrix of ordinary processes through which chronic pain becomes experience and contributes to the further "becoming" of experience.

Resistance and Its Modes

I must narrow the focus of this analysis because of the requirements for a chapter-length treatment of a still-too-large subject. I discuss chronic pain only with regard to how the relationship between pain and moral world is illumined by two rather different aspects of *resistance,* a current interest of many anthropologists that I find both promising and problematic. I employ the notion of resistance in the widely shared political sense of resistance to authority and in another somewhat special sense that emerges from my own theorizing about suffering.[4]

RESISTANCE AS AN EXISTENTIAL PROCESS

In the course of experience, people come up against *resistance* to their life plans and practical actions (Scheler 1971:46). Resources are limited, often desperately so. The mobilization of force is inadequate, insufficient to achieve success in critical negotiations. And, most predictable of all, misfortune strikes. Loved ones die; others fall seriously ill or become incapacitated. Crops or businesses or marriages fail. Aspirations give way gradually or, following a catastrophe, in a moment. Demoralization becomes desperate and poisons relationships. Loss, fear, menace derail life projects. For many, too many, vicious cycles of deprivation and oppression make misery the routine local condition. For those in the lowest socioeconomic strata, life is brutal. Persons are rendered wretched as a normal, day-to-day condition.

Bearing afflictions of the body, of the spirit, and of the social network and working through their distressing consequences are the shared existential lot of those whose life is lived at the edge of resistance.[5] To this dark side of experience we give the name *suffering*, with all its moral and somatic resonances. Suffering, then, is the result of processes of resistance (routinized or catastrophic) to the flow of experience. Suffering itself is both an existential signifier of human conditions *and* a form of practical and, therefore, novel experience that undergoes extensive social elaboration (Kleinman 1988a, 1986).[6]

RESISTANCE TO POLITICAL POWER

In its more usual sense, resistance has the rather different meaning of resisting the imposition of dominating definitions (diagnoses), norms defining how we should behave (prescriptions), and official accounts (records) of what has happened.[7] We resist, in the micropolitical structure, oppressive relationships. Such resistance may take the form of active struggle against dominant forces or a more passive form of noncompliance. The historical idea of resistance, such as that of the struggle of subordinate social groups with superordinate ones, conveys images of hidden motives, false compliance, malicious gossip, passive hostility, even sabotage (see Scott 1985:xvi, 290–291). I believe this idea of resistance, though seemingly greatly distant from the domain of health, can be, with appropriate modifications, applied to less dramatic daily experiences of suffering, including that of chronic pain patients. Most patients with chronic illness, which by definition cannot be cured but must be endured, do not comply entirely with their doctor's prescription. There is little doubt that this "weapon of the weak" may be at times one of the few forms of resistance to medical authority that is feasible, even though it is often self-defeating.

With this discussion as background, I turn to examine both types of resistance among patients with chronic pain who were interviewed in the Harvard chronic pain research projects.[8] My purpose is to see how useful this approach is in deepening our understanding of the experience of chronic pain as human suffering.

The Delegitimation and Relegitimation of Experience

CASE 1

Stella Hoff is a thirty-one-year-old Ph.D. biochemistry researcher in medicine who has suffered severe pain for four years following a car accident.

I could be dead or quadriplegic. As it was, I was totally, totally stunned. Shocked. I sat there and shook. At the hospital they diagnosed a concussion, and I had broken a few small bones in my foot. . . . Otherwise, there was nothing else injured. But right away I could feel pain. . . . And that started the whole process. Four years of pain, surgeries, casts, more pain, more tests, more drugs, more surgeries, bad surgical effects, and now this constant pain. . . . And me, us—our lives ruined. All for what?

Dr. Hoff is tall, angular, intense. A woman of few words, clipped accent, she is often bitingly sarcastic about others and herself. Dr. Hoff is elegantly but simply dressed; her movements represent her persona: quick, controlled, assured. In her white laboratory coat, surrounded by her research equipment and assistants, she looks the very epitome of precision and efficacy. A competent and conscientious scientist, she has also something distant, formal, even cold in her bearing. You need to meet her only once to appreciate a fixed expression of tension in her hyperalert eyes and thin, drawn mouth. The intensity of expression seems contentless: it could be fear, it could be hurt, it could be vulnerability. Once you know her story, there is little question what the intensity is about, however. It is her pain—constant, severe, dominating. Dr. Hoff is fighting each moment to remain in control, fighting not to give in, not to scream.

If I have gotten anything positive out of this terrible experience it is to be more sensitive to the experience of others, especially patients. I don't think doctors have any sense of how to deal with pain patients. . . . I was infuriated by an orthopedist who told me, "Well, it's just pain."

The words she uses to describe her pain are "exhausting, wretched, unbearable, agonizing." Nothing relieves this continuous pain. It is usually a five on a scale of ten in the morning, gets to seven of ten in the late afternoon when she leaves the laboratory, and in the evening is "at least" an eight. When the pain is greatly exacerbated, "it can be a twelve out of ten." The pain is much worse than any pain she experienced before and is regularly "excruciating." For her pain symptoms and the related problems, Dr. Hoff sees a primary care physician once every ten days on the average and specialist surgeons and pain experts. She has also consulted psychiatrists and several practitioners of alternative healing systems.

The pain and associated weakness affect most of her activities. It is extremely painful to work in the laboratory, though she does it. It is too painful to do yard work, clean the house, or cook anything involved or elaborate; she cannot play sports; and because of pain she avoids social activities. Pain keeps her in bed for most weekends each month. Over the eighteen months of follow-up interviews, Dr. Hoff's pain waxed and waned. On one occasion she had "very little pain" and reported "it is not interfering with my life very much." On another occasion the pain was "torturing and grueling," though it lasted at this intensity only a few days.

Dr. Hoff has insight into the personal meaning of her pain: "It has been totally devastating to me. Losses and what they have meant to me." She recognizes the pain has made her irritable, fearful, and overly attentive to bodily change.

Formal psychological testing showed Dr. Hoff to be experiencing considerable anxiety, irritability, and fear. She felt blocked in getting things accomplished, joyless, and she experienced rage, a desire to smash things, and a strong suspiciousness that others treated her badly, could not be trusted, and would take advantage of her if she did not exercise vigilance. Her psychiatric assessment was consistent with recurrent major depressive disorders for the past three years, for which she had received clinical trials of various antidepressants and psychotherapy, which had, in her words, "improved the depression but scarcely affected the pain."

Dr. Hoff's primary care physician felt frustrated by her care. He estimated seeing her a hundred times or more over the previous four years. He regarded her as a "classical chronic pain syndrome" patient, and noted that her marital life, work, and problematic experiences with the medical system had placed her in a situation of chronic stress, depression, and "self destructive" anger. He thought there was a strongly psychosomatic component to her pain. He thought of her as one of the most difficult patients he had treated in a very busy practice. He took that to be the reason that led doctors to "drop her." "Let's face it, Arthur," he said, "she is a problem patient. She's just extremely demanding, and she doesn't get better. I feel I need all my skills and then some to stay in the office with her when things are bad. Also being a biological researcher doesn't help."

Other physicians she consulted complained of the same problems. "You know," said one of the pain specialists,

she is an academic researcher. She knows the language, the medicines. She's read more of the papers on this thing than I have. And she has had so many negative experiences already that she's wary. And then again she has this way of coming across like an intellectual machine rather than a person. I mean she is cold, no emotions, watching you all the time. I find myself trying to avoid treatment interventions that might possibly lead to bad side effects. . . . I mean it just makes the whole thing so much more complicated . . . difficult. When I see her name on my list of patients for that day I feel on edge myself.

Dr. Hoff, in contradistinction, sees herself as the almost silent bearer of a misery only she and her husband know. "I have worked when the pain is a ten," she states emphatically through lips drawn tightly together.

Pain is too much for physicians to deal with. Most of us can't tolerate listening to people in pain. We want patients who get better, or better yet if they don't they shouldn't complain. Pain patients like me are a sign of the failure of the medical care system, of something terribly wrong at the core.

Dr. Hoff's anger at her professional colleagues is the other side of her anger at the pain and at herself.

Look what I lost because of it, and where I am now. I get angry with myself, but I can't express it, never could. I get very quiet, others learn to leave me alone—thus, I don't address it. My anger is even too much for Everett [her husband] to address. I lose confidence that I can control this damn thing, go on with it, have confidence in the future . . . get better.

Dr. Hoff is a laboratory researcher, an academic who does full-time medical research, who says she likes her work and is good at it,

but I have missed so much time because of the pain and the surgery that I still have to prove myself. I've lost time. My generation of researchers has moved on: they direct their own labs, have their own research program, some have tenure. I'm starting all over again. I've lost three or four years. I have to prove that I can put in a full research day, complete projects, that I'm like everyone else.

She describes lab life as hectic, pressured.

Previously I brought all my work home with me. It was bad for my family life and my own peace of mind. I felt driven, and would continue to work late into the night. I felt something tormenting me, driving me on.

Because of the time she has missed, Dr. Hoff has not received the promotion she believes she deserves, and she feels she has also missed out on professional opportunities, getting her name on papers coming out of the lab, traveling to meetings, and that even her salary has lagged behind.

It's distressing to be viewed as a risk. I used to be seen as a rising star. . . . There is the constant stress of producing, no matter how I feel, to be productive, act successful, present myself as healthy. But I'm not healthy; yet I can't be honest about how I do feel. Have to pretend. Also, I don't know myself how far I can go. . . . I've never had a chance to find out. I've got to be successful in this job: there aren't better ones available. And I've got my grant and am turning out the papers, "cutting the meat" as we say around here. But it isn't a single objective—I need to do the whole thing, to be a steadily productive, day in, day out, investigator—no matter how much pain I feel.

Dr. Hoff is presently negotiating a more stable position:

They still don't have the confidence in me. I ought to be head of my laboratory—the current head is someone who started after I did. I taught her techniques. I'm a perfectionist in everything I do and always have been. That's why it's so hard for me to accept [the effects of the pain]. . . . Even in writing up the data it takes me longer. I've got to do it my own way. It's overwhelming to do the research, analyze the data, present it, keep publishing, stay up-to-date with the literature, do my part in the marriage, in keeping up the house, and still be myself. I once thought I could do it all . . . but now I know I can't.

Accomplished in academic studies, Stella Hoff expected success at a high level. "I had very romantic fantasies of being world famous." The harsh realization set in and was intensified after the accident.

I recognized for the first time that I wasn't necessarily going to be famous or successful. I had given up writing . . . and in biochemistry I had my doubts. I didn't think I had the toughness to be a great researcher: to do something original and significant. That's why I worked so hard, spent all those hours. I kind of doubted I could "naturally" develop as a researcher. I started out well, but I soon began to have trouble. It is one thing completing a single study and quite another to undertake an entire project. The summer before the accident I began to get very serious doubts. Things were not going well. I began to think of other jobs; something to fall back on. I had driven to job interviews . . . I was chagrined—almost in a trance of unreality. I didn't like the places I visited and couldn't conceive of myself as simply . . . as simply a practicing [technician]. . . . I know it sounds terribly snobby, but I had always thought of myself as a scientist . . . it was a blow to my ego to interview for that job.

Perhaps this illness has prevented or rather delayed a coming to terms with success. So far I have been potential, not actual, success. I think of not succeeding because of the illness . . . but thinking through this condition . . . I'm beginning to wonder whether . . . [it] is not a disguised form of avoiding failure. I don't think I really believe that, but this set of interviews has set off all sorts of associations I haven't made before. I know there are times when stress makes my symptoms worse—lots of times—but then again I can name several very stressful times in the last year or so when my pain did not seem to be affected at all. I know that psychosomatic relations means in some way my mind should be influencing my illness. Strange to say, my experience is almost the reverse. I don't seem to be able through will or feeling or desire to influence my body. In fact my body seems to determine how I feel.

Regarding her family, Dr. Hoff says with a mixture of sadness and bitterness:

Now, they [her family] get pretty angry at me. They simply don't understand what is going on. In fact, my mother can't bear to talk about my illness. She reminds me how much illness she had, and still had five children, worked, got on with her life. My sickness has really affected them.

In the course of many hours of interviews, Stella Hoff told me about another side of her illness experience, a side she said she had never spoken about with her practitioners.

Do you believe in evil? I mean, we don't use the term in biomedicine, but it does describe experience. Suffering is an evil. I mean suffering that has no meaning, that brings nothing good with it. There is a spiritual side of my pain. That is what I mean by evil. My spirit is hurt, wounded. There is no transcendence. I have found no creativity, no meaning in this . . . this entirely horrible experience. There is no God in it. . . . It shatters all I took for granted and believed in. I came from a religious family, French Protestants. I was taught to put faith in God. All I was taught . . . all my family and personal life . . . has been shattered, taken away.

Dr. Stella Hoff's experience of chronic pain spills over the frame of any single analytic focus. The richly human echoes and protean complexities quite obviously can (and probably should) be analyzed from a number of different perspectives.[9] From the one advanced in this chapter, I note that the catastrophic onset of her misfortune delegitimates a world of experience that she associates with confidence, control, and success. It is a standard suburban, North American upper-middle-class world of academic achievement and promising professional career. Ambition, competition, and competence are personal dispositions structured within a moral terrain in which progress is regarded as only natural and the actual range of life choices in fact appears almost limitless. (Dr. Hoff came of age in the 1960s and 1970s, before the invention of the new tradition of American decline.) In this post–World War II era of great American wealth and empire, the social reality of the "people of plenty" structures the habitus (embodied cognition, affect, facial appearance, stance, and movement) of expectation of great success which reaffirms and recreates a social world preoccupied with winning—all components of the American upper-middle-class cycle of self-improvement and self-promotion. Winsome personality, speed of movement, blemishless skin, directness in speech, "standing tall," and gestures of power define this cultural habitus as an icon of the American way.

Yet, there is also the hidden fear of "falling from grace," which helps to focus attention on what is culturally most at stake: economic advancement and social mobility, a secularized soteriology (Newman 1989). Not to rise is a threat to social persona and social esteem; it is often experienced by members of the American middle class as a shameful moral weakness. Dr. Hoff, even before her catastrophic accident, had a gnawing uncertainty about whether she would in fact make it in the high-pressure, high-status stakes of science. She had looked into an alternative applied career as a technician, even though it was close to unacceptable to her disposition and the actual values of her world.

The accident, the injuries, the awful pain, and even the iatrogenic and frustrating medical care turned that world of experience on its head. In this single sense only, hers is like the experience of the multigenerational, inner-city poor, whose intersubjective world is structured by vicious, brutalized cycles of misery, where dispositions of hopelessness and hatefulness recreate and normalize the on-the-ground social reality—though her far greater resources and memory of a very different background augur for a vastly different future. Nonetheless, Stella Hoff does descend into a world of suffering whose bodily and affective processes become, and structure the further "becoming" of, painful social relationships in workplace and family setting. She exchanges a world of aspiration for a world of despair, but unlike the truly disadvantaged, she retains the possibility of reemerging. Stella Hoff loses one world to enter another. Her experience of delegitimation is intensified by the responses of practitioners, who contribute to the disconfirming sense that the symptoms are somehow too extreme, too troubling, too difficult to control. There is the suspicion of amplification or exaggeration owing to psychological problems and "stress." This latent, and at times even voiced, accusation challenges the validity of her illness experience and threatens to add the stigma of mental illness or even malingering. To demonstrate the serious burden of her suffering, the desperate desolation, Stella Hoff, like most other chronic pain patients, feels pressed to dramatize her symptoms. Her pain is twelve out of ten. This patently melodramatic device in turn confirms the suspicions of practitioners. The outcome is a poisoned clinical atmosphere in which trust and support—so central to the healing process—are replaced by suspicion, accusation, and ultimately a pervasive, mutually frustrating resentment that makes empathetic care virtually impossible.

The reverberations of this downward spiral include notably Dr. Hoff's literal experience of a spiritual fall from grace.[10] Demoralization as an intersubjective process of suffering shared by patient, family, and practitioners eventually resonates in existential and teleological language. Here the technical rationality and scientific intellectual devices of biomedicine cannot contain the participatory reasoning of the patient who seeks to understand not how but why, not causal mechanism but ultimate meaning, not reason for treatment failure but chance for salvation (see Tambiah 1990:101–110). Thus, Dr. Hoff's story underlines the capacity of suffering as a transpersonal experience to cross the artificial divides between values and practice, religion and medicine, which have become so dysfunctional in the American health care system. Pain, then, almost becomes an icon of cultural delegitimation of our society's priorities and practices. Perhaps this is why the image chronic pain patients present is viewed as so menacing, why pain patients are cast so often as modern pariahs.

Can we fit the image of resistance into this analysis too? Resistance, in the sense of barrier or opposition to the flow of lived experience, clearly applies to Stella Hoff's traumatic injury and its desperate consequences. Yet I would argue that the other meaning of resistance— active or passive counterresponse to micropolitical dynamics and the macro-level forces that either intensify or moderate their effect—also can be made to apply. The trajectory of Dr. Hoff's pain, a particularizing *social course* of illness experience that is inimical to the biomedical claim of a *natural course* that unfolds from the disease process itself, spirals around her research work and the pressures of her academic career. Once in place, complaints of pain are readily absorbed into a language of complaint about the enormous pressures and perceived injustices of academic life. Pain is experienced as bridging somatic and social space. To a certain, limited extent, embodied pain sanctions opposition to the way the research experience is constructed, which provides an incremental gain in time and autonomy. Yet obviously these "gains" are small compared to the losses that Dr. Hoff experiences on account of her chronic pain. More impressively, her chronic pain offers Dr. Hoff an occasion to oppose medical practices that routinely disaffirm her experience of complaints as genuine and serious. And taking up an oppositional stance to authority also obviously resonates with her Huguenot heritage and her personality style. She has become, in the eyes of her professional caregivers, a "problem patient": a derogatory, even stigmatizing label, that in my experience often means the patient is making demands that the practitioner will not or cannot meet. In Stella Hoff's case, more than one hundred visits to a primary care physician over four years may well be so extensive a resort to medical care that few would see her needs as reasonable. But the source of the problem, notwithstanding the claims of her practitioners to the contrary, may well be the system of care and the actual experience of the care they provide. Dr. Hoff is insistent that her pain, including the fullness of her experience, be taken seriously. Her demands confront the inadequacy of the biomedical, including the psychiatric and psychological, approach to chronic pain. The recipient of iatrogenic treatment, she fights back, mobilizing knowledge and professional and financial resources that most pain patients do not have available. She turns even her spiritual crisis into an assault on the dehumanizing language of a treatment system that addresses neither ethical nor teleological questions. She resists the inappropriate extension of biomedicine's rational technical manipulations into the domain of deeply intimate human experience that calls for compassion and witnessing.

And ultimately her suffering challenges simplistic American cultural orientations about youth, health, and freedom.

And yet, as much as the metaphor of resistance reveals those sides of the chronic pain experience that are often hidden under other social science rhetorics, other aspects of suffering seem obscured or perhaps even distorted by this analytic schema. There is a definite limitation to the applicability of this perspective, and that limitation indicates a more general problem with the anthropology of suffering. Before I examine that problem, however, I will provide a brief account of another exemplary experience of chronic pain from the Harvard study. I will then adumbrate, again briefly, chronic pain patients' experiences from the research I have conducted in China, to draw a cross-cultural comparison.

CASE 2

Mary Catherine Mullen is a thirty-year-old married woman from a poor Irish American family in Boston's South End, a bastion of Irish working-class culture. She has suffered from severe "migraine" headaches for five years. Greatly overweight, with a strong family history of headaches and diabetes, Mrs. Mullen fears that her headaches are not getting better, in spite of various medical treatments, and that she will have to endure them for the rest of her life, as has her mother. Her headaches are associated with a depressed and angry mood for which she sees a counselor weekly, and which has transformed her, she holds, into someone quite different from the shy, smiling, self-effacing person she was as a child and adolescent. Mrs. Mullen attributes the onset of her headaches to her husband's alcohol abuse and the subsequent verbal and physical violence he directed at her, which made him, in her words, "a real Jekyll and Hyde."

When the headaches began, Mrs. Mullen was contemplating divorcing her husband. She was desperate to protect herself, and her then five-year-old daughter, from her husband's violence. She also felt trapped by her lifelong diffidence and incapacity to express her needs. Her husband's inability to find or hold good employment meant that they "lived from one paycheck to the next." The feeling of financial insecurity infiltrated other aspects of their life. There were no medical benefits; they were forced to stay in a room in her mother's house, which was undesirable to all, and Mrs. Mullen had to continue to work in a low-level, dead-end job in a local department store which she detested. Finally, she had the terrible apprehension that her husband would end up physically abusing their daughter, just as she had been abused by her own mother.

Her response to this intolerable life situation was a cycle of dysphoria, from desolate depression to explosive anger. When depressed, usually at a time her husband was drunk, she became deeply hopeless and virtually immobile—unable to speak out or even act preventively to protect herself or her daughter. When angry, usually when her husband was sober, she would "lose control": scream, throw things, and shout out a litany of wrongs that oppressed her. She even feared that she herself would eventually batter her daughter, thereby copying her own mother, for whom she had come to have an inexhaustible well of anger.

Mary Catherine Mullen was the illegitimate first child of Maggie O'Leary, described by Mary Catherine as an "irresponsible, rebellious" teenager who had run away from a large family of hard-drinking Irish immigrants, and a much older man, who passed through Maggie's life in several intense weeks and then disappeared utterly. Her mother, whom Mary Catherine claims vehemently was "incompetent to care for me," virtually abandoned Mary Catherine, placing her with her own mother, while she wandered in a near alcoholic delirium from man to man. Finally, when Mary Catherine was six, Maggie O'Leary reappeared suddenly, without prior notice, one evening and demanded that her child be returned to her. Despite Mary Catherine's pleas that she remain with her grandmother, whom she had come to regard as her mother, she was forcibly repossessed and immediately entered into her mother's unstable, peripatetic life. She remembers these years of childhood and early adolescence as lacking in all security. She felt unloved and dangerously threatened by her mother's physical abuse. From this time onward, Mary Catherine felt a deep hatred for her mother. At age fifteen she had a sexual affair with an older laborer, which resulted in an abortion, about which she continues to feel guilt. She now believes that she undertook this relationship and dropped out of school in order to break away from her mother and at the same time "to get back at her for all she had done to me." Soon after the abortion, she began to date and quickly married her current husband.

It is an abiding source of shame for Mrs. Mullen that the young couple eventually had to "beg" her mother to permit them to move into her house because of lack of funds to live on their own. At the time she felt trapped in her marriage, her work, and in her mother's home. She watched impotently as her mother took advantage of the situation, treating her like a maid and allowing Mary Catherine and her family no privacy. In spite of her growing anger, she felt incapable of defending herself by talking back to her mother or husband. "If something is on my mind, I can't say it, fear hurting someone's feelings. Can't say no to people."

Over the course of months, Mrs. Mullen descended into despair. She thought of her life as hopeless, and increasingly she felt inadequate and worthless. At one point she thought seriously of suicide. Then the headaches began. So severe were they that she felt compelled to withdraw to her bedroom, where she locked the door, lay on her bed, and remained in the dark until sleep obliterated her pain. Because of her pain, and in spite of the serious financial repercussion and in the face of angry protests from her husband and her mother, Mrs. Mullen quit her job. Within weeks, she determined that the headaches were so severe that she could no longer do housework or cook for her family either. Her husband took over these activities grudgingly, but over time he became more solicitous and helpful. Despite the absence of health insurance, Mrs. Mullen insisted on visiting physicians, including pain experts, who diagnosed migraine, tried her on various treatments, none of which has controlled the pain, and prescribed bed rest and avoidance of "stressful" activities. She further insisted that her husband and mother assume financial responsibility for these medical visits.

As Mrs. Mullen's pain experience deepened, her mother, like her husband, became sympathetic and began to help with the housework. Her husband quit drinking. Her mother showed her affection, Mary Catherine asserts, "for the first time in my life."

They treat me the way I have to be treated [because of the headaches]—considerate. If they are not, I'll kill somebody! . . . Everyone stays out of my way when I have a headache and that's what I want them to do.

Although the headaches have continued over the five years, they have slowly begun to diminish in intensity and to become more "tolerable," though at times, particularly when Mrs. Mullen is "under stress," they return to the former level of severity. The depression has lightened, but the sense remains of a deep pool of hate that erupts into angry outbursts. At these times, Mrs. Mullen will "throw up" to her mother accusations about the past. This is the first time in her life, she says, that she has been able to say the things she always needed to say to her mother but couldn't: namely, how she grew up terrified, feeling unloved, and greatly vulnerable. When, at the times she is not in pain, she tries to discuss these problems, her mother still turns away from her, "she can't handle it." But during Mrs. Mullen's explosions of rage, her mother is forced to listen.

The analytic language of delegitimation, relegitimation, and resistance in the interpersonal world of experience seems particularly apt in interpreting Mary Catherine Mullen's experience of chronic pain. Of course, the literature on chronic pain contains numerous accounts of the influence of family processes on the onset and course of symptoms. In fact, this is arguably the major causal pattern that behavioral psychologists diagnose and treat (Sternbach 1978; Turk et al. 1983). Psychoanalytically oriented practitioners and family researchers speak of the "gains" of illness and include in that category the explanation that pain and other chronic symptoms can restructure family relations and communication patterns, which clearly has taken place in Mrs. Mullen's household. Yet, the implication is often that either the circumstances are determinative as behavioral operants conditioning individual behavior, out of awareness of the sick person, or that there is a rational calculus by means of which individual decisions are made that reflect a shift in cost/benefit, a kind of malingering (see relevant chapter in Burrows et al. 1987 and also Turk et al. 1983). I find these implications unsatisfactory and am disturbed by the behaviorist language that would have us believe that Mrs. Mullen is either an ingenuous automaton or a blatant manipulator. Ten hours of interviews with Mrs. Mullen, corroborated by research and clinical work with many patients with chronic pain, make me greatly suspicious of the behaviorist discourse, which I find stereotyped, overly focused on pain as a problem of an *individual*, and dehumanizing.

In the perspective I have advanced in this chapter, Mary Catherine Mullen is born into a delegitimated world. Illegitimate, abandoned by her mother, raised by her grandmother in a family setting where she was viewed as tainted by her mother's sinful ways, Mary Catherine's early socialization disaffirmed her person and placed her in an anomalous relationship with her grandmother and others. She bore a sense of shame and also carried the idea that she was not good enough to receive her mother's love. When her mother precipitously removed her from her grandmother's home, she experienced a major loss and second transformation of her world. That transformation again encouraged an experience of delegitimation. Her mother abused her emotionally and physically. She also forced Mary Catherine to accept the name of the man to whom her mother was then married. For a while Mary Catherine had two family names: her mother's and her stepfather's. The confusion in identity was a simulacrum of her growing sense of tangentiality to her world. In that world, she repeatedly heard her mother excoriate her origin and personality. Disaffirmed and disaffected, she grew into adolescence feeling worthless. She felt a lack of efficacy with others and alienated from her family.

A common idiom of distress was her mother's headache. When her mother had headaches, which were frequent, Mary Catherine was expected to take care of the other children and her stepfather. Her mother's withdrawal and lack of affection were justified by the headaches, as were her irascible disposition and angry outbursts. Thus, Mary Catherine experienced headaches as a rhetoric of complaint for expressing hostility and controlling others.

The experience of delegitimation was reproduced in her relationship, in the early part of the marriage, with her husband. She seemed unable to control his drunken behavior and its violent consequences. She also seemed unable to effectively negotiate with him over their limited resources, much of which supported his alcohol abuse. After the birth of their daughter, she felt more intensely still the disaffirmation of her experience as wife and mother. Forced to move into her own mother's home, owing to her husband's failure as a provider, she saw herself as coming full circle in a lifelong cycle of despair. Mary Catherine's great obesity, about which she felt helpless and ashamed, became a bodily index of her alienated social status, a habitus structured out of the stigmatized position, poor self-esteem, and a self-defeating sense of inefficacy in her world. This alienation of habitus in turn creates the negative dispositions and interactions that perpetuate that world.

The experience of pain in a world without security (in family, job, finances, or neighborhood) is what distinguishes chronic pain among the poor and the oppressed. When one cannot marshal resources, symbolic and instrumental, because they do not exist or one's access to them is obstructed, the very idea of control becomes untenable. The normal, everyday routinization of misery, furthermore, can be experienced as bodily pain. As a result, the confluence of this source of pain and bodily pathology makes it impossible for the afflicted person to determine what "causes" pain to worsen and what will limit or remove it. Pain cannot be made meaningful any more than can the rest of life. The absence of control as well as legitimacy means that to survive, those patients who lack resources yet are exposed to great pressures must conduct the moral equivalent of a life-and-death struggle. Pain becomes the bodily component of so fundamental an experience of suffering that the local world is in effect a world of suffering. Pushed up against the limits of control and meaning making, poor and oppressed patients may take up whatever is at hand to respond to adversity that can no longer be easily assigned to either medical or nonmedical sources. Thus, Mrs. Mullen's pain also represents a kind of solution, albeit compromised, to the consequences of dwelling in a world of suffering.

The development of chronic pain, whatever its sources, sanctions a transformation in her experience. The pain becomes a means of resisting her husband's irresponsibility and her mother's cruel manipulations. Her sense that her world is not her own, that she has no central, secure place in it, is replaced by illness behavior through which Mrs. Mullen, with surprising energy and efficacy, moves to the center of that world and even comes to dominate its flow. The severe migraine headaches authorize a relegitimation of intersubjective experience. They are in fact emblems of a new way of engaging in the stream of experience. Mary Catherine Mullen's episodes of headache might even be thought of as a kind of social dissociation, from a hesitant, marginal orientation to her world, in which she is absorbed into the flow of practical actions effected by others, toward an assertive, central orientation, from which she reorients the flow of aggrieved sentiments and practices. The relegitimation of the world authorizes her access to the moral devices of accusation and restitution.[11] Of course, there is also evidence that Mrs. Mullen's resistance has certain negative effects, real and potential, such as expensive medical bills, unemployment, and perpetuation of a cycle of somatized distress and greatly disruptive explosions of rage into which her daughter may become the next conscript. Also, it is unclear how long such a newly invented ritual of behavioral reversal can keep going without straining the social ethos to the point of breakdown. For these reasons, it is difficult to know, at this point, if Mrs. Mullen's form of resistance in the politics of family should be regarded as effective. What is more certain is that for poor working people from deprived backgrounds with few life chances and greatly limited resources, who lack reserves to respond to crises, even the dubious efficacy of embodied resistance may mean the difference between enduring and succumbing. In the exigency of routinized hurt and grievance and demoralization, simply to continue not to be overwhelmed may be a kind of desperate victory. Pain, like other forms of suffering, is resisted (Scott 1990).

CASE 3

An even clearer example of the possibilities, and limits, of the moral efficacy and practical uses of resistance via chronic illness is provided by the research I have conducted in China among those deeply affected by the Cultural Revolution (Kleinman 1986; Kleinman and Kleinman 1991). In this research, Joan Kleinman and I encountered such frequent examples of neurasthenia symptoms sanctioning major changes in work and family, in relation to the local Communist authority structure, that we concluded that chronic, disabling bodily complaints were a source of power in Chinese work units. But it was also obvious that social categories of individuals—those with bad class backgrounds, women, youths who had been Red Guards and had been "sent down" to remote rural areas—strongly influenced who had need for such power and who could exercise it under particular conditions. Moreover, delegitimation meant something very different in the Chinese context. Our research subjects, like tens of millions of their Chinese compatriots, experienced the moral delegitimation of Communism in the fiery chaos of the Cultural Revolution. Their communities, and the societal political system of which these are part, had lost moral legitimacy, and even the sources of social efficacy were undergoing dramatic change.

The ancient spine of Chinese society, the bureaucratic order, dislocated; factions fought each other in large and small work units, sometimes creating civil wars in the cities; families were broken; systems of communication, transportation, justice, public safety, health, and welfare fragmented. Parents were attacked by children; teachers were assaulted by students; Red Guards broke into homes, looted their contents, beat their occupants, at times to death, and destroyed precious objects such as ancestral tablets, heirlooms, and books. By the late 1970s, though order was restored by the army and the party, cynicism, demoralization, and alienation were widespread. Delegitimation spread from a crisis of confidence in the political system to a wholesale questioning of indigenous cultural institutions.[12]

From the end of the Cultural Revolution until the beginning of the 1980s, the state allowed expression of public loss and anger. Yet, when these popular expressions began to coalesce into the early phase of a movement for democratization, they were attacked. Thus, the social memory of the Cultural Revolution was silenced or reworked in an authorized version, a "public transcript" that located blame in the Gang of Four and their ultra-leftist associates, while exonerating the party, the state, and their local representatives. Each urban work unit, each rural village was left to rebuild its tattered social structure. Bitter memories, hatred of leaders and coworkers, burning grievances, and inflamed traumas were all officially suppressed. A single authorized version of the past was fabricated, collective grieving was brought to an end, and the people were ordered to get on with the projects of socialist reconstruction and, later on, economic reform.

By 1980, the delegitimation crisis in China had reached epidemic proportions; it challenged the social organization of communalized work, the foundational Confucian code, even the family—the cultural grounds of trust and achievement. This political and cultural crisis of delegitimation intensified during the economic reforms of the 1980s, especially with the brutal suppression of the Democracy Movement at the end of the decade. Underneath the rosy picture of China's economic successes, the crisis persists up to the present as the dark and dangerous side of China's "modernization."[13]

Between the late 1970s and 1980, there was a brief period of national preoccupation with victims' accounts of their trauma—a brief literary flowering that is called the literature of wounds or scars. As noted, by 1980, China's political leaders had determined that these morbid stories, many of which had a critical edge, had gotten out of hand. Yet another campaign was initiated, and the crackdown ended expressions of social criticism through biographies of the traumatic effects of terror and loss. Thus, in the early 1980s when we were conducting our research, we were impressed by the way that retelling narratives of sickness, especially of neurasthenia—a common syndrome of chronic pain, sleeplessness, fatigue, dizziness, and related physical symptoms, as well as sadness, anxiety, and anger—authorized social memory and thereby enabled oblique criticism of the Cultural Revolution and the political process generally, which our informants regarded to be the origin of the complaints.

In their narratives of illness, patients' remembrance of bodily complaints broadened into more general stories of suffering that integrated memories of menace and loss with their traumatic effects (demoralization, fear, desperation) and with their sources (criticism sessions, beatings, prison, exile). Bodily memory, biography, and social history merged. The bodily axis of moral processes of social experience aggregated historical event, symbolic meaning, and social situations. The memory of bodily complaints evoked social complaints that were not so much "represented" as lived and relived (remembered through experience) in the body.

Relegitimation has failed at the macrosocial level in China, both through the brutal repression of the Democracy Movement and in the failure of the Chinese Communist Party to reform. Yet, at the regional and local levels, various kinds of relegitimation efforts have occurred, with varying degrees of success. Hence, in Guangdong and Fujian provinces, and elsewhere along the coastal edge, "market reform" has continued virtually unchanged, substituting material success, "getting rich," for erstwhile values, whereas in other, poorer, more violated provinces a Communist counterreformation was under way in 1992. Most notably, in many work units and villages, there is a unified opposition to central and regional directives, and informing on others and collaborating with the entrenched political leaders are much less prevalent than during the Cultural Revolution. This is the case, it seems, even within the Communist Party itself. In this sense, the breakdown of moral authority is so pervasive that China, even in the midst of enormous economic growth, can be said to be in an advanced stage of a cultural delegitimation crisis, and it is uncertain what will follow.[14] Yet what is certain is that resistance through somatic symptoms and disability has not been an effective means for either expressing collective opposition or ushering in new forms in the moral order. Even on the personal level it has been more self-defeating and socially unavailing than effective in reconstructing the order of experience.[15]

For example, a middle-aged teacher in a rural town in Hunan had withdrawn into reclusive existence, mourning her losses in the political devastation of the whirlwind, under the authorization of her neurasthenic complaints. Her withdrawal had no effect on the local political situation, but in fact worsened her family problems and deepened her own feeling of desolation. Another neurasthenic patient, a very competent Hunanese school administrator, carried her neurasthenic depression and pain as publicly recognized scars of her personal losses in the Cultural Revolution. Because of her complaints, she had been engaged in negotiations with the leaders of her work unit to either take early retirement or have removed an old cadre who blocked her administrative reforms. Yet her symptoms only made her situation more desperate and did not alter the political impasse in the work unit. A third sufferer of headaches, Hu Chengyeh, responded to a lifetime of discrimination because of his stepfather's landlord status, worsened for him personally by the Maoist political campaigns, by developing a defiant isolation and irascible persistence in seeking retribution for his chronic pain. Behind the physical pain the sense of bitter injustice was so strong as to be unmistakable. While his obsessive quest for "remedy" ultimately improved his work situation, it greatly worsened his family life and his hatred. The result was a corrosive political silence replaced by louder and louder physical complaints that deepened his alienation. (These and other stories of Chinese survivors of the Cultural Revolution who suffered from neurasthenia are described at greater length in Kleinman 1986:105–142.)

The Limits of Resistance as an Anthropological Interpretation of Suffering

Perhaps I have not done full justice to the model of resistance. Because the research I conducted in Boston involved the elicitation of personal and family narratives of pain and did not include participant observation in their communities, my access to worlds of pain was constrained. This is an important constraint for an interpretation of intersubjective experience, inasmuch as I have had to assemble that interpretation from personal accounts and brief home visits with family members. In spite of this methodological restriction, I do feel this chapter contains evidence of the utility of the analytic framework in the anthropological study of the social experience of chronic illness. Its chief value is as an operational device, which, as I have tried to illustrate, can facilitate analyses of the local mediation between microsocial psychological processes and the macrosociopolitical context. Johnathon Parry and Maurice Bloch (1989:1–32) contend that the short-term cycle of transactions that individuals undergo parallels the long-term cycle of transactions at the societal level: together they *reproduce* cultural forms and social structures. In the perspective that I am advancing, the connection between these short- and long-term cycles occurs within the medium of intersubjective space where moral order, affective ties, and bodily processes are integrated into a form of experience. The model of resistance, and the closely related concepts of moral delegitimation and relegitimation, offers only one perspective on this psychocultural mediation.[16] Yet the limitation of this model, I believe, can be generalized to other anthropological approaches to the study of human suffering.

I characterize that limitation in the following terms. Just as anthropological accounts fault biomedicine for its failure to respond to the teleological requirements of suffering—those existential and spiritual questions of what is most at stake in human experience which query the ultimate purpose of living—so, too, do culturalist accounts, which are so effective in diagnosing the inadequacy of natural science renditions of human conditions, fall prey to a type of social scientific appropriation of suffering. Thus, interpreting chronic pain as resistance, or for that matter as discourse, gives primacy to the search for meaning over the rest of experience. The interpretive requirements of suffering for theodicy—namely, the struggle of rebuilding a coherent account of why misery should exist in the world (see Weber 1978:518–529)—are viewed by many anthropologists as the core reality of suffering. But, as Veena Das (1994) demonstrates in accounts of the tragedy-filled lives of Indian survivors of the Hindu-Sikh ethnic conflict and the Bhopal disaster, most of those who encounter deep suffering experience a chaotic, aleatory world. The wrenching process of having to bear the awful consequences of loss, menace, and the brutality of everyday deprivation are experienced not as theodicy but as terror and desolation and, for all too many, as the abulia of alienation. Whatever its particular features, the intersubjective experience of suffering is so various, so multileveled, so open to original inventions that interpreting it solely as an existential quest for meaning, or as disguised popular critique of dominant ideology, notwithstanding the moral resonance of those foci, is inadequate. It may distort this most deeply human of conditions.

For an ethnography of experience, the challenge is to describe the processual elaboration of the undergoing, the enduring, the bearing of pain (or loss or other tribulation) in the flux of intersubjective engagements. The ethnographer needs to fasten onto the overriding practical relevance of experience for those who engage in it, for whom something (though not necessarily the physical complaint) is almost always exigent. At the same time, the ethnographer must struggle not to dehumanize the stream of experience through professional deconstructions that are totalistic and thereby claim an authoritative knowledge of determinants and effects. Such an interpretation must be invalid because it denies the uncertainty and indeterminacy and sheer novelty of human engagements. Experience is emergent, not preformed. It changes. It goes on and on. The ethnographer must be cautious about creating an end that is artificial, an illusion of a finality that is not to be found in intersubjective space, where the echoes of embodied memories reverberate even after a death. The cultural constructionist's icon can be as inhumanely artifactual a characterization of experience, then, as is the pathologist's histological slide.

Properly deployed, the model of resistance must avoid these misuses and abuses of anthropological interpretation. That means that it probably can never be entirely satisfying as an explanatory account of human suffering. And perhaps that is as it should be. For when pain is configured as suffering, it evokes intractable, inexhaustible existential questions. These questions are worth pursuing to the extent that we can better understand human conditions or provide assistance to sufferers but are as vulnerable to reductionist social scientific accounts as to biomedical ones. And here anthropologists of pain find themselves in an ethical position roughly similar to that of the clinician. For both, it is essential first to do no harm. For both, the moral requirement of engaging people who suffer is to struggle to transcend limited and limiting explanatory models so as to witness, to affirm their humanity. Anthropologists, of course, are professionally trained to engage religious themes; clinicians are not. Yet that professional training can also distance the ethnographer from this existential obligation of human conditions. For both anthropologists and clinicians there may come a time when, like the grieving author of the ancient *Lamentations over the Destruction of Sumer and Ur* (Mintz 1984:22), they need to admit, "There are no words!" It is in this spirit that I adumbrate resistance, delegitimation, and relegitimation of local worlds—admittedly inelegant yet useful words—as *figures* to bring forward aspects out of the complex, collective *ground* of chronic pain that have heretofore been obscured. This is yet another side of a subject that is best dealt with, not by insisting on a single "objective" interpretation, but by juxtaposing multiple, positioned, intersubjective perspectives.

7

The Social Course of Epilepsy

Chronic Illness as Social Experience in Interior China

Epilepsy is a relatively new focus for research in international health. With increased recognition of the importance of chronic disease and disability in the health status of communities in Asia, Africa, and Latin America, attention is shifting to those conditions that create a heavy burden of perduring suffering for patients and families (Chen, Kleinman, and Ware 1994; Frenk et al. 1989). Epilepsy, a disorder of recurrent unprovoked seizures, has a prevalence of 4 to 8 per 1,000 in Europe and North America, with rates three to five times higher in low-income societies (Desjarlais et al. 1995). These higher rates are due to conditions of deprivation that enable perinatal problems, promote higher rates of injury and infections, and seriously limit treatment. The same conditions intensify the consequences of epilepsy, such as serious burns and other injuries, and abridge the aspirations and life chances of sufferers and their families. Epilepsy patients are frequently denied schooling, shunned by their peers, find it difficult to marry, and meet active discrimination when they seek employment. Remarkably, in spite of effective biomedical treatments that can

This chapter is a revised version of an article published in *Social Science and Medicine* (40 [10]: 1319–1330) in 1995, by Arthur Kleinman, Wen-zhi Wang (Beijing Neurosurgical Institute), Shi-chuo Li (Ministry of Public Health, Beijing), Xue-ming Cheng (Beijing Neurosurgical Institute), Xiu-ying Dai (Ningxia Medical College Hospital), Kun-tun Li (Changzhi Medical College, Shanxi, China), and Joan Kleinman (Departments of Social Medicine and Anthropology, Harvard University). Reprinted with kind permission from Elsevier Science Ltd., The Boulevard, Langford Lane, Kidlington OX5 1GB, UK.[1]

substantially reduce and even prevent seizures entirely, few epileptics are in biomedical care. In Pakistan and the Philippines, more than 90 percent of those with epilepsy are not receiving biomedical treatment (Desjarlais et al. 1995: chap. 8). Were there evidence that various traditional healing methods or alternative lay therapies can control seizures, this finding might be less troubling. Because there is no such evidence, economic, cultural, and other local social forces must be regarded as crucial.

Given this background, it is not surprising that epilepsy has attracted the interest of social scientists. The leading social theory applied in epilepsy research globally is still, more than thirty years after its formulation, the model of *stigma* introduced by the sociologist Erving Goffman (Goffman 1963). This model has been modified only modestly by sociologists and social psychologists (Jones 1984; Ainlay, Becker, and Coleman 1986; Westerbrook, Bauman, and Skinner 1992). Stigma theory holds that epilepsy is a culturally devalued condition. Once this negative label is applied to a person with seizures, that person bears the brunt of societal reactions that lower the sufferer's self-esteem, creating the inner sense of being discredited or discreditable, which over time spoils his or her identity.

Temkin's classic account of epilepsy in the West, from ancient Greece to the mid–nineteenth century, also emphasizes stigma (Temkin 1945: 8, 11). Temkin, writing well before Goffman crystalized his model out of the symbolic interactionist tradition's concepts of labeling and deviance, viewed the stigma that attached to epilepsy patients as derived from ideas about its contagiousness, its "disgraceful" loss of bodily control and self-control, its religious interpretation as sign of sin, and its association with demonic possession and witchcraft (ibid.:8, 84, 90). Yet Temkin also points out that the historical record is complex. In ancient times, epileptics were regarded as sacred, and in the Renaissance, "pity, compassion, and special consideration" for sufferers of the "falling sickness" were urged upon the public (ibid.:156). The early nineteenth-century movement to hospitalize epileptics, which would probably now be widely viewed in a Foucaldian sense as yet another instance of the modern state's project of social control, is viewed by Temkin in a more benign way (ibid.:245). As with leprosy, an even more deeply stigmatized disease, any disorder in the Western Christian tradition could be associated with seemingly incompatible ideas of damnation and grace (Gussow and Tracy 1970).

The long and vicious wave of interest in hereditary degeneracy which followed the triumph of the evolutionary paradigm in the latter part of the nineteenth century and continued right up until World War II, a story that Temkin did not tell in his historical account, appears to have intensified the stigma of epilepsy, which was then framed as a condition of inherited physical *and* moral degeneracy. In her "Stories of Epilepsy," Ellen Dwyer (1992) records this construction of epilepsy from 1880 to 1930 in North America. Physicians showed a marked "antipathy" toward their epileptic patients, who were held to be personality disordered, congenitally predisposed to criminality, and therefore an appropriate object of eugenic policies.[2] Epilepsy patients saw their admission as immigrants to the United States restricted and their right to marry abridged by certain states. There were even cases of involuntary sterilization. Dwyer tells the sad story of an effort in New York State to create an "isolated colony" to confine sufferers of epilepsy. She makes the strong claim that because of their frustration with the failure of medical therapy, medical experts were attracted to social isolation and eugenic practices as social treatments. With the advent of effective drugs, Dwyer also claims, medical writings on epilepsy as a public problem declined as did the search for social solutions and also the hostility directed toward patients.

Cross-cultural studies of epileptic patients emphasize high rates of psychological and social problems. Studies of epilepsy in as disparate a set of nations as Chile, the Cameroons, Ethiopia, and Kuwait emphasize stigma as commonplace and traumatizing.[3] Negative attitudes about marriage, sharing accommodations, schooling, and even physical contact abound. Accusations of possession and witchcraft and actual social deprivation and ostracism are also frequent. Louis Alvarado and colleagues (1992) draw attention to the importance of financial problems in coping with epilepsy in Chile. Another study (Jilek-Aall and Rwiza 1992), one of the few long-term longitudinal studies of epilepsy patients in a low-income society, followed up 164 outpatients treated in Tanzania thirty years earlier. Sixty-seven precent of the sample had died, half of them owing to seizures that caused drowning, severe burns, or other trauma. This mortality rate is twice that of their age cohort in the same rural population. Suicide also occurs among epilepsy sufferers (Stagna 1993:1149–1161). Thus, mortality as well as morbidity is a serious social consequence.

Medical anthropological accounts of epilepsy have sought to go beyond the stigma model to develop a social theory of the contextual processes within which it is experienced. For example, based upon extensive research in Tanzania, Susan Reynolds Whyte shows that social devaluation of epileptics, though widespread, is constructed and expressed in locally distinctive ways (Whyte 1995:226–245). It is true, she points out, that in certain East African settings epilepsy patients eat and sleep apart, cannot pass on inheritance, and can become outcasts. Ideas of pollution and contamination create deep difficulties for patients and for families, as do accusations of witchcraft and sorcery. But when seen from the perspective of social actors, the situation is more complicated and uncertain. Families feel a powerful need to protect their members with epilepsy from others' fear of contamination and from those who will not help; they protect epileptics by keeping them isolated at home. This is a greater abridgment of life chances than stigma per se. Nor are families passive. Traditional healers are sought out because of accusations of witchcraft. Patients and families do not actively avoid biomedical treatment. They are all too often unaware of the availability of effective medicine. Many respondents have no idea what (indigenous or biomedical agency) causes epilepsy. Families and patients struggle in these complex local contexts to make sense of a serious chronic disorder and to provide security for yet another emergency for which inadequate resources are already seriously strained. And yet, Whyte argues, families assist rural patients to maintain a social persona that is not limited to their devalued affliction. Thus, Whyte concludes, stigma, which is indeed present, is not a straightforward determinant of the social experience of epilepsy patients. Stigma theory, she contends, is not the only or even the most relevant social theory.

Byron Good and Mary-Jo DelVecchio Good draw upon the findings of a study of the illness narratives of epilepsy among patients and family members in Turkey to delineate the complexity and uncertainty of the social processes involved in the construction of illness experiences. They demonstrate how the lived experience of the chronically ill is represented and shaped through narrative devices that present illness as open to mystery, potency, and change (Good and Good 1994). Possibilities for transformation in the conditions of the afflicted are kept alive. Multiple perspectives and divergent interpretations are encouraged. Alternate sources of power for potential transformations are conjured; social actors reject the anticipated; hope is engendered. The storytellers of epilepsy—patients and family members—guide the imaginative responses of others. This is not so much resistance to dominant moral meanings of illness—popular or professional—as it is a subtle reframing of experience by those who are most affected on behalf of different issues at stake in their lives and local contexts.

Stigma theory is indirectly critiqued for the passivity it ascribes to patients who become the oversocialized victims of too determinative labels and inflexible societal discrimination. Patients and families are given the single option of disavowal. In place of the inadequacies of this brittle model, a more ethnographically grounded view is installed. Patients and families are viewed in all the complex uncertainty of social experience, where irony, passion, and contradiction—all elements in the subjunctive mode of creating sickness stories—foster the remaking of moral meanings and the reframing of the ontology of suffering. This may be one of the more valuable contributions of experience-near studies in medical anthropology.

James Trostle, another anthropologist who studies epilepsy, takes a different but complementary tack (Trostle 1988; Trostle, Hauser, and Susser 1988). He demonstrates that the biomedical and behavioral medicine models of noncompliance, analogous to stigma, also privilege passivity and paternalism. Noncompliance, which is as extensive in epilepsy as it is in other chronic conditions, can be replaced with an ethnographic interpretation of drug-taking behavior that makes cultural and personal sense of choices that these other models treat as ignorant, irrational, or perverse. This is the orientation of much of medical anthropology, which insists that the only valid grounds for understanding illness and treatment are the microcultural worlds in which patients and families engage in everyday social activities. In those worlds, culture is realized in daily rhythms, rituals, and relationships; suffering is always a mode of a culturally particular form of social experience; illness has social consequences; and chronic illness and disability take a social course. That course is organized as much by what matters for the participants in a local world as it is by the biology of the condition. Indeed, over time the continuous sociosomatic interaction between both processes creates a local ontology of illness.[4]

Epilepsy in Chinese Society

In urban Chinese society, the prevalence rate of epilepsy is 4.4 per 1,000; the overall rate is 3.7 per 1,000 (Li et al. 1985; Yang and Cao 1989).[5] Thus, there are close to 4 million Chinese with epilepsy.

A study of public awareness of epilepsy conducted among 1,278 respondents in Henan Province in 1988 found that 93 percent had

heard of epilepsy; more than three-quarters of the sample knew someone with epilepsy; and almost three-quarters had seen someone have a
seizure (Lai et al. 1990). Negative attitudes were extensive. More
than half of the sample said they would object to having their children
associate at school or play with persons with epilepsy; more than half
also believed epileptics should not be employed in the same jobs as
others. Notably, 87 percent, irrespective of their education level, would
object to having their children marry a person with epilepsy; while
one out of six were so uncertain about the condition that they said
they would have nothing to recommend should a family member or
friend develop epilepsy.

The Study

The current study was initiated as a collaboration between medical anthropologists and epilepsy researchers. Its goal was
to examine the collective experience of epilepsy sufferers in poor interior regions of China that reflect the social conditions of most of
China's peoples. Individuals with epilepsy in urban and rural areas of
Ningxia and Shanxi provinces were asked to participate in the study,
along with a few who attended local epilepsy clinics. Ningxia and
Shanxi are two of China's poorer provinces, where a nationwide
community-based epidemiological survey of epilepsy in 1985 had demonstrated high prevalence and good case records. Eighty participants
were enlisted: twenty rural and twenty urban patients from each province. They and their family members were interviewed during home
visits by local research teams who had been jointly trained in the use
of a semi-structured interview schedule in training workshops. The interview canvassed demographics, experiences of illness and treatment,
and both family and patient perspectives on local social responses to
and consequences of the illness. The interview format used open-ended
questions to encourage extended responses. Patients and family members were interviewed both together and apart to make it more feasible for differing views to be expressed.

The sample is roughly representative of the local demographics of
epilepsy sufferers (see tables 1 and 2). In the Ningxia rural sample, most
patients (70 percent) belong to the Hui nationality; Ningxia urban
sample, Hui (15 percent). The Hui are a Muslim ethnic minority, a

Table 1 *Sample: Age, Gender, Occupation*

		Gender		Age	Occupation[a]						
	Number	*Female*	*Male*	*Mean*	*1*	*2*	*3*	*4*	*5*	*6*	*7*
Ningxia											
Urban	20	12	8	30		13	1	2	1	1	2
Rural	20	8	12	28	16				2		2
Shanxi											
Urban	20	9	11	47		11	1	4	1	1	2
Rural	20	9	11	39	19			1			
Total	80	38	42	36[b]							

[a]Occupations: (1) peasant farmer, (2) unskilled worker, (3) office worker/cadre, (4) technician, (5) student, (6) retired, (7) other (rural factory worker, unemployed).
[b]Range = 15–70.

Table 2 *Sample: Marital Status, Education, Family Income (N = 80)*

	N	Percentage
Marital Status		
Single	20	25
Married	59	74
Divorced	1	1
Education[a]		
Elementary school	23	29
High school (middle and senior)	34	43
Technical school	5	6
College	3	4
Illiterate or minimal literacy	15	19
Family income (in *yuan*: $1 = 5.6 yuan)[a]		
<100	11	14
100–200	23	29
200–400	27	34
400–600	17	21
>600	2	3

[a]Total adds to more than 100% due to rounding.

group that predominates in the province (Gladney 1993). Most rural respondents are peasant farmers; most urban patients are workers. One-fifth of the sample is illiterate, and few have more than a junior high school education. Three-quarters are married and only one is formally divorced, though several are separated. In these characteristics and in income the sample is similar to the local populations among which they reside.

Results

Patients (and families) varied in the names applied to their condition. The technical name for "epilepsy," *dian-xian-bing* (colloquial, *dian-jian-bing*) in standard Chinese, was used by a minority of respondents (see table 3). The term "attacks," *fan-bing-le,* was

Table 3 *Name of Illness Reported by Patients and Family Members (N = 80)*

	Ningxia		Shanxi		Total			
	Urban	*Rural*	*Urban*	*Rural*	*Urban*	*Percentage*	*Rural*	*Percentage*
"Epilepsy" (*Dian-xian-bing*, colloquial, *Dian-jian-bing*)	2	0	14	11	16	33	11	19
"Convulsion" (*Chou-feng-bing*)	3	5	2	1	5	10	6	10
"Sheep convulsions" (*Yang-jiao-feng*)	1	8	4	8	5	10	16	28
"Attacks" (*Fan-bing-le*)	15	12	3	1	18	37	13	22
Other	1	4	0	8	1	2	12	21
Don't know	1	0	3	0	4	8	0	0
Total[a]					49		58	

[a]Adds to more than 80 because some respondents gave more than one name.

most commonly used. It is nonspecific, even ambiguous; it does not convey as clearly the stigma of the other terms.

Expenditure on prescribed medicine as a percentage of monthly family income averaged 16 percent, forty-four yuan, with a range that reached 44 percent among the most impoverished. A few families spent between five hundred and six hundred yuan per month. If expenditures for special foods given to strengthen sick persons, clinic visits, use of alternative healers, transportation, and time taken off for help seeking are added to this figure, we estimated very roughly that families may have averaged close to 25 percent of monthly family income in expenditures for treatment of their epileptic members. Owing to the great transformation that has taken place in the 1980s and 1990s in China's health care system, for most families relatively little of this cost—usually a percentage of the cost of medications—is reimbursed by work units or other health insurance schemes. Most rural patients had no health insurance.

Great variation exists in lay ideas of the cause of epilepsy, ranging from heredity, head injury, possession, geomancy, poverty, and overwork to anger and fright. (Pluralism has always been commonplace in Chinese perspectives on illness [Kleinman 1980].) In interpreting the cause of first and subsequent attacks, patients and family members showed a tendency to increasingly use overwork, strong affects, and a wide range of new explanations to account for why seizures continued (see table 4). Possession and head injury were less frequently named as likely causes.

Help seeking, from the initial to subsequent seizures, showed a tendency both in rural and urban areas for patients and families to increasingly consult practitioners of traditional Chinese medicine and various folk healers as well as to use folk remedies. In rural areas, reliance on low-level primary care practitioners decreased, and there was overall a slight diminution in relying on treatment approaches provided by family members and neighbors, which were, surprisingly, very limited to begin with (see table 5).

A survey of respondents' perception of the chief effects of epilepsy on the patients and their families showed emotional, financial, and family/marital burdens to be extensive. Relations with others and overall quality of life also were reported as strongly affected. These effects appear to be somewhat greater in rural areas. Stigma (affecting both the family and the person), "loss of face," *diulian* (conveying the embodied sense of shameful loss of moral status), and diminished

Table 4 *Perceived Cause of First Attack and Subsequent Attacks*
(N = 80 epilepsy patients; parentheses indicate subsequent attacks)

	Ningxia		Shanxi		Total			
	Urban	Rural	Urban	Rural	Urban	Rural	Total	Percentage
Heredity	1 (0)	0 (1)	1 (0)	1 (1)	2 (0)	1 (2)	3 (2)	4 (3)
Congenital	1 (1)	0 (0)	0 (0)	0 (0)	1 (1)	0 (0)	1 (1)	1 (1)
Head injury	6 (3)	4 (0)	2 (0)	1 (0)	8 (3)	5 (0)	13 (3)	18 (4)
Infection	1 (0)	0 (0)	0 (0)	1 (0)	1 (0)	1 (0)	2 (0)	3 (0)
Retribution	0 (0)	1 (0)	1 (0)	2 (0)	1 (0)	3 (0)	4 (0)	6 (0)
Possession	4 (1)	6 (4)	3 (0)	2 (0)	7 (1)	8 (4)	15 (5)	21 (7)
God's will	0 (0)	0 (1)	1 (0)	2 (0)	1 (0)	2 (1)	3 (1)	4 (1)
Negative geomancy	1 (0)	0 (2)	1 (0)	4 (0)	2 (0)	4 (2)	6 (2)	8 (3)
Poverty	0 (0)	1 (3)	2 (3)	3 (3)	2 (3)	4 (6)	6 (9)	8 (12)
Wrong food	1 (1)	1 (2)	2 (2)	0 (2)	3 (3)	1 (4)	4 (7)	6 (10)
Overwork	1 (8)	1 (9)	1 (9)	3 (4)	2 (17)	4 (13)	6 (30)	8 (31)
Anger	3 (13)	1 (17)	8 (14)	6 (11)	11 (27)	7 (28)	18 (55)	25 (75)
Fright or anxiety	3 (7)	3 (6)	5 (13)	2 (4)	8 (20)	5 (10)	13 (30)	18 (41)
Other[a]	7 (9)	4 (9)	4 (2)	5 (2)	11 (11)	9 (11)	20 (32)	28 (30)

[a] Weather, menstruation, smoking, febrile seizures, carbon monoxide poisoning, etc.

Table 5 *Help Seeking for First and Subsequent Attacks*
(*N* = 80 epilepsy patients; parentheses indicate help seeking for subsequent attacks)

	Ningxia		Shanxi		Total			
	Urban	Rural	Urban	Rural	Urban	Rural	Total	Percentage
Hospital	14 (15)	4 (13)	5 (17)	0 (15)	19 (32)	4 (28)	23 (60)	29 (75)
Clinic	3 (11)	9 (9)	8 (6)	4 (19)	11 (17)	13 (28)	29 (45)	30 (56)
Rural doctor	1 (0)	3 (7)	0 (0)	8 (1)	1 (0)	11 (8)	12 (8)	15 (10)
Family or neighbors	0 (2)	1 (2)	3 (2)	4 (0)	3 (4)	5 (2)	8 (6)	10 (8)
Folk prescription	0 (8)	0 (5)	0 (3)	0 (4)	0 (11)	0 (9)	0 (20)	0 (25)
Traditional Chinese medicine (TCM) practitioner/prescription	1 (12)	2 (10)	1 (10)	1 (6)	1 (22)	3 (16)	5 (38)	6 (48)
Folk or TCM surgery	0 (8)	0 (4)	0 (7)	0 (0)	0 (15)	0 (4)	0 (19)	0 (24)
Shaman, other religious healer	1 (5)	1 (8)	2 (3)	3 (5)	3 (8)	3 (13)	6 (21)	8 (26)
Itinerant practitioner	0 (2)	0 (6)	0 (0)	0 (3)	0 (2)	0 (9)	0 (11)	0 (14)
Prayer	0 (0)	0 (4)	0 (0)	0 (7)	0 (0)	0 (11)	0 (11)	0 (14)
No treatment	0 (0)	0 (0)	1 (0)	1 (0)	1 (0)	1 (0)	2 (0)	3 (0)

self-esteem (represented by several of the categories listed) are wide-spread. (See tables 6 and 7.) We shall discuss these social effects be-low, when we develop key themes that emerged in respondents' ac-counts of their experiences of epilepsy.

The Social Experience of Suffering: The Social Course of Illness

Epidemiologists in North America indicate that among epilepsy patients in biomedical treatment who are followed for twenty years, two-thirds will have become seizure-free for five years or more (Annegers, Hauser, and Celoeback 1979; Hauser 1993:165–169; Com-mission on Epilepsy, Risks, and Insurance 1993). They also report that seizures recur in 25 percent of patients who continue medication, whereas they occur in 45 percent of those who cease taking medica-tion. Clinical epidemiological research shows that if seizures are not controlled in the first year following onset, only 60 percent of patients can be expected to enter remission; and after four years of uncon-trolled seizures, this figure drops precipitously to 10 percent. China's epilepsy experts have not published data on each of these prognostic is-sues. Chinese findings do show that in retrospective assessment 40 per-cent of 448 patients with epilepsy who had received no anti-epileptic drugs had gone into remission for two years and 27 percent had done so for five years (Zhou 1989). If the North American findings are also relevant for the experience of Chinese patients, then we can see why there is a large difference between the relative optimism of health pro-fessionals and the somewhat more pessimistic view of families and patients. For the professional the effect of treatment is much better than no treatment, and the earlier the treatment is begun the higher the rate of success. For patients and families the situation is less clear-cut, because they can see for themselves, in their own experience and that of others, that seizures may continue in spite of treatment, and during periods of no treatment there may be no seizures. Thus, in the absolutist idiom of the local world of sufferers, as opposed to the probability-based world of professionals, the efficacy of the treatment of epilepsy is ambiguous.

In our Chinese sample, relatively few patients had experienced re-mission (in the technical biomedical definition, become seizure-free

Table 6 *Effects on Family* ($N = 80$)

	Ningxia		Shanxi		Total			
	Urban	Rural	Urban	Rural	Urban	Rural	Total	Percentage
Stigma	19	19	13	10	32	29	61	76
"Loss of face," *diulian*	13	11	5	5	18	16	34	43
Emotional burden	20	20	19	20	39	40	79	99
Family and marital conflict	16	14	10	6	26	20	46	58
Financial problems	19	20	12	14	31	34	65	81
Work problems	9	6	10	0	19	6	25	31
Children's problems	10	4	2	2	12	6	18	23
School failure	2	0	0	1	2	1	3	4
Relations with others	15	15	10	5	25	20	45	56
Quality of life	18	20	10	6	28	26	54	68

Table 7 *Effects on Sick Person* ($N = 80$)

	Ningxia		Shanxi		Total			
	Urban	*Rural*	*Urban*	*Rural*	*Urban*	*Rural*	*Total*	*Percentage*
Stigma	20	16	17	18	37	34	71	89
"Loss of face," *dianlian*	15	13	15	10	39	23	53	66
Self-esteem	19	14	18	17	37	31	68	85
Emotional burden	20	19	19	20	39	39	78	98
School failure	6	11	4	0	10	11	21	26
Marital and family conflict	16	17	8	7	24	24	48	60
Arranging marriage	7	8	2	4	9	12	21	26
Work problems	18	14	16	12	34	26	60	75
Financial problems	14	19	14	14	28	33	61	76
Relations with others	17	17	15	9	32	26	58	73
Quality of life	17	17	16	13	33	30	63	79

for five years); many had frequent seizures in spite of taking biomedical drugs (mean: four seizures each month). Half did regard their current treatment as "effective," but most assessed efficacy only over a period of weeks or months, a notion that is markedly different from the biomedical category of remission. Thus, "efficacy," in medical anthropological terms, involves different and even contested formulations.

Our evaluation of compliance with biomedical recommendations was limited to asking patients and family members if they had stopped using prescribed medication. Because Chinese for a variety of reasons, like people elsewhere, may not wish to tell professionals if they have discontinued or altered the prescribed regimen, our evaluation, if anything, is likely to seriously underestimate noncompliance. More than one quarter of our respondents, nonetheless, told us that they had stopped their treatment overall. The figure increases for specific treatments. When asked about Dilantin, a common anti-epilepsy drug, twenty-four of sixty-one (39 percent) for whom it was prescribed had ceased taking it on their own: ten because they evaluated it as ineffective, six because of side effects, one because it was too expensive, and seven for other reasons. Similarly, out of twenty-eight patients who were prescribed phenobarbital, another commonly used drug, seven stopped taking it because they thought it was ineffective, five because of side effects, one because of its expense, and six for other reasons. Thus, most (nineteen out of twenty-eight, or 68 percent) had decided not to continue the recommended medication. This is a common finding cross-culturally; it is a powerful corrective to the biomedical bias that the doctor controls the treatment. To understand why patients and families decide to do what they do, it is essential to understand their experiences of illness and of treatment.

Numbers do not provide an adequate account of what those experiences are like. What they do show is that the course of this chronic condition is complex and plural, and often uncertain. Patients and families grapple with many difficulties. The resources that they require to be successful in coping with a chronic condition, especially in times of exigency, are usually greatly limited, constrained by what their work units are ready to support, which is often the minimum they can get away with paying, by their own marginal reserves, and by other demands and opportunities of their local settings. Those local settings include both formal and informal sectors of health care, and networks of connections (*guanxi wang*) that can mobilize needed resources, or further drain reserves. Interpersonal networks, work units, and the sectors of care may combine in one case of epilepsy to lighten financial and emotional burdens and to minimize the effects of bias so that disability is avoided. In another case, the local world of social experience may deepen the suffering of patient and family. Epilepsy, in turn, can effect changes in those worlds, altering the experience of families, networks, and work units, as, for example, when the social and financial relations of network members are placed under great pressure by a serious recrudescence of seizures such that reciprocity is broken and bitter resentment results.

Examining the themes that emerge from patient and family accounts, we focus on several that illustrate the social experience of epilepsy in local worlds and how the course of epilepsy affects and is affected by those local contexts. In a society of more than 1.1 billion people there are thousands of local contexts and very substantial diversity. It would hardly be acceptable to generalize to this multitudinousness from a small sample. That is not our intention. Instead, we seek to illustrate key types of interpersonal issues that are at stake in the contexts of our respondents.

Suffering as Social Experience

The Western tradition's emphasis on the subjective feelings of the afflicted individual, often viewed as isolated and forlorn, is the dominant analytic paradigm for understanding the suffering that results from serious chronic illness and disability (Kleinman 1988a:3–30, 100–200; Morris 1991:244–266). So framed, suffering becomes the pain, hurt, loss, and search for meaning of a unique person who alone must bear the deep burden of his or her troubles. From Greek tragedy through the Bible to the works of Shakespeare and the rest of the Western literary canon, and onward to contemporary literature, the paradigmatic locus of suffering is the private space of the person with the problem: the fallen hero, the sinner, the leper, the bereaved spouse, the epileptic, the victim. Chinese culture too has many examples in its poetry and painting of the individual sufferer (Elvin 1985: 156–189), but to a greater extent the Chinese tradition has taken the locus of suffering to be the intersubjective space of interactions, especially in families (Kleinman and Kleinman 1991). Viewed this way, suffering is a mode of social experience. The point is not to minimize the seriousness of the problems faced by individual patients with epilepsy in our study but rather to appreciate the importance that they and their families attribute to the interpersonal, relational locus of hardship among the members of the family. Indeed, this intersubjective sensibility frequently leads family members to emphasize their own adversity as equivalent to or even greater than the patient's experience.

His disease brings our family lots of trouble. The heaviest burden is in our minds. I'm always crying about it. I have no money to give our son treatment. Wouldn't it be better for me to die? Others raise sons in order to have blessings in their old age. But what do I have? I'll only reap hardships and worry as long as I live. There is no one in my family to look after him.

Mother of a twenty-five-year-old son with epilepsy

I'm afraid I will not live too long, so my children will endure hardships.

Thirty-seven-year-old woman with epilepsy

For her mother and me, the illness is like a heavy stone.

Father of a fifteen-year-old epileptic girl

To have someone sick in the family is the greatest burden any family can bear. . . . This is extremely bitter for him [husband]. For his child to have a disease that can't be cured . . . As for me, I couldn't be more saddened either . . .

Mother of a twenty-year-old epileptic son

My life depends on him and his support. Because of this disease, my sons and their wives don't treat us well. This saddens me, makes me feel depressed and disheartened.

Wife of a sixty-six-year-old peasant farmer with epilepsy

But my burden how heavy, how heavy it is.

Husband of a forty-six-year-old woman with epilepsy

The focus of concern is on the family and its members. What is most at stake in suffering is the abridgment of the family's aspirations, the threat to the life chances of its members, the loss and hurt of the others. Fei Xiaotong, China's doyen of anthropology, reasons that Chinese society is based upon relational ties of the self (Fei 1992:24–25). The family's success is as much the means of fulfillment of its individual members as it is the furtherance of the long collective project of ancestors and descendants. The self is its roles and relations with others in the family (and in turn with their collective and individual networks). Suffering, therefore, is as much the intersubjective experience of parents, spouses, siblings, and children as that of the sick person. As Fei puts it: "Your relatives and you are from the same blood; you have all sprouted from one root. In principle, you share the same fate; your pains and sorrows are interconnected, and so you should help meet each other's needs" (ibid.:124–125).

The construction of suffering as social experience is neither un-known nor unimportant in the West (Bowker 1970); that it is privi-leged in Chinese society should make us sensitive to its significance elsewhere as well. Appreciating the implications of the intersubjective experience of suffering begins with understanding its epistemological and moral basis but eventually requires that we understand suffering as a different way of living with illness in the social world, a different ontology of epilepsy.

Epilepsy, Marriage, and the Social Obligation of Caregiving

For Chinese parents the presence of a child disabled by sickness means that they are responsible for his or her care until they or the child dies, or until that son or daughter marries (Xiong et al. 1994). With marriage, the responsibility for care is shifted to the spouse and their future children. Thus, there is great pressure to arrange mar-riage. To do so, parents try to disguise that their child has epilepsy. If they can't do that, they will barter for a spouse with promises of an urban residence permit or a job. Illness and disability restrict the pool of potential marriageable partners to those who also have illness or disability and to those who are poorer, more rural, less educated, and physically less attractive. The consequences of disguise and barter are fraught with interpersonal tensions that parents, patient, and spouse must negotiate over the long term. But not to marry is still worse: it threatens the centrality of family in Chinese society.

My mother introduced my husband to me. . . . I did not tell him I had epilepsy. I cheated him. But during the wedding ceremony I had a convulsion and shouted out. Afterwards, I explained to him . . . now he is always angry.
Forty-one-year-old woman with epilepsy

. . . my family has to pay a lot of money to get a groom to move into our house.
Twenty-two-year-old unmarried woman with epilepsy

Her future has been destroyed. This illness must affect her marriage prospects.
Mother of nineteen-year-old unmarried epileptic

With an illness like this, no one wants to marry me. . . . I dare not think about my future prospects. . . . The greatest effect this illness has on me is that I no longer have any hope about my future. . . . I cannot get married.
Her daughter

"He would be better after he married," we said. So we found him a wife. After he married he went to see his father-in-law. At their home he had a convulsion. They were frightened out of their wits! His father-in-law asked me, "What's happened?" But I did not dare tell him the truth about it. I was afraid his daughter would divorce my son. I told him, "It's the first attack. I don't know what happened."

                    Father of twenty-two-year-old with epilepsy

If I weren't sick . . . I wouldn't have had to marry a husband like this one. I'm not satisfied with him even now.

                    Thirty-three-year-old woman with epilepsy

If his illness cannot be cured, and he remains unmarried, his mother and me will worry about him our whole life.

                    Father of twenty-nine-year-old epileptic son

Financial Burdens

Many respondents hold that the financial consequences of epilepsy are serious and even ruinous. Perhaps no other aspect of social life so clearly shows the power of chronic illness to affect social worlds and reciprocally of those worlds to influence the course of illness and treatment. The current economic transformation of Chinese society marks finances as a major issue of the times, especially so in very poor regions where our study was conducted.

As the following excerpts disclose, some peasant farmers and laborers in our sample lived at the very brink of financial catastrophe. The social welfare net of communalized life is no longer available to prevent the poorest in China from falling into extreme poverty. In low-income societies in Asia, Africa, and Latin America and among the poor in high-income societies, all that it takes to push families off their thin perch is a serious illness. The economic constraints on the social course of epilepsy and other chronic illnesses often mean the difference between receiving treatment and not, between remission and relapse. The illness, in turn, transforms the economic conditions of everyday life, using up meager reserves, creating or deepening debt, forcing families into humiliating and often unavailing negotiations with creditors, who are themselves under financial pressure. The outcome is illness as the precipitant of end-stage destitution. This is a powerful social consequence of illness that deserves far more attention in medical anthropology.

Our economic condition has become worse. I have not found any way to make money, and spend all my time with him; each day I look after him. We couldn't buy what we want to buy because we have to save money to treat the disease for my son.

Father of a young patient

Now our living standards are lower than ever. We have no money to buy vegetables and meat. We eat only rice and flour. We eat meat only once a month or every two weeks. Before we bought lots of apples. But not now. Even during the summer months, watermelons, other melons, we scarcely buy any at all. Even our children's clothes, we haven't money to buy them.

Fifty-five-year-old male patient

For his illness, we have spent over ten thousand yuan, most of which is borrowed from other families. Usually we would be saving money. We don't dare to think of what will happen later on. We have no way out.

Father of epilepsy patient

Sometimes when he wants to borrow money from his older brother, he won't give him any, and the elder brother says, "You're strong enough, but you can't make money, and can't even support yourself!" His wife also complains about him and says, "You're a disabled fellow who can't make money! No money, there's nothing for you." He can't even afford to buy chemical fertilizer from the production team.

Father of twenty-five-year-old peasant farmer

There are eight people in my family who count on me. I could do whatever I wanted if I were not ill. Now I have this disease. I can't go outside and earn our living, so our economic situation is very bad. Our children have no clothes to wear, you can see their backsides. It is not like this for other people's children. I have two children who cannot afford to pay the school fees. It is very embarrasing to ask for a subsidy from the school. I cannot do farm work. I don't have enough strength to do it. The administration did not give me any subsidy. Now our life is filled with bitter hardships. The more children there are, the worse it is. My wife also has an illness. She is very weak and hasn't enough strength to work either. Each day we eat only two meals. We eat no fish or meat or even eggs during the year, because we cannot afford to buy them. We are satisfied if we eat only rice. . . . There was no one to do the farm work. No one to help me. I was so worried I cried. I could not go out to make money. . . . Nowadays everything takes money.

Fifty-six-year-old peasant farmer with epilepsy

Sometimes my unit doesn't give me reimbursement for the costs of the medicine. I have to pay by myself. Each time when I ask for reimbursement, I must speak many nice and flattering words to them. If they are happy that day perhaps they will reimburse me. This disease needs a lot of money; it is as if it were a bottomless pit that can never be filled.

Thirty-three-year-old woman with epilepsy

To avoid such catastrophic consequences, families offer what *resistance* they can muster to the local pressures that threaten to overwhelm them. Such resistance might include "noncompliance" or foot-dragging with treatment for seizures which is unacceptably costly, and also concealment and disguise to reduce the abridgment of life chances, the use of euphemism, protective ingratiation, defaulting on debts, manipulation of strangers and members of social networks, and even the employment of local idioms of fate and victimization—all strategic actions in the struggle to cope. Resistance to stigmatization is also a strategic action to keep a family's place in the social order, a cultural performance with the objective of maintaining respectability and holding on to moral, as well as financial, capital.[6]

Stigma, Face, and Delegitimation: The Moral Experience of Epilepsy

Recent research in the West challenges the idea that the stigma of epilepsy is unrelenting and its effects always devastating (Jensen and Dam 1992). In those whose seizures are in remission, psychosocial functioning has been reported as high, with low levels of distress (Jacoby 1992). In the early phase of epilepsy, the diagnosis itself, *pace* labeling theorists, does not seem to create distress (Chaplin et al. 1992). Severity and chronicity of seizures seem to best predict psychosocial responses. Most epileptics avoid serious psychosocial problems. Public information campaigns in Western societies have improved public attitudes toward epilepsy sufferers. In the United States, the Americans with Disabilities Act of 1989, a watershed in the legal protection of the rights of the disabled, has benefitted epilepsy sufferers' quest for employment and insurance by reducing institutional discrimination.[7]

The situation of epilepsy in interior China, and in other low-income regions, is altogether different. Even though Deng Xiaoping's paraplegic son, Deng Pufang, has popularized the plight of the disabled generally, investing political capital in a domain that had previously received almost no national attention, the public response to epilepsy, especially in the impoverished region where our research was conducted, is unchanged. Those with seizures routinely experience discrimination in schools, in the workplace, and in the community.

Most patients in our sample are in a chronic phase with frequent seizures. For them and for their families, the serious consequences of epilepsy are intensified by Chinese society's prioritizing of social control as the chief concern in the societal response to this and to other chronic conditions (e.g., schizophrenia, mental retardation, substance abuse) in which behavior is affected (Phillips 1993; Fei 1992:28). The emphasis on social control, rather than patient rights, means that students with epilepsy may be removed from the classroom, workers with epilepsy may not be permitted to carry on with their jobs, and work units may discriminate against patients and families who are requesting more resources for treatment.

Social control also works through stigma. Because of their fear that the entire family will be disgraced, family members conceal the diagnosis, patients may drop out of treatment, and often families sequester their epileptic members at home. As already noted, they resist the negative effects of social control. Overprotection of sufferers, a form of intra-familial social control aimed at preventing epileptic family members from being publicly shamed and protecting them from potential physical harm, is too often the chief constraint on patients' life chances.[8] Spouses and parents may stop working and give up all other activities so that they can constantly attend affected kin. Well intentioned though it be, overprotection may convert impairment into disability and handicap.

As in the West, stigma is a moral category. Yet in the Chinese context, moral blame is not applied to the patient alone but extends to the entire family. Ideas that attribute the cause of epilepsy to bad fate, heredity, negative geomantic forces, and the malign influences of gods, ghosts, or ancestors—all are accusations about the moral status of the family. Inasmuch as Chinese society turns on the individual's kinship circle and social network, families and networks that are morally compromised are perceived as ineffective and indeed actually can become so as members drop out and their social-relational power is lost. The moral effects of epilepsy cross from the social body to the physical body. The moral status of the person is his or her face (*lianmian*); social relations "give face" or "save face." To "lose face" is to carry the social experience of shame into the inner experience of the body-self (Kleinman and Kleinman 1994). The indigenous Chinese model of stigma, however, is a sociosomatic one that frames intersubjective *delegitimation*, not spoiled personal identity, as the central process. Since the person is constructed in Chinese culture as a relational self, delegitimation is the most fundamental assault the person can experience (Fei 1992:24–25).

The moral crisis of epilepsy occurs because of the delegitimation of the person and the family in a structure of social relationships that affects marriage, livelihood, and all aspects of social intercourse. The moral capital of the family and the network is spent down. Over the long term, delegitimation is routinized, so that patient and family are regarded as morally bankrupt and capable of bankrupting others. The ruins of social relations ruin lives. *Renqing,* favor, the affect central to social exchange, can neither be given nor received. To lose face, to be unable to allocate *renqing,* to experience delegitimation means that the social course of epilepsy for patients and families is potentially a form of social death (Hwang 1987; King 1991). Just as loss of vitality (*qi*), in indigenous common sense, leads to death of the body, so too devitalized interpersonal networks, believed to be contaminated by bad fate and therefore feared to be contagious, can also lead to the death of connections, the very essence of social death among Chinese. It is not at all surprising, therefore, to what extent families will go to ward off, to resist, delegitimacy.

We don't want others to know about his disease. He's grown up now. It is not good that others know about this kind of illness. Now the four of us think that other people all look down on us. We only tell our family . . . things are well with us, and don't tell them about our problems. They all think that everything is well with us and that we are lucky.

> Mother of nineteen-year-old epileptic son

I think this illness makes me lose face.

> Twenty-two-year-old female with epilepsy

I don't want anyone to talk about my disease. When I'm sick, I think I'm inferior to others.

> Twenty-year-old female patient

I always feel I am inferior to others. I can't raise my head in front of others.

> Forty-eight-year-old male patient

Because my wife has this illness, I have lost jobs. I don't like to mention this matter to my friends and coworkers. I'm afraid others will ask me about it, and I wouldn't know how to respond. I don't like to go out with her, or see a film. I'm afraid of what others will say. And I'm afraid that she will have an attack in front of others.

> Husband of a thirty-year-old patient

Conclusion

Our findings, limited though they be, support the idea that epilepsy is best regarded as possessing a *social course* (Ware and Kleinman 1992). We use these words to draw a specific contrast with the biomedical idea of the natural course of disease, including epilepsy. The social course of epilepsy indicates that epilepsy develops in a local context where economic, moral, and social institutional factors powerfully affect the lived experience of seizures, treatment, and their social consequences. The social course of epilepsy, furthermore, is plural, heterogeneous, and changing. It is as distinctive as are different moral worlds, different social networks, different social histories.

To understand that lived experience, the suffering associated with epilepsy has to be viewed as occupying an interpersonal space, a world of situated *social experience* that connects moral status with bodily status, family with afflicted person, perhaps even social networks with neural networks. The social experience of epilepsy is multitudinous, yet difference is also constrained by powerful factors such as deprivation and delegitimation (Kleinman 1992:169–197). Relevant social theories are needed to better understand the social life of illness and the ill. In addition to stigma theory, we suggest other pertinent social theoretical issues that are emergent in the worlds of the patients and families in our study: delegitimation, sociosomatics, efficacy and compliance as socially contested evaluations, different social ontologies of suffering, and coping as resistance. Together these concepts begin, in a small way, to fill in the map of the *social course of disease*. What we have said about epilepsy can be applied to other chronic conditions. Perhaps no domain of health is more ripe for the development of social theory.

Treatment of epilepsy in low-income societies like China currently centers on pharmacology. The central issues for public health policy have been to provide access to health services that can deliver effective treatment, and to focus on preventable causes. Framing epilepsy in terms of its social course suggests that to improve the quality of life and reduce disability, it is essential that health and social policy address the context of social experience. Stigma, institutional discrimination, the relatively high cost of care in a setting of chronic deprivation, and the other specific social consequences we have delineated, including the social resistance put up by sufferers, are as important for health and health policy as is basic medical services. Indeed, they are as salient for the content of medical care as are diagnosis and pharmacology. The social course of illness constitutes much of what is meant by prognosis. Health education, disability laws and services, community action projects, and work- and family-based rehabilitation programs are essential to this orientation.

Epilepsy in China indicates that health policy is inseparable from social policy, and that social policy is inseparable from social theory. Social theoretical innovations are necessary if policy is to address the large variety of local communities and collective experiences. Especially salient is the powerful constraint of circumstances of deep deprivation, which affect so many globally. To bring together social and health policy, narratives as well as numbers, social services along with health services, and social theory with health science perspectives should be the challenge for policy formulation.

8

Violence, Culture, and the Politics of Trauma

Violence is now a major preoccupation in the media and in academic circles. Scholars, journalists, physicians, and politicians draw upon images of violence to discuss subjects as various as international security, public health policy, the moral status of television programs, and national and local politics. In writing the report *World Mental Health: Problems and Priorities in Low-Income Countries* (Desjarlais et al. 1995), we have become specially interested in the appropriation of the images of violence and the uses to which the traumatic consequences of violence are put by professionals, the media, and laypersons. In this chapter, we try to think through a few of the key questions on this topic, particularly regarding the trauma that results from political violence. What sort of *problem* is such trauma? What do the health professions have to say about it? Why is it being medicalized? And what are the consequences of making a *victim* (or a victimizer) into a *patient*?

Political violence carries the most ancient provenance. Wars, executions, and torture have been the authorized forms of asserting state power throughout the historical record. Although it is tempting to see the current level of political violence as a pandemic, political violence has been endemic over the centuries. Enormous eruptions of violence

The original version of this chapter was written with Robert Desjarlais; I have expanded and rewritten that version for this collection of essays. I presented the original paper at the Scientific Institute on Ethnocultural Aspects of Posttraumatic Stress and Related Disorders held in Honolulu in June 1993. Another related paper on political violence with Robert Desjarlais appeared in *Anthropology Today* (Desjarlais and Kleinman 1994).

such as this century's two world wars have punctuated an already dev-astating record. It is chastening to remember that as violent as our times seem to be because of the close coverage of "low-intensity" con-flicts (a troubling euphemism), the terrible conflicts of the Second World War led to 50 million deaths and the uprooting of hundreds of millions of people (Gilbert 1989). Although the killing fields of the Great War were more narrowly bounded in geography and resulted in less than half the carnage that would mount so gruesomely and wantonly in the 1940s, the trench battles between 1914 and 1918 marked—physically and psychologically—almost an entire generation (Fussell 1975; Keegan 1976).

Nonetheless, the end of the twentieth century is a bloody time. The insurgencies in Angola and Mozambique, the repressive regimes in Guatemala, El Salvador, South Africa, and China, the "dirty wars" in South America, the civil wars in Cambodia and Sri Lanka, and eth-nic, religious, and civil strife in the Balkans, the Middle East, South Asia, and much of Africa have all contributed to the grim statistics on mutilation, death, displacement, and societal breakdown. The suffer-ing that results from political violence includes a range of traumas: pain, anguish, fear, loss, grief, and the destruction of a coherent and meaningful reality. "Low-intensity" warfare, for instance, expressly aims at control of populations through the application of terror and de-struction to entire communities. State violence is meant to control people through fear and suffering, a fact that much of social scientific analysis has focused on. The leading social theories have been heavily influenced by a long-standing continental critique of the abuses of au-thoritarian states. Yet, in this period we are also increasingly aware of the violence that accompanies social disorganization and political dis-solution. Liberia, Somalia, Bosnia, and Rwanda are examples of the horrendous consequences of violence when there is no state author-ity capable of maintaining order and assuring security. The frailty of the nation-state and of the transnational world in which we now live suggests that violence and terror will mark any new world order that might ensue.

Images of violence are taken into the process, so that pictures of mutilation and destruction are used to terrorize and control. Daniel Santiago writes of the "aesthetics of terror" in El Salvador:

People are not just killed by death squads . . . they are decapitated and then their heads are placed on pikes and used to dot the landscape. . . . It is not enough to kill children; they are dragged over barbed wire until the flesh falls from their bones while parents are forced to watch. (1990:293)

The mass use of rape in Balkan villages occupied by Serbian Chetniks, the burning of whole families in South Asia, the mutilation of corpses in Liberia, the "disappearances" favored in Argentina, terrorist actions in the Middle East, the necklacing of those labeled informers in South African townships—all of these performances affect populations through direct observation and through the symbolic imagery of the popular culture. Images of torture, destruction, and dislocation, as well as the abandonment and orphaning of children, are calculated to demoralize and to intimidate. Thus, human trauma is a planned and desired outcome. (See also Keen 1994 on the political uses of famine in Africa.) Its significance is manipulated through control of the cultural apparatuses of meaning making. For example, during the worst days of China's great famine from 1959 to 1961, the state-controlled newspapers reported bumper harvests at the very moment that 30 million were starving to death. In this way, a moral critique of the immense failure of the Chinese Communist Party's policies of the Great Leap Forward was preempted, but also, the state ruthlessly conveyed the idea that it could authorize or deny any reality. It did so again in the aftermath of the Tiananmen Massacre, when dissident workers were executed with special silver bullets, a bill for the cost of which was later sent to their families. The message: we (the Chinese government) hold all the political as well as moral power.

Cultures of fear have been created by other repressive regimes in the former Soviet Union, Cambodia, South Africa, Cuba, Chile, and Guatemala. Creating helplessness and mistrust through images of suffering is also a traumatic (and, at times, calculated) consequence of political violence. These techniques of violence are meant to intimidate witnesses, to suppress criticism, and to prevent resistance. They seek to propagate pusillanimity. They continue to break bodies long after the political situation that produced them has changed, as in the case of the persistent toll of traumatic amputations owing to the millions of land mines that combatants planted during the active phase of the Cambodian wars. These techniques of violence are intended to tyrannize through the development of cultural sensibilities and forms of social interaction that keep secret histories of criticism secret and hidden transcripts of resistance hidden (Scott 1990). That is, trauma is used systematically to silence people through suffering.

When those who experience violence escape to places of refuge, they must submit to yet another type of violation.[1] Their memories of violation, their *trauma stories* become the currency with which they enter exchanges for physical resources and achieve the new status of political refugee. Increasingly, those complicated stories, based in real events, yet reduced to a core cultural image of victimization, are used by health professionals to rewrite social experience in medical terms. The person who undergoes torture first becomes a victim—a quintessential image of innocence and passivity who cannot represent him- or herself—and then becomes a patient with posttraumatic stress syndrome. Indeed, to receive even modest public assistance it may be necessary to undergo a transformation from one who has lived through the greatly heterogeneous experiences of political terror, to stereotyped victim, to standardized sufferer of a textbook sickness. Given the political and economic import of such transformations, the violated themselves may want, and may even seek out, the moral as well as the financial consequences of being ill. We need to ask what kind of cultural transformations they undergo, and what the implications of these transformations might be. What does it mean to invest those who are traumatized by political violence with the moral status of a victim or a patient?

There is a troubling issue. The countries of the North, in their applaudable quest to support solidarity for human rights and offer sanctuary and protection, appropriate trauma stories and images of violation from political upheaval and oppression in Asia, Africa, the Middle East, Latin America, and the Caribbean. Yet these places of refuge in North America and Western Europe include societies in which violence is a crucial part of commercial culture. The danger is that tales of human misery from abroad will become part of that commercial culture as "infotainment" on the nightly news. Spectacular forms of foreign trauma disguise routinized domestic misery. This cultural representation even carries the self-satisfying message that in spite of all the degradation in our midst we are "above" that kind of abuse which we associate with the incorrigible failings of the "old world" and with a Conradian view of the barbaric side of the formerly colonized nations. It is a comforting myth that obscures our nation's role in the major economic and political transformations that have intensified violence in the South. Stories of untamed violence in the so-called third world are then used to domesticate our own forms of oppression. Images of violent political events are of *crises* that disguise the everydayness of *routine* violence. Paul Weaver (1994) talks of the media's validation of crises as collusion between journalists, public officials, and narrow interest groups in the selling of stories.

The Medicalization of Suffering:
Posttraumatic Stress Disorder

Given the economic, cultural, and political forces that exert pressure on health care in the United States, the medicalization of violence can at least partially be understood as integral to the troubling irony we have just described. To wit, the way in which professionals in health institutions think and talk about trauma situates it as an *essential* category of human existence, rooted in individual rather than social dynamics, and reflective more of medical *pathology* than of religious or moral happenings. Psychologists and psychiatrists construct violence as an *event* that can be studied outside of its particular context because of its putative universal effects on individuals. They place it in an overly simple stress model, as the distress produced in a person who has undergone a traumatic episode. Collective trauma is not mentioned. Personification has always been a preferred means of representing the trauma of suffering, as in the Bible and in writing today (Mintz 1984). A group's trauma is pictured in the bodies and words of individuals. The voices and facial expressions of individual victims or patients, which can so vividly portray the trauma of the person, do not show the interpersonal and community-wide effects of violence. Let us turn to the professional personification of political violence as posttraumatic stress disorder (PTSD) in the American Psychiatric Association's diagnostic system, *DSM-IIIR,* the official version at the time this chapter was written, for an illustration of how social problems are transformed into the problems of individuals, how collective experiences of suffering are made over into personal experiences of suffering, and how, thereby, social traumas are refigured, for policy and intervention programs, as psychological and medical pathologies. (The ideas presented here on PTSD have been influenced by the writings of Allan Young [1990; and see chapter 9 below].)

DSM-IIIR states that PTSD's essential feature

is the development of characteristic symptoms following a psychologically distressing event that is outside the range of usual human experience (i.e., outside the range of such common experiences as simple bereavement, chronic illness, business losses, and marital conflict). The stressor producing the syndrome would be markedly distressing to almost anyone, and is usually experienced with intense fear, terror, and helplessness. The characteristic symptoms involve re-experiencing the traumatic event, avoidance of stimuli associated with the event or numbing of general responsiveness, and increased arousal. (American Psychiatric Association 1987:247–250)

The *DSM* enumerates trauma-inducing stressors, and then describes the variety of traumatic experiences:

Commonly the person has recurrent and intrusive recollections of the event or recurrent distressing dreams during which the event is reexperienced. In rare instances, there are dissociative states . . . during which components of the event are relived, and the person behaves as though experiencing the event at that moment. There is often intense psychological distress when the person is exposed to events that resemble an aspect of the traumatic event or that symbolize the traumatic event, such as anniversaries of the event. (American Psychiatric Association 1987:248)

The *DSM* description continues with a list of additional features of the experience: persistent avoidance of the stimuli associated with the trauma; numbing or diminished responsiveness to the external world; persistent symptoms of arousal; symptoms of depression, anxiety, difficulty concentrating, emotional lability, headache, vertigo; and muteness or nightmares in children. Notably, the official text points out that "studies indicate that preexisting psychopathological conditions predispose to the development of this disorder." The differential diagnosis includes anxiety, depressive, adjustment, and organic mental disorders. The *DSM* section ends with its classic presentation of diagnostic criteria as a forced choice among listed symptoms. The minimal criteria include one out of four forms of persistent reexperience of the trauma, three out of seven types of persistent avoidance, and three out of six persistent symptoms of increased arousal. The draft text for the next edition of the *DSM*, *DSM-IV*, which appeared in 1994, proposes several useful changes in the diagnostic criteria. However, the comments here are confined to the official document that guides current practice.[2] Among the hundreds of studies that have applied these criteria to special populations are reports of high rates of PTSD among political refugees, victims of ethnic conflict, survivors of natural and industrial disasters, and those who have experienced serious domestic violence (see Desjarlais et al. 1995).

A cultural critique of the official text (*DSM-IIIR*) is revealing in several respects. First, the differential diagnosis does not mention the possibility of ruling out normal responses to trauma. The expectation seems to be that response to trauma, no matter how appalling that trauma, should not lead to persistent reexperience, avoidance, or arousal. The prose emphasizes that the traumatic event is outside the range of "usual human experience" such as bereavement, illness, business loss, marital conflict. But given the downright common, even routine experience of political trauma in many parts of the world, the idea of what is usual sounds suspiciously ethnocentric, even provincially middle class and middle Western. Indeed, the text itself says that "stress . . . would be markedly distressing to almost anyone." But what is a common stressor under conditions that obtain in Bosnia, Haiti, Colombia, or even South Central Los Angeles may seem remarkably uncommon in Cambridge or the upper eastside of Manhattan. We have no doubt that political violence has physiological, psychological, and social effects that can be devastating, but why call these effects, even the worst of them that are experienced by only a minority of sufferers, a disease?

Just as Vietnam War veterans claim serious effects of PTSD, the diagnosis could be seen as covering the effects of warfare that formerly were labeled "shell shock," "battle fatigue," and the like. As Samuel Andrew Stouffer (1949) and his colleagues showed in their research on American soldiers in the Second World War, the longer a soldier—any soldier—was in battle, the more likely it became that he would suffer these traumatic effects. After more than six months in active combat without relief, most soldiers in a unit would experience such symptoms, which made them unfit for battle. As John Keegan (1976) suggests, these symptoms are probably normative for soldiers, at least since Waterloo when diary accounts of the effects of warfare became available. If this is a disease, then it is one that has a protective consequence—namely, removal from the killing fields—and direct origins in the "normal" terror of battle.

Second, strong emphasis is placed on the "psychological" effects of the traumata: "a psychologically distressing event" that is "usually experienced with intense fear, terror, and helplessness." As with the rest of the *DSM*, the locus of the experience is taken to be the mind of the individual. The criteria for PTSD do include those of physiological arousal, but the text's emphasis seems very much on emotional responses. The problem with mapping distress in the mind of the individual is that such a cartography tends to overlook the fact that the causes, locus, and consequences of collective violence are predominantly social. Political violence devastates families and communities and destroys the routines of everyday life; the physiology of trauma is as much a result of social trauma as it is an entity unto itself. The experience of suffering is interpersonal, involving lost relationships, the brutal breaking of intimate bonds, collective fear, and an assault on loyalty and respect among family and friends.

A third point worth noting is that PTSD's diagnostic criteria repeatedly emphasize *persistence* of symptoms. The idea is that the experience is pathological because it persists. The implication is that a normal response to trauma does not involve continuation of complaints. This is very much the way bereavement is handled too. Uncomplicated bereavement ends, psychiatrists claimed in the past, usually by six months, nearly always by one year. Bereavement lasting more than thirteen months is prolonged, even pathological. In the *DSM-IV* draft criteria, a bereaved person's sadness, agitation, guilt, difficulty concentrating and sleeping, and thoughts about death, if they last more than *two months,* can be diagnosed as a major depressive episode. The bereaved person is expected to get on with it—get back to work, get into a new relationship. In much of the world and still for many in America, fidelity to the dead lasts more than two or even thirteen months, even for a lifetime. (See Nadia Seremetakis's [1991] description of grieving in Greece, which, like grieving in many societies, is for the long term.) The idea in the *DSM* is that suffering can not and should not be endured. It should be brought to an end. This is central to the ideology of America: there is nothing that needs to be endured. Even memories can be "worked through." It is sadly wrong. Most poor people worldwide and in the United States must endure the often unendurable; not even the middle class can escape certain forms of suffering. And key memories of trauma—collective and individual—are not to be erased but to be worked with, even commemorated. Indeed, commemoration of collective trauma is one of the means by which societies remember (Connerton 1989).

Not surprisingly, the authors of this influential text have very little, almost nothing really, to say about human suffering; yet, the examples that are given—natural disasters, accidents, combat, rape, torture, death camps—are exactly what most of us would take to be quintessential examples of suffering. John Bowker (1970), who writes about how the world's major religions deal with problems of human suffering, canvasses some of the same problems, but from an entirely different

point of view. In Christianity, Judaism, Islam, Hinduism, and Bud-
dhism the experience of human misery, from sickness, natural disasters, accidents, violent death, and atrocity is taken to be a defining
condition of people's existential plight. With more than one hundred
conflicts in societies in the North and South and violent repression as
a policy of state control in many nations, the brutal experience of violence including combat, torture, and rape is fairly ubiquitous on our
planet in our time. Add natural disasters and injury from automobile
and other serious accidents, and it is arguable that most people in the
world dwell in settings in which such events are commonplace, even
routine. Clearly the *DSM*'s authors have a very different set of normative social experiences in mind. Suffering in North America is thought
of as perhaps no longer normative, or it would seem, normal.

And that is one of our chief complaints about PTSD: it medicalizes
problems as psychiatric conditions that elsewhere and for much of human history in the West have been appreciated as religious or social
problems. All told, the ideology underlying the notion of PTSD re-
produces a very specific ontology of the person—that of upper middle-
class society in the United States. As the moral and political philosopher Charles Taylor (1990) has noted, that human beings are radically
detached from their social environments, are defined by a rich and
"inward" depth of emotions, and are driven by zeal to change and
remake themselves is an idea quite recent to the West. The commonsensical force of the idea of deep indwelling subjectivity is helping to
shape the discourse on PTSD. The situation is straight out of Michel
Foucault: a series of statements, like those found in the *DSM*, create
a certain reality or "visibility" (Deleuze 1988) that effects a form of
being that "can and must be thought" (Foucault 1985:7). As anthropologists, however, we must advocate that there are other ways to
think about trauma (Das 1994).

The social construction of human misery as PTSD is just the latest
example of what Max Weber (Wrong 1976) had in mind as the increasing application of the technical rationality of bureaucratic institutions to spheres of life that were previously handled by the religious
and moral idioms of everyday experience. It is a colonization of the
lifeworld by professional discourse. Professionals may not (probably do
not) explicitly aim at advancing professional power and the division of
labor of the bureaucratic state. Indeed, they often regard themselves
as resisting the interests of social control. Yet with several hundred
thousand well-meaning social workers, psychologists, and psychiatrists

in North America competing for a limited number of patients, PTSD certainly has to be seen as a form of medicalization that is influenced, at least in part, by the interest of economically hard-pressed professions to increase jobs and income in an era when health care is faced with shrinking resources. You cannot bill third-party payers for coming to the aid of those who have experienced political trauma. You can bill them for major depressive disorder, any one of the anxiety disorders, or PTSD. Every conceivable psychological problem is listed in the *DSM* as a disease, precisely because treating disease is authorized for remuneration, whereas responding to distress is not. Thus, there is a political economy to the use of the disease concept (see Kirk and Kutchins 1992). Don't misunderstand our point. We do not deny that those who are traumatized are genuinely suffering or that mental health professionals are working with competence and compassion to aid them. Treating persons with PTSD may improve symptoms and limit distress. We do not deny this or derogate its significance. We are, however, asking mental health professionals, patients, and laypersons to attend more fully to PTSD's implicit cultural, political, and economic implications. What constraints do (or should) those implications place on clinical practice?

Violence and the Local Setting of Social Experience

Yet this is not the only, or even the chief, thrust of our critique of the way political violence is being turned into a health problem. Rather we seek to argue that the medicalization of political trauma violates the experience of that trauma. As a result, purely medical phrasings distort and neglect the social experiences that sufferers undergo. Included in these experiences are moral, religious, and social processes that contribute to the most egregious human effects of violence. A call to "experience" is, of course, yet another discourse, but one that attends more closely, and with more reflexivity, to the local complexities that pattern any form of suffering. Simply put, medicalizing political violence removes the human context of trauma as the chief focus for understanding violence. It treats the person as a patient, the host of a universal disease process, victim of inner pathology. Many persons who experience political violence are the victims of intentional and systematic harm that is motivated by issues of power, not pathology. They may develop a posttraumatic syndrome. Do they have a disease? Or are they experiencing a greatly distressing, yet normal, psychobiological reaction? The disease model tends to remove agency. Yet, even when faced with the vast machinery of state power, human agency continues to operate (Levi 1988). Some contribute to their own problems owing to the dynamics of their local world. A firmer ground for analysis is an understanding of how that local world mediates between broader political forces and the responses of individuals. Let us consider a case example.

On the Fourth of July, 1991, Mrs. Fang, a woman from a rural county town in an interior province of the People's Republic of China, traveled several hundred kilometers to undergo a series of medical evaluations in a major urban medical center, where she was interviewed by Arthur and Joan Kleinman. Complaining of headaches, dizziness, visual symptoms, numbness, and whole body pain that had incapacitated her for two years, Mrs. Fang told a story—a familiar tale of political oppression in China—with which she has for many months been preoccupied, perhaps even obsessed. In 1989, when pregnant with her second child, she was forced to have an abortion in the third trimester of pregnancy. It was her third abortion since 1986. Each abortion, she claims, was forced upon her by the leaders of her work unit. Since 1989, she has been grieving and in a state of continuous, pervasive anger. She is openly critical of the forced abortions and of the acquiescence of local bureaucrats in an oppressive policy. The doctors in the medical center heard her out, but ended by diagnosing a long-term personality problem and short-term stress-related psychosomatic syndrome and by prescribing various medications.

Told this way, the story could easily appear in a North American newspaper to illustrate the trauma of routinized political oppression in an authoritarian Communist country whose one-child-per-family policy has become a focus of criticism by human rights advocates and has also received recent notoriety in the media as a common reason given for seeking political refuge by Chinese who have illegally entered the United States. That is the way stories like Mrs. Fang's are most often appropriated. The stress-related condition is seen as the traumatic effects of a form of political violence: the inscription into the female body of the social memory of state control.

However, there is much more to Mrs. Fang's story as told by her and the cadre who accompanied her on the long journey of medical help seeking. To understand that narrative, we must position ourselves in her world: a factory in a modest-sized rural county town in a poor and remote region. The factory has been repeatedly criticized by the local population control authority for failing to assiduously enforce the one-child policy. Mrs. Fang had come to believe that owing to that local campaign of criticism, the leaders of her work unit, whom she otherwise liked and regarded as reasonably tolerant and supportive, would be unwilling to accept her pregnancy. (Indeed, she had been requested to undergo her first abortions early in two previous pregnancies.) But precisely because she and her husband had a good relationship with them, and found their unit's cadres to be sympathetic, she believed that once the baby was born, the unit's cadres would have no recourse but to accept the reality of a second child in their family. Therefore, she hid her pregnancy. She did so, moreover, even though her friends and coworkers, who also wanted more than one child, had agreed collectively to avoid pregnancy for a limited time, while the work unit was trying to get out of the spotlight of political criticism. After a while, workers and cadres had agreed, the intensity of the political campaign would abate, as it had so often in the past, and it would be possible to secretly negotiate additional births in the work unit.

When Mrs. Fang, now so evidently pregnant that she could no longer avoid public disclosure, revealed her pregnancy, the entire work unit—workers and leaders—were deeply angered. They accused her of being selfish and reckless. She was also accused of breaking the social compact, and thereby threatening the entire community, including those women who had not yet had even a single pregnancy. When she brazenly responded that all of the accusations were unfortunately true but beside the point, since she would soon be delivering a baby, she created pandemonium in her unit. Both cadres and workers told her that her behavior was unacceptable. Why should she be given special license, they demanded, especially when she had betrayed a social strategy aimed at assisting all the women in the unit and had lied to them all to boot? The general sentiment was strongly against her. Mrs. Fang's response was like pouring cooking oil on an open fire. She agreed with all the accusations, but, "smiling" at her "comrades," as she herself told the story, while the accompanying cadre shook her head in amazement at the brazenness of the act, Mrs. Fang told them that they would just have to accept it, whether they liked it or not, since they were now stuck with the result.

The members of the work unit were outraged. Furthermore, when the population control cadres learned of the pregnancy, the work unit's leaders confronted a crisis that had gone beyond the boundaries of their domain of control. The dramatic consequences are a story to be told at length in another place, but among the results were a collective demand for abortion, a suicide attempt by Mrs. Fang's husband that was precipitated by her accusation that he was too weak to protect her and the fetus, suicidal behavior by Mrs. Fang herself (which was held by her coworkers to be manipulative and insincere), the forced abortion, grieving. Then came a pendulum swing in accusation from the accusers to the accused, with demands for financial restitution, various failures at compromise, and Mrs. Fang's illness career that first met grudging acceptance, but after two years of help seeking that had seriously depleted the work unit's medical insurance fund, was now causing a recrudescence of accusation and conflict.

The point we seek to illustrate is that to understand Mrs. Fang's suffering, we must enter her world and attend to its complex array of discourses, sensibilities, and competing demands. That world is not a passive recipient of the vector of macrosocial forces, such as the one-child-per-family national policy, any more than is Mrs. Fang. Rather, the local world actively mediates the effect of political pressure on persons. In the interactions between positioned participants that make up that world, the dynamics between victims and victimizers turn on what is locally at stake. There is social and individual agency. While the biographical details of Mrs. Fang's life and the description of the setting assist us to understand the nature of the political trauma Mrs. Fang suffered, the diagnosis of a stress-based psychosomatic condition does not. Nonetheless, that diagnosis will become consequential in the social process of suffering itself. It creates an interpersonal experience of which Mrs. Fang is the central (but not the only) part.[3]

Suffering is interpersonal; political trauma is more than and different from a disease condition even though it has physiological effects; and the political process is as central to the appropriation of the images of suffering as it is to the experience of suffering. The experience itself is characteristically cultural, elaborated in ways that differ from its development in other societies. That is the lesson of Mrs. Fang's case.

Mrs. Fang has persisted in her reexperience of trauma, in the disabling complaints she associates with that trauma, and in yet other ways that would allow a diagnosis of PTSD, were it used in China, which it is not. But in our view PTSD would be an inappropriate formulation of this case, for several reasons. Mrs. Fang is not a passive sufferer of traumatic stress. There is no single trauma story for her case either. Each positioned participant tells a different, even conflicting story. Mrs. Fang's persistent symptoms are in part the result of Mrs. Fang's persistence. The trauma itself is social in consequence, and Mrs. Fang helps to create it. Is she pathological? If so, is her pathology the consequence or cause of the trauma? And what kind of pathology is it? (PTSD is not the only label that might be applied to Mrs. Fang's experience that would seem problematic. Resistance to political authority would be equally problematic. So too would be the imagery of innocent victimization. And while personality disorder will come to mind for psychotherapists, does that contested label solve or deepen the problem?) How then should we engage the problem of the traumatic consequences of political violence?[4]

Toward an Ethnography of Political Violence

From our perspective, the epidemiological statistics, comparative psychometric surveys, and high-level discussion of political violence as a public health or clinical condition provide an inadequate basis to understand its sources, forms, and consequences. In the ethnographic view, political violence is situated in native social spaces: a home, a street, a park. These are the contexts of ethnic conflict and religious riots in Sri Lanka and India where, as Stanley Tambiah notes (1993), the police may decide in one community to pull back and forgo their responsibilities for protecting the public, while in another they hold the line against aggressors. These are contexts where, as Veena Das (1994) shows for religious conflicts in India, crowds do not spontaneously lose control but rather are mobilized, armed, and incited to violence by political activists and thugs who want particular persons to be "taught a lesson"; contexts where neighbors on one block kill one another, while those on another with a different history of interests and relationships shield one another (Das 1995).

The description of the dynamics of political violence in distinctive life contexts clarifies how large-scale forces alter interpersonal relations. Certain categories of persons and certain individuals are placed at great risk, while local worlds protect or even strengthen the position of others. The parochial world is the setting where violence is taken up in networks of relationships that either intensify or dampen its effects, networks that have a genealogy, a concrete configuration of events and stories. Violence qua violence is a difficult category to understand, whereas particular contexts and histories of violence can be studied and compared. Instead of focusing our analyses on the psychological reactions of victims, or the putative "essential," "inherent" aspects of violence as a phenomenon, we would do much better to attend to political violence and its consequences as *processes* that are motivated by the layered specificities and inexpediencies of social and political forces. The focus on local worlds enables us to examine the social processes that underwrite the targeting, implementation, and response to violent actions. In this way, violent actions at the community and even neighborhood level, and discourses on those actions at the national and international level, pattern one another.

In the ethnographic perspective, those who suffer the traumatic consequences of political violence are more effectively approached as a greatly heterogeneous category of social sufferers, rather than as patients or victims. The violated need not be romanticized or cynically deconstructed. There should be no problem in acknowledging that those who experience violence have physiological as well as psychological responses. Those reactions can be studied collectively as well as individually. Those responses tell us as much about the moral quality of our interpersonal worlds as about inner worlds; moral-somatic worlds are inseparable from the experience of trauma. Trauma links inextricably the social and psychobiological processes that animate human experience. Experience, so conceived, can be (and really is) as readily dehumanized by social science perspectives that attend only to the social side of that dialectic as by health sciences ones that permit only biological explanations. Sufferers of social trauma can also actively participate in victimization, their own and others. It is understandable that health care institutions, to the extent that they must provide rapid and effective treatment, think of sufferers more as patients. A problem arises, however, when the medicalization of distress goes beyond the hospital wards and forms part of the standard public discourse on violence and its consequences. The idea of "victim" is also problematic, and shows that medicalization is not the only discourse on violence that creates difficulties. The cultural codes of our age appropriate the imagery of victimization to serve a variety of political purposes. "Victim" is a highly politicized and even commodified category. Victim has come to mean authorization for indemnification. We also listen to the voices of victims for their moral uses in the commercial culture. We are supposed to feel morally improved, even uplifted, having heard their cries and seen their anguish; we, in turn, at times appropriate their misery to authorize our own criticisms and demands. The cultural dynamics of witnessing have become ethically murky; witnessing sells TV programs! Victims have become cultural capital. Their outrage is compromised by commercial interests, so that indifference and complicity unmake moral responses, which must be one of the more appalling commercializations of human experience.[5]

Emphasis on the microcultural context of violence should assure that the complex ironies of atrocity and routinized oppression can be examined without disaffirming the human experiences at stake in trauma. The ethnography of political violence, for all its ethical ironies, is still at best an engagement that can describe a native place in which violence is distinctly human. Political trauma is interwoven with moral-somatic processes that bring social memory into the body and that project the individuality of persons into social space. Thereby, context and event, process and person are inseparable. That space of social experience in which violence is a way of living (in Wittgenstein's terminology, a form of life) needs to become the focus of research, if ethnography is to advance understanding of the actualizing of violence.

The ethnographic gaze must attend also to the appropriation of images of violence. Those images are powerful sources of motivation for reprisal, revenge, and recurrent cycles of assault. They are also potential means for local prevention. The images tell us about the dynamics of both macro and micro political processes. Narratives and pictures of torture are appropriated by those in national and international agencies who are engaged in managing the outcomes, and political capital, of collective violence. Here the labels applied to the process, as well as to the participants and the outcomes, carry with them entire technologies and rationalities of which medicalization is only one (albeit a major) example. The professional appropriation of violence in narratives and images of terror extends to the various academic constructions, none of which can any longer be permitted to pose as "objective" and lacking self-interest.

The objectification of political violence as a "problem" for national and international security, as a social "crisis," or as a public health and mental health "epidemic" is also amenable to ethnography, this time focused on the appropriations (and appropriators) of violence. How an identified public problem gets created out of the complex uncertainty of everyday life is the story of culture in the making, the *realization*, or emergence, of cultural patterns out of the everyday processes of social interaction and interpersonal experience that include class, ethnic, factional, and gender differences. The story of how our local or wider worlds come to be is the story of those who possess the authority to legitimize certain narratives while silencing others. The problem of violence and its traumatic effects must be articulated in this broader context if we are to identify the major junctions for intervention (compare Gusfield 1981).

Our argument is not that clinical and public health formulations of trauma do not have appropriate uses. They do. Nor do we think that witnessing misery and acting to assist sufferers is bad faith. It is not. Rather we seek to place clinical, public health, and social policy problem frameworks in a wider discourse on violence as a cultural problem, one in which, moreover, the analysts, the experts, and the observers participate. We all should, indeed we must, respond to trauma as a form of social suffering. Yet we must all also be aware of the way our language, actions, and professional competences are caught up in cultural and political forces that contribute to the very problem we seek to remedy. So powerful are the technologies and accompanying technical rationalities that we use to diagnose, treat, and evaluate mental health problems that we must be sure that sufferers of violence are not exposed to potentially disruptive or unnecessary interventions. The first goal of cultural analysis should be to assess how the dominant policy frameworks contribute to the burden and abridge the prospects for repair. That is in large part a question of how those frameworks themselves are taken up in much larger cultural-political economic processes that make up our world.

Where a diagnosis of PTSD can assist in directing humane, effective care to people with real needs, it should be applied. Where it can guide preventive programs, it also deserves to be tried. But we should also keep in mind that any articulation of "trauma" effects a specific and limited social-political reality. Given the tenuous balance between therapy and violence, the diagnosis of PTSD should be avoided whenever it is an encumbrance or irrelevance. That same reflexive approach should extend to concerns for the way those who have undergone political violence are at times labeled as "victims," an oversimplification. That category will be valid for many, perhaps most, but not for all; it needs to be understood, moreover, as an active category of social agency in a moral and political process.[6]

PART THREE

The State of Medical Anthropology

9

The New Wave
of Ethnographies in
Medical Anthropology

In the past few years more ethnographies on subjects squarely in medical anthropology, or relevant to it, have been published as book-length volumes than in the previous four decades. That many of these books are also written at a high level of scholarship and are attracting attention from many outside the field makes their significance all the greater. Whereas articles in academic journals and book chapters once were the chief means of publishing academic work, even as recently as five years ago, now book-length monographs are appearing so frequently that they are transforming the very way we think about medical anthropology as a scholarly field. Though impressive in sheer number, the appearance of a gathering wave of ethnographies in medical anthropology should not come as a surprise. The field has grown; scholars who have devoted their careers to it are publishing their magna opera; and the field has attracted excellent students, many of whom are now publishing revised versions of their dissertations at the very outset of their careers. Anthropologists from outside the subdiscipline have been drawn to its subject matter to a degree they could not have imagined in the days when medical anthropology was perceived by other social anthropologists as theory-averse. How could they not be attracted when so many of its topics—from the body-self as a site for contesting ethnic identity, through the human consequences of violence and forced displacement, and on to the project to develop technological control of the human genome—have come to rank among the most challenging intellectual and policy questions of

our era. And, of course, the presence of book series—especially the pro-
lific and long-running University of California Press series—has opened
a special space for publications by medical anthropologists.

Even as recently as the mid-1980s, it was far from clear that publications in medical anthropology would take this crucial turn. At that
time, there was substantial pressure for researchers to publish in a variety of types of academic journals. These included new journals in
medical anthropology which were actively competing for high-quality
articles; journals in general anthropology, where academic editors, sometimes grudgingly, were coming to recognize that medical anthropologists were engaging issues of theoretical importance to the discipline
as a whole; and, not least of all, journals in biomedicine, mental health,
and international public health which were "discovering," yet again,
the salience of anthropological contributions. Applied anthropologists
had long been effective at getting their research across in the format
of the short article. Biological anthropologists, doing what I imagine
now would be called biomedical anthropology, also have followed that
model. But social anthropologists have had a much harder time of it.
Not only did ethnographers write much longer articles—short ethnographic papers being something of an oxymoron—but even long articles could not easily encompass the ethnographer's theoretical excursions, detailed descriptions of context, and discursively interpretive
prose. The result was highly unsatisfactory.

Ethnography, like biography and social history, requires space, a lot
of it. The book-length monograph provides that, and more. It enables
the ethnographer to find an intellectual horizon that is appropriate to
the subject matter. It offers the possibility of engaging different scholarly literatures and of presenting research findings—masses of them—
by different means. In order to build the scaffolding of scholarly
materials that makes cultural analysis convincing and authorizes the
ethnographer to apply that analysis to different problems and special
themes, the author composes an iterative process that goes back and
forth across ethnographic context, social theory, and key issues. The
sedulous reader of ethnography, being a devotee of detail, expects
to become absorbed in the intricacies of thought and experience that
represent an alternative way of being-in-the-world. While coherence
and analytic power count for something, so too do reflexive voice,
style, thickly described ethnographic materials, and *aperçus* that illuminate a local world, often in order to challenge a putative universal or

to critique the world of the ethnographer, a not-so-silent subject in many ethnographic monographs.

If all of this sounds old-fashioned, that is one of the arresting charms of ethnography. In place of our era's egregious emphasis on minimalist interpretation, ethnography develops, meanders, even circles back; it goes on and on. Ethnography's very format attests to its marginality to the rest of social science. From the perspective of biomedical science, it is, together with historical narrative and philosophical argument, part of the humanities, not the sciences. And yet physicians and many other professionals are often attracted to ethnographies for that very reason; these genres greatly widen the scope of intellectual possibilities and they put one in touch with different modes of experience, different life worlds, including novel ways of regarding one's own experience.

In keeping with the idea of the margin that I used in the Introduction to describe my own work, I would press this image further as a means of understanding why ethnographies are effective, at least in the realm of health and healing. The ethnography book challenges the basic conventions; it offers an alternative construction in an alternative style. It creates another world and compares it with the taken-for-granted one in order to obtain critical leverage. And it does so with thoroughness. That it is principally (though by no means entirely) qualitative sets it off from almost all other methods used in the health sciences. It belongs to the no-man's-land that runs between science and the humanities. Because it does not fit with the other forms of knowledge construction in the health field, ethnography has been well positioned to represent other things that are also at the margin of medicine, such as lay perspectives, the experiential aspects of illness and care, alternative medicine, the local community context of policy and practice, deviance, and the myriad problems, ordinary and extreme, that are constantly passing into and out of biomedical authorization. The marginality of ethnography has made it a more appropriate means of representing pluralism, reflexivity, and uncertainty, and of drawing upon those aspects of health and suffering to resist the positivism, the reductionism, and the naturalism that biomedicine and, regrettably, the wider society privilege. That ethnography also comes in a book-length form with the proviso that talking and living with people are crucial to research practice and that theories and facts are inseparably linked in a constructionist circle is an irony still so challenging to the way the health professions do their everyday business that it concentrates the power (to threaten and to liberate) of the medical margin.

Because dozens of first-rate ethnographies have been published in recent years, medical anthropologists need to come to terms with the possibilities, and of course the limitations, of ethnography as a genre. What sorts of things does it do best? What sorts of things does it not do well? In this chapter, I review examples from the new wave of medical ethnographies in order to evaluate their contribution. I spent several years reading these works, teaching a number of them in a graduate seminar, and sifting the still larger pile of monographs for appropriate examples. I came away from these exercises with a new appreciation of the extraordinary intellectual energy in medical anthropology today. This essay will not provide a comprehensive sense of the field. Rather it represents how I see medical anthropology through the lens of ethnography.

I think these books open to readers what is most interesting in this field in this era. On the whole, their effects have been remarkably positive. That there is also reason for disquiet, or at least uncertainty, is a sign that these works are effective enough at carving the imagery of the field to project even those surfaces that represent ethnography's and medical anthropology's limits.

While most of the books are written by medical anthropologists on subjects that are central to the field, a few are included for other reasons. The overlap between psychological anthropology and medical anthropology can be (and often has been) considerable. I include several works that belong as much to the former as to the latter. I also include ethnographic works in general anthropology because the theme of suffering they address is so relevant that whatever their authors intended, they have taken on a life of their own in medical anthropology.

These volumes address long-standing questions in the intersection of society and health, some already prefigured in preceding sections of this book, as well as new subjects that I take to be of related interest. Thus, I come back to the culture of biomedicine through studies of menopause, aging, and traumatic memories as well as through the counterexamples offered by Asian medical systems. And I press further the discussion of sociosomatic relationships in normality and pathology with the assistance of ethnomusicological, performance-based, and aesthetic studies. The strategy of reviewing the work of others greatly extends my own competences and materials, making it possible to return to old subjects via new routes, and to explore new ones in old ways. This chapter can be read, then, in light of what has gone before, as a colloquy between the work of others and my own work in medical anthropology.

By ending with a review of books, I also seek to promote a different kind of *reading* of ethnographies than is usually published. As I complained in the Introduction, too often in reviews of the scholarly literature, treatment of even a major book is published as a one- or two-sentence summary that ends up caricaturing a work that is complex and multifaceted. Because cultural interpretation is itself so concerned with the thick description of difference, this treatment is at the very least a dismaying irony. To overcome this practice, a review of books that devotes time and space to the authors' words and their effect upon a long-term student of the subject seems the right thing to do. It also allows me to emphasize the process of partaking in scholarly engagement with the literature as the crucial intersubjective practice of participation in the building of an academic field.

Medicine as a Social Idiom

Libbet Crandon-Malamud (1991) organizes a useful ethnography of medical pluralism in the highlands of Bolivia around a single idea that seems so implausibly simple at first, the reader is alarmed that it may not be adequate to support an entire volume. Her research takes origin from Paul Unschuld's (1975) radical suggestion that we turn the professional commonsense idea that medicine is an end in itself on its head, and in its place come to view medicine as a primary resource—like capital—which because it is fungible can be used to acquire (or create) a secondary resource that is even more significant in local social life. When medical pluralism exists, explains the author, medicine can be used to obtain secondary resources such as social relations and material goods that can support social mobility. Even in talking about medicine, villagers are redefining and negotiating social identities. Boundaries in the village she studies are relatively fluid across social status and even ethnic identity. Ultimately, the force responsible for maintaining and altering their permeability is the political economy. Medicine is only one of the pores in the boundary layer through which social entrances and exits are arranged. Thus, even people's evaluation of medical efficacy, surely much to the consternation of health professionals and health services researchers, is subordinated to other more central processes in the social context. Doctors may think patients are visiting their clinics because of symptoms and treatments, but in fact the visits are bound up in a much larger and more fundamental social process.

The reader's initial skepticism over the simplicity of the central idea is only deepened by the author's tendency to treat the concept rather woodenly and to repeat it, as if she herself harbored some unexpressed doubt for which the repetition of this explanation provided reassurance. In fact, the analysis is impressive and would be even more convincing if the author let the ethnography roam outside the tight confines of the analytic framework. The Bolivian highlands are populated by three overlapping groups: mestizos, formerly of high status and now, four decades after the revolution, well on the way toward impoverishment; Aymara Indians, many of whom are peasants; and Methodist Aymara, a relatively recent urban group who are engaged in commerce and rising in status. Between these groups ethnicity masks class relations and becomes a mode for negotiating the meaning of social identity. Local medical traditions are open to this social mosaic. Choice of a healer can be analyzed in extra-medical terms of solidarity, resistance, accommodation, empowerment; so can clinical work: "etiology is a metaphor of history, and use of . . . metaphors in medical dialogue is an attempt to change history" (p. 46).

Four key metaphors of social life are deployed in diagnosis and treatment: insatiable hunger, vulnerability of subordination, victimization, exploitation. These metaphors participate as social idioms in the expression and working out of mestizo and Aymara and Methodist antagonisms. To the outsider's surprise, medicine is the most effective method for conversion from one social position to another.

Crandon-Malamud interprets the etiological agency of *kharisiri*—a phantom who magically removes the fat from the kidneys of victims. In an earlier historical period, the phantom was popularly held to be a Franciscan priest who gave the fat to the bishop to make holy oil. By 1977, the phantom was believed to be a mestizo who traded in human fat. Thus, the insatiable hunger of the supernaturals for human beings represents the changing history of Bolivian elites, all of whom, it seems, exploit Aymara Indians.

Through medical dialogue and curative strategies, they [the Indians] make alliances, disassociate themselves from others, exchange resources, and try to forge new identities that will open opportunities and improve their lives under

conditions of extreme and seemingly unrelenting national economic contrac-
tion, regional peripheralization, and local marginalization. (p. 138)

It may sound repetitive, but the argument—a more complex one than
was originally articulated—is effectively put.

Now the author turns to ethnographic case illustrations to convince
us that her conclusions are founded in the vicissitudes of the local
world. The narratives are well turned out, the writing is fluid, and the
detail exquisitely concrete, yet the presence of a nearly omniscient in-
terpreter who has control over all sides in the medical encounters is
disconcerting, as is the deterministic analytic line that leaves little room
for novelty and uncertainty (p. 146).

For example, how can Crandon-Malamud be so sure that

the social order to which Gladis [a mestizo] belonged was impotent in a universe that had become, for her cultural group, chaotic and uncontrollable, and
for which one could not prepare. Her illness and death may be interpreted as
having resulted from the strain of her inability to make order of and control
events in that universe. (p. 188)

Does the ethnographer, in the face of such chaos, feel the need to provide the missing order? What follows are subtle case descriptions, at
times illustrated with great sensitivity with drawings by the author's
daughter, an impressive artist, who seems to want to evoke the forlorn
silence of a more ambiguous and perhaps even more dangerous setting than that which her mother presents. Although the author seems
preoccupied with making her case airtight, it is the large space of the
ethnography itself which allows readers to become so involved in the
indigenous world in the first place that they can begin to question
the strict limits the author places on the interpretation.

Wisely, the author comments: "Diagnosis is subjected to dialogue;
dialogue opens diagnosis to debate" (p. 204). We in fact do come to
appreciate that "people compete and negotiate to monopolize the control of the consumption of opinions and thereby gain some power,
which can later be used to get something else: resources, legal protection, loyalty, or security" (p. 207). Yet, the reader might well ask, don't
highland Bolivians ever go to practitioners because they want to feel
better or receive medications? Don't they ever go just because they
are faced with troubling symptoms, which must at least sometimes be
symbols that stand for themselves (Wagner 1986)? Or because whatever medical practice they choose at the end-stage of sickness is indeed

the ultimate resource? Readers who can put aside such questions will find important conclusions.

Without doubt, the author convinces us that at least for certain residents of the village she calls Kachitu, the evaluation of medical efficacy takes place neither in the idiom of symptoms nor in that of practitioners' interventions, but rather "within the context of interests in such secondary resources." *From the Fat of Our Souls* may be one of the clearest demonstrations of this *cultural construction of efficacy,* one of the most difficult issues in all of medical anthropology. Land, agricultural goods, jobs, privileges, power—any or all may be implicated in the question of efficacy. Making this point with impressively concrete detail is a major achievement, and one that could not have been accomplished without the scope and the depth of the book-length ethnography.

And this is the note the volume could and should have ended on. Instead, we get a final, clearly unintended, shock. Notwithstanding an earlier critique of positivism, we come across page after page of tables in appendixes, which register the quantitative data from a survey that is too small and unsystematic to be statistically significant, but is filled with a simplistic categorization of illness beliefs: "magical," "natural," "psychological" (none of which is central to the core theme of the book). Could it be that in spite of the frequent repetition of the interpretive model, the author still feels the need to convince us that the conclusion is really valid because the survey demonstrates consensus on the folk categories? If so, the demonstration is both unnecessary and beside the point of the ethnography. Thus, this otherwise useful ethnography ends with a final, surprising irony. This is after all a modernist volume filled with a deft certainty about what is at stake and a dogged determination to come to one overwhelming point; it eschews the uncertainty and paradox of postmodernist prose. And yet, the irony of the ending lends itself to a postmodernist critique of the uses of ethnography. Crandon-Malamud needs to make the point that medicine is taken up in much broader social processes, certain of which have almost nothing to do with sickness and therapeutic remedies per se, and which cannot therefore be understood if the focus on illness and care is too narrowly that of the medical professionals. In so doing, she tells us (inadvertently) about the ethnographer's need to appropriate medical themes for the purposes of social theory, so that we come to see that the social anthropologist too is taken up in much broader social processes, certain of which may seem to have little to do with her subject matter, but which become consequential. If Crandon-Malamud had made the suffering of the leading characters in her story as various and plural as she makes their health care system, whose description is indeed impressive, doubtless the theory would have been less tightly integrated, but the ethnography would have been more compelling.*

A rather different approach to medicine as social idiom is taken by Christopher Taylor (1992), whose *Milk, Honey, and Money: Changing Concepts in Rwandan Healing* takes its intellectual origins from the French ethnographer and sometime medical anthropologist Marc Augé's distinction between three "socio-logics" in ethnographic analysis and from gift exchange theory. Augé's Gallic tripartite organization of social analysis includes (1) the logic of difference in symbolic phenomena, (2) the logic of reference that relates symbolic difference and difference in the social order, and (3) the logic of events, which relates the first two levels of analysis to their historical genealogy. As we shall see, Taylor applies this framework both to Rwandan society's culture of healing and to specific healing "events." These logics of the social world also enable Taylor to draw upon the society-wide transformation of the socio-logic of the gift to the socio-logic of the commodity as a basic turn in the cultural history of healing in Rwanda. Subsequent tragic events in Rwanda—genocide, massive displacement of populations, starvation, deadly epidemics—make the reader wonder if Taylor's peaceful account could possibly be of the same Hutu and Tutsi groups. The fate of his ethnography will be forever affected by this immense, historical transformation, almost as if his book belonged to the prehistory of the Rwanda we have all come to see on the nightly news, an archetype of the inhumanity and death of a broken society. We need to put aside these images to engage this ethnography, but at last we must return to the juxtaposition to bring Taylor's work into historical perspective.

The term for "man" in Kinyarwanda, *umugabo,* derives from *kugabo,* "to give." Thus, the idea of gift giving is built into the cultural category of the person, both as generosity in personality and as reciprocation in social relationships. The Rwandan gift-exchange relationship also "embodies spiritual power" (p. 5). Taylor follows Marcel

---

*I was saddened to learn from the *Anthropology Newsletter* of April 1995 of Libbet Crandon-Malamud's death from cancer at age 47 earlier in the year.

Mauss's classical formulation fairly closely. Similarly, he stays close to Chris Gregory's (1982) reformulation of the Marxist notion of the commodity as an alienable object from whose exchange no social bond necessarily results and which "appears" to operate independent of human agency, lending commodities their "animate capacity" to be "fetishized."

In Rwanda, under the system *ubuhake* (abolished in 1954), a Tutsi cattle patron gave a cow to a Hutu client in exchange for prestations of beer, agricultural goods, labor, and loyalty in warfare. In turn, the patron protected his clients from the exactions of other Tutsi. The client possessed usufruct rights to the cow's milk and in its male offspring, but female offspring had to be returned to the patron. This feudal political scaffolding extended from Tutsi king to vassals and down to Hutu cultivators.

Taylor uses these concepts as well as those of reciprocity and redistribution to understand the transformation of socio-logics in Rwandan society from personal domination in the regime of gift exchange to abstracted domination in the regime of commodity exchange.

A crucial part of socio-logic for Rwandan healing is the dialectic between flow and blockage, which carries the exchange logic from the social body into the physical body. Fluids flow or are blocked. *Isibo*, flow as a noun, connotes the flowing of cattle and warriors and the flow of force or élan; the verb *gusibo*, from which it derives, means "to plug, fill up, obstruct." The one implies the other. Flow is openness, continuity, but it also implies blockage, interruption, closure. In this symbolic system, a key role is played by liquid gifts: honey, beer, porridge, but also milk, semen, blood, and even rain.

Pathology is depicted as blocked flow or hemorrhagic flow. Witches and poisoners, agents of pathology, block flow. "Illness is often seen as a perturbation in the movement of one or more bodily humors, a movement whose cause comes from outside the self—from witches and spirits" (p. 21). The same symbolic dialectic carries over into Rwandan political discourse and into the spiritual sphere in the relationship of human, bovine, and divine fertility and well-being. Power is flow, of rain, rivers, blood, semen, milk, honey, and so on. Problems arise when flow is arrested. Conflict in "social life perennially disrupts orderly fluid movement" (p. 75).

Healing techniques work within the socio-logic of removing blockage and enabling flow. Through extended case studies, Taylor shows how the female body comes to be viewed both as the site of blockage in gift exchange and under the socio-logic of commodity exchange. Yet, in the latter the problem and the treatment turn more on issues of individual fulfillment than on those of social reproduction of the kinship group. Thus, the changing political economy works through the symbolic system to alter the understanding of pathology and treatment outcome. Money is not like other things that flow; it changes the very nature of the social process.

> Confession has become institutionalized as a central activity and as a "core symbol" in modern rituals of political repression. . . . Confession has also thrived as a therapeutic technique. . . . But confession could also be viewed . . . as the manifestation in the therapeutic and religious domain of a society's transition to capitalism, for part of this transition involves a "monadization" of the person (Augé 1975). (Taylor 1992: 197)

Taylor's analysis is enriched by his readings in Francophone medical anthropology, especially the work of Augé, Françoise Heritier, and René Devisch. Across the three socio-logics, Taylor shows that the flow/blockage symbolic idiom creates a homology between cosmological, ecological, political, and medical concepts and practices that together form a sociosomatic reticulum for society-mind-body interactions. Whereas the homology is impressively elaborated under the gift exchange regimen, when Taylor attempts to deploy it to criticize capitalist practices, the dualistic analysis gets exaggerated.

"If Rwandan gift logic is characterized by the flow/blockage dialectic, capitalist culture appears to reverse the relation between flow and blockage. Blockage (project making, accumulation) becomes positively valued" (p. 203). It is simply not convincing either as conclusion or methodology when Taylor states that internal causation is to the body as supply/demand is to the market, or that autonomy is to the person as the market is to society (p. 212).

But in spite of somewhat overdoing the rhetoric, Taylor's contribution is to show that symbolic analysis can be used to illuminate ordered historical transformation in a healing system and in its relationship to politics and the economy, at least prior to 1994, a year of disorder and horror. The ethnographic stories he tells of therapy sessions are effective in illustrating the symbolic terms of his analytic model. Taylor shows himself to be the intellectual heir of Victor Turner (1967), whose depiction of an entire symbolic system of healing is perhaps still the most formidable undertaking in this tradition of anthropological analysis. Moreover, unlike Lévi-Strauss, Taylor does not misapply psychoanalysis as a quick and dirty fix, deus ex machina, to shore up the account of how symbols heal. Rather he stays with the micropolitics of relationships, where his data are grounded and his analysis is most convincing, leaving psychosomatic issues for other researchers who possess ethnographic materials that are more appropriate for such interpretation.

Taylor's volume also is rich enough in detail to let the reader see the limits of this revivification of the program of symbolic analysis. Current anthropological sensibility makes it increasingly difficult to support the idea of shared symbolic systems whose logic is so tight and extensions are so visible that they can be traced directly from cosmology through politics to therapeutic practices. In order to maintain this position, the complexities of everyday social life, the uncertainties basic to social transactions, and the openness of politics and history to novel developments have to be discounted, while the unity of symbolic meanings has to be overvalued and a blind eye turned to instances where the system breaks down, simply does not apply, or is contested from within. Taylor's work, like Crandon-Malamud's, is backward-looking toward a time of greater confidence in social determinacy and in the uniformity of social systems. At the end the reader is left with an analytic strategy that claims too much, and that is unable to encompass the serious complexities in how social change relates to health and health care. Nonetheless, in pressing the symbolic program to its limits, Taylor shows us just what that approach can and cannot accomplish in medical anthropology.

More troubling still is the dismaying juxtaposition between Taylor's Rwanda of the past and the nightmarish Rwanda of the present. The very word conjures imagery of extreme dislocation; the contemporary reader is mortified by an account of balance and stability. The interpretation of social change as the transformation of gifts into commodities and the relationship of blockage and flow is not likely to help much in making sense of the political catastrophe. That truly enormous human disaster has changed the very conditions of health and health care, as it has of so much else. It has likely also changed the relationships of Tutsi and Hutu for generations to come, making much of the cultural analysis obsolete, perhaps anachronistic. The horrors of 1994 also make writing about Rwanda a wholly different genre. Symbolic analysis clearly is not an adequate approach to the chaos of societal disintegration, where the cultural universe itself is either shattered or seemingly irrelevant. This suggests that perhaps Taylor's analysis also inverts the picture of earlier social upheavals in Rwanda by providing much more coherence than social experience is likely to have possessed.

One almost wants to say that after the Rwandan nightmare, modernist accounts of social order seem improbable at best and perhaps in future will be regarded as impossible. But this is unfair because it is ahistorical. Taylor wrote about, and in his own small way contributed to, the intellectual construction of an era in Rwanda that is gone, a world that no longer exists. The new era requires a theory of extreme upheaval, a semiotics of violent chaos, a phenomenology of desperate failure. While even those accounts will require cultural grounding and symbolic exegesis, their vector, we must assume, will be toward the ethnography of disordered states.

Medical Ethnography

Since W. H. R. Rivers, a psychiatrist, pioneered ethnographic fieldwork early in this century, a number of anthropologist-physicians have conducted ethnographies (e.g., Fabrega 1974; Field 1960; Kleinman 1980, 1986; Lewis 1975, 1980; Taussig 1980; and more recently Cohen 1992; Farmer 1992; Littlewood 1993, among others); yet, perhaps none, including Rivers, has come closer than Stephen Frankel (1986) to writing what I shall call a medical ethnography. A medical ethnography is a description of a society through a medical lens, a systematic focus on the health-relevant aspects of social life. Frankel, who earlier had practiced general medicine among the Huli of the Southern Highlands of Papua New Guinea, returned as a Cambridge-trained social anthropologist to write *The Huli Response to Illness*. His general description of the social context fairly quickly settles on diagnosis, illness experience, and treatment. Indeed, Frankel includes a survey of morbidity (pp. 60–72), even though he never departs from an ethnographic mode of writing. Yet, that mode of writing is as much medical (particularly British medical cadences resonate in the ear) as anthropological. The style is concise, direct, and crisply pragmatic, even when Frankel discusses Huli cosmology, social organization, or symbolic meanings of life and death and the spirits. That Frankel also includes ecology, the history of epidemics, and the Huli's conceptual underpinnings of ideas of risk and resilience fits in well with an effort to canvass all the dimensions of the Huli life world that are relevant to health.

The Huli cosmology contrasts rather fundamentally with the mainstream views of experts in social development and international health; it all but mocks the deep faith in secular progress:

The Huli preoccupations with entropy, with decreasing yields, with a recent upsurge of human and porcine disease and with increasing strife are expressed in the *dindi gamu* lore in terms of a predestined progression towards devastation that can only be averted by prescribed ritual acts. These afflictions that the Huli interpret as indicative of a fundamental deterioration in the ritual forces that maintain the natural and moral order can also be seen as the products of recent ecological changes that have affected horticulture and disease patterns. (p. 26)

Indeed, the Huli, not tongue-in-cheek but accurately, blame recent decline on the coming of Europeans. Over the past decades, social change has brought epidemics of venereal diseases and malaria, deterioration of the soil, and worsening of other ecological conditions.

As with many anthropological descriptions of New Guinea communities, Frankel emphasizes the ethos of individualism, person-based social networks, and tensions between the sexes. Fully one-third of marriages, for example, end in divorce. Every ethnographer eventually shows the colors of his "school." Frankel does not waste much time in getting down to classic interests of British social anthropology: Huli illness categories represent the social order, Frankel announces:

Diagnoses may be based upon breeches of norms, for example of hospitality, of sexual conduct or of religious observance. Such illnesses can thus become strategies of social control which in these instances could lead to generosity, sexual restraint or deference to a pastor respectively.

Just because the point has been so well established that it reads today like a cliché should not lessen its significance, as is the case with the news that the Huli practice prevention through protective rituals and regard health as a social as well as a physical state, a fragile quality to strive for. These are widely shared aspects of ethnomedicine that must be telling us about central facts in social responses to illness. Nonetheless, if this were all there was to the ethnography, the reader, dutifully educated, would find the book tedious. But beneath the cool prose and dour, even somber medical outlook the ethnographic gaze twinkles and occasionally sparkles; Frankel has much more to tell us. Some authors need only a few sentences to warm up, others require a few pages. Frankel finally gets to the subjects that excite him on page 55. Interestingly, the first of these is literally a subject on the surface, not in the depths, which brings out his multiple skills as a medical ethnographer: "The skin, as the visible aspect of the body, mediates between an individual's inner state and others' appreciation of him" (p. 55). The quality of the inner state is visible in the appearance of the skin. The shine or luster of the skin forms a semantic network with social effectiveness, good health, and resilience. "Bad skin," in contrast, is a physical-moral state of "dirt," "defect," "decrepitude" in the body and in social states. Health is personified as the beautiful skin, vigor, and striving of young men; ill health is incarnated as a "shabby," sickly, impoverished "recluse." The description reminded me of Kenneth Read's (1955) writing on the moral-somatic status of "skin" for the Gahuku-Gama, elsewhere in Papua New Guinea (see chap. 3 in this volume). That the Huli suffer greatly from skin diseases overcodes this category.

For Frankel particularly noteworthy is the association between illness and death, which is not at all inappropriate in a setting of high child mortality where adults too may succumb quickly to a serious infectious disease. "Some who feel ill from any cause, when asked how they are, may simply reply, '*homedo*' (I am dying)." For the Huli, "dying is a vulnerable condition in continuity with demise, from which recovery is likely. *Homayo*, he died, can be said of a corpse, or of someone who was very ill but is now all right" (p. 59).

The Huli must now be counted among that vast cross-continental arc of peoples for whom a concept of vitality or life force is central. *Bu*, life force, refers to "breath," the pulsation of the heart, and also to "the drive which activates all other functions" (p. 83). In serious illness, *bu* is "smothered."

"He is dead. There is only *bu* left now . . ." The distinction here is similar to the one that we make between cerebral and cardiac death. Such a person is regarded as dead despite their continuing breathing and heartbeat. (p. 83)

So much for the idea that the debate on "brain death" is an issue unique to technologically advanced societies.

It is also impressive that even within this medicocentric study, Frankel finds that the social processes of litigation and retribution and compensation are more important than medical treatment for the members of Huli society. "The presence of illness may constitute evidence of a legitimate grievance, and the resolution of the conflict represents treatment of the illness" (p. 134). Huli women, we are told, "use" illness strategically to draw attention to grievance and to resolve its sources—a finding that again comes close to a universal in medical anthropology, though it can be generalized to other categories of the powerless.

In the final pages, Frankel shows how the social idiom of balance, reciprocity, and compensation works its way through the actions of the patient's therapy management group, is involved in responses to violence, and connects a view of the fragility of society to a view of the impermanence of personal health and well-being. Frankel ends on a grand theme common to studies in medical anthropology, as we have already seen in Crandon-Malamud's book, namely, medical pluralism. Diversity, he shows, is of long standing in Huli society, where the indigenous medical culture has plural aspects and alternatives.

Here, then, in the space of a thin monograph, with much insight into social process but limited elaboration of theoretical models, many of the traditional concerns in medical anthropology are addressed. Ethnography is appropriated to the interests of medicine, and narratives and numbers are combined in the text. This is best seen in the survey of morbidity, which shifts the perspective and the language of description from anthropology to clinical epidemiology. Viewed from the vantage of the 1990s, Frankel's work seems to harken back to an earlier era, much as Taylor's and Crandon-Malamud's do, but for a different reason. The alignment of subject matter is overbalanced toward traditional public health and clinical concerns. The appropriate contrast is with a more recent ethnography by the physician-anthropologist Paul Farmer.

Farmer's *AIDS and Accusation: Haiti and the Geography of Blame* (1992) is a large-scale effort to combine history, epidemiology, and social experience within a thick description of suffering in rural Haiti. It largely succeeds. Farmer's objective is to narrate the meanings of the AIDS epidemic in Haiti against a daunting set of backdrops: the depressing cycles of Haitian history, the equally depressing history of the AIDS epidemic, the epidemiology of AIDS in Haiti, and the local experiences of Haitians in the impoverished village of "water refugees," Do Kay, where he has conducted both field research and medical assistance projects. The "geography of blame" adds an additional backdrop: the international relations of Haiti with the United States and with the international political economic order. Like Frankel, Farmer moves fluidly between ethnography and clinical epidemiology, but he also is just as deft in crossing the boundaries with history and political economy.

AIDS, Farmer makes chillingly clear, was "the last thing" for the people of Do Kay. Forced out of their ancestral homes when their valley was flooded for a hydroelectric development project that provided them neither water nor electricity, villagers have been able to barely survive in a setting of great privation. The HIV infection for many has intensified that world of poverty into an ethos of desperation. Farmer's ethnography of suffering insists that to understand the meaning of AIDS, the ethnographer needs to continually relate the long cycle of political economic oppression with the short cycle of illness.

In the Kay region, as elsewhere in rural Haiti, suffering is indeed an expected condition. It may well be true that "we're always sick around here," as several villagers stated, and familiarity with serious illness, especially tuberculosis, certainly conditioned the response of the villagers to a previously unknown sickness. Haitian structures of feeling about suffering, in which are embedded a deep respect for the role of human agency in human affliction, were equally formative to the nascent model of *sida* [AIDS]. Serious illness is as often the result of injustice or malice as it is of "accident" or "fate." (p. 47)

What is at stake for the villagers? Farmer indicates that this is a complex issue that touches on the interpenetration of moral and religious experience with intergenerational poverty and political oppression. When asked "How are you?" the villagers of Do Kay answer, "I'm fighting with life." Farmer does not present a picture of passive victims. Rather his account is about struggling, coping, resisting, and the complex mix of deeply human practices that make both rational choice theory and vulgar Marxist melodramas of the socially determined lives of the oppressed seem serious distortions. By the late 1980s, Haitian peasants were "intentionally politicizing their discourse" (p. 58). Farmer argues that this reorganization in the uses of narratives "revolved around *questions of agency in suffering.*"

Is it the infertility of the soil, or the heartless machinations of the urban bourgeoisie that are invoked in discussions of poverty? Is infant diarrhea caused by microbes, or by microbes caused by dirty water, which in turn is caused by an irresponsible government? Is *sida* caused by sorcery, or by the bitterness that drives the poor to "send illness" on one another? The illness narratives collected in Do Kay posit several different kinds of cause. And underlying these is a series of oppositions: personal/impersonal, just/unjust, invented/unmerited, necessary/unavoidable, endurable/unendurable, inside/ outside, and others not yet uncovered. Equally important categories—and somewhat different from that of cause—are local undertakings of recrimination and appeal and the assignment of blame. (p. 58)

Farmer transits from the large picture to the village and then again to the backdrop through three chapters that each present the illness narratives of a different *sida* sufferer. These are examples of what might be called, in line with Farmer's dual role as ethnographer and clinician, witnessing individual suffering in a space of social suffering. Indeed, Farmer's skill is to make the transition between macrosocietal and microvillage levels of suffering fluid and compelling. Dieudonne, one of the subjects of these chapters, observes: "*sida* is a jealousy sickness" (p. 106). He goes on, "What I see is that poor people catch it more easily. They say the rich get *sida*; I don't see that. But what I do see is that one poor person sends it to another poor person. It's like the army: brothers shooting brothers. The little soldier (*ti solda*) is really one of us, one of the people. But he is made to do the bidding of the State, and so shoots his own brother when they yell 'Fire!' Perhaps they are at last coming to understand this."

Farmer tells the shameful story of the erroneous yet disastrous blame placed on Haiti early in the epidemic as its source. This story also played down the contribution to dissemination of this deadly sexually transmitted disease by gay men from North America who frequented Haiti for sex tourism. Farmer also narrates the equally sad story of the way WHO and CDC models of AIDS at first obscured the chief current form of transmission of HIV in Haiti, heterosexual sex, most efficiently from male to female. Both stories are about the larger economic, political, and historical sources of vulnerability in the West Atlantic system.

"Turning and turning in the widening gyre," Farmer analyzes AIDS and sorcery, AIDS and racism, and AIDS and empire (the Western Atlantic system). In each domain, he shows that the established center does not hold; things as they are—as they are usually presented in culturally authorized discourses, medical and popular, that is—do fall apart. There are really two epidemics: AIDS and blame. The latter, concerned with sorcery, AIDS-related discrimination, and conspiracy theories, arises as "one social group attributes unsavory motives to another" (p. 245). These epidemics are also heterogeneous with different dynamics and effects. Farmer sketches those effects as they devastate lives. The anthropology of suffering, he concludes, is an amalgam of the historical, political, economic, and cultural sources and consequences of affliction: overlapping circles that can arrest one at a specific point but need to be visualized as an intersecting whole. Farmer succeeds better than any other author of a medical ethnography at illustrating this canonical conception in the discipline.

It is a sign of cumulative strength shared among the younger generation of ethnographers that Farmer is not hampered by factional differences over "biomedical" and "critical" anthropology labels, but freely passes between questions in virology and political history. The accessibility of his writing to a wider audience in the social *and* health sciences also, it is to be hoped, is a sign of the intentions of the new cohort of physician-anthropologists. This accessibility is gained at a cost, however; a cost that that cohort should consider. Farmer's engagement with social theory is less extensive than it could have been, and the historical critique, written with such obvious passion, is less nuanced than the past—so uncertain when it is lived, so clear when it is "history"—deserves. Haiti, to be sure, is a grossly flagrant case of imperialism, racism, and not-so-benign neglect. And yet as Farmer's three illness narratives so poignantly show, the depiction of human complexity can only enrich our appreciation of the social processes at work in the systemization of suffering.

Yet another strategy for conducting a medical ethnography is to write from within another cultural form of medicine, and to do so by explicitly eschewing comparison with biomedicine. Judith Farquhar's *Knowing Practice: The Clinical Encounter of Chinese Medicine* (1994) is a strong version of such a strategy. Her account results from study of the practice of traditional Chinese medicine (TCM) in the Guangzhou College of TCM in China.

Farquhar seeks to get at indigenous clinical priorities in medical work (p. 2; what I have elsewhere called "clinical reality," Kleinman 1980:120, 132). "In close relation to this everyday practical form, the collective accumulation of expertise through scholarship, teaching, and healing generates doctors as embodiment of virtuosity, a form of experience that links practice to history and practitioners to knowledge" (p. 2). The object of enquiry is *kanbing,* "looking at the illness," which doctor and patient do together in a clinical encounter in which "the doctor does not have the power to reject any sign reported by the patient; patients . . . retain a sense of being the experts, the authority of last resort, on their own illness."

Dissecting the cultural practice of *kanbing* leads Farquhar to center

her ethnography on the indigenous model of practice from classification to prescription. Although she often buttresses her interpretation
with information from observations of clinical practice, most of her
scholarly material is textbook descriptions written by and for practitioners. Rather than emphasize the classics, however, Farquhar works
with recent publications from the Guangzhou College of TCM and
from other traditional medical schools in China. A cornerstone of
her analysis is her description of *bianzheng lunzhi*—the practical rationality guiding differentiation of symptoms/signs into a syndrome and
determination of therapy. Entire chapters are devoted to the diverse
components of the diagnostic process, including: *ba gang* (the eight
rubrics—cold/hot, interior/exterior, depletion/repletion, yin/yang),
bingyin (illness factors), *zangfu* (visceral systems of function), *wei qi
ying xue* (the Warm Illness school's four-sector theory), *liu jing* (the
Cold Damage school's six warps). For illustration, the author returns
from time to time to three paradigmatic textbook cases that she discusses from these differing angles, but she also draws upon much direct quotation from published texts.

It is simply not feasible in a short space to recreate the elaborately
detailed evocation of practice that this ethnographer-sinologist describes. There is nothing comparable in the English language literature. For each of the elements in the diagnostic process, for example,
she offers a precise cultural interpretation of its expedience. Thus, for
chuanhua (transmission and transformation of pathology through the
four temporal sectors of a syndrome's defensive *qi,* active *qi,* constructive *qi,* and blood sector), she takes the reader on a journey through
the "complex entailments . . . space, time, and quality" in which theory and practical action are "inseparable" (p. 118). Or to take an example from the therapeutic aim of the indigenous model of clinical
practice, treatment methods (*zhifa*) are presented not simply as therapies—herbal remedies, acupuncture, breathing exercises—but much
more tellingly as an integrated process of knowing and acting:

A centering process that acts by drawing in deviations and filling up gaps in a
continuing flow of "physiological activity" (*shengli hudong*) appears here as
the pattern of medical action. The course of medical intervention is not determined with reference to any predetermined goal; rather, the physician must
maintain a sense of the location of the center at each stage, evening out the
excesses and deficiencies that constitute deviations from this shifting middle
path. Chinese medical action is thus intrinsically temporal and activist; intervention is required in every pathological yinyang situation as the illness develops, and the state of play must often be reevaluated in the expectation that

new excesses and deficiencies will develop. Treatment seldom departs far from concrete illnesses, which are not helpfully thought of as if they were tokens of a type. For Chinese medicine, contingency is not what threatens a course of treatment but rather what shapes it. (pp. 167–168)

Thus, *linghuo*, connoting both efficacy and virtuosity, flexibility and sensitivity, is presented as a form of clinical judgment in action that relates the collective experience of the medical archive and the personal experience of the practitioner in the process of healing (p. 168). Is it any wonder then that Farquhar never saw "two experienced doctors mobilize precisely the same protocol in their clinical work" (pp. 133–134)? Rather than nature, truth, or law, "the social values of effectiveness, responsiveness, and service and the personal values of virtuosity and connoisseurship—goodness in several senses of the word—dominate Chinese medical texts" (p. 174).

Thus, a drug prescription treats kinds of activity that are in this situation pathological (excessive or inadequate) with opposite kinds of activity that can be wholesome in the situation by virtue, not of their essence, but of their opposition. The functional efficacies of the materia medica are literally incorporated in the person of the sufferer, cooling her Heat, replenishing her depletion. (p. 203)

Given the Chinese perspective that the world undergoes relentless transformation, that all things are fluid, it is not at all surprising that TCM's therapeutic orientation is the management of recovery—a continuous constraining of change toward healthier directions. Drawing upon "a coordinated use of 'logically inconsistent' methods to produce a nuanced specificity" (p. 222), Farquhar's analysis of therapeutics is as detailed as her analysis of syndromal classification. Her gaze never leaves the core clinical process. This is very much an internalist account. Though much of what Farquhar covers could be understood as relating to anthropological debates about technical and performative rationality, the culture of institutions and professions, "biopower," and long-standing medical anthropological comparisons of Asian and Western "science," she maintains a strict discipline, avoiding these larger issues, with only a few exceptions, including an unfortunate defense of falsifiability and a useful examination of the relationship of knowledge to social life. Otherwise, the ethnography sticks to *kanbing*.

Because of the fidelity to the description of the clinical encounter, it is astonishing that we learn so little about particular practitioners, particular patients, or particular encounters. Rather her concern is the ideal-typical. Thus, the cases that get her attention are from text-books, not from her participant observation. The diversity and com-plexity of actual clinical encounters is not her interest. Nor is she espe-cially interested in the influence on practice of changing institutional, political, or economic realities, which in the case of Guangzhou has been extensive in recent years. There are points in the analysis when one feels almost suspended in a timeless ethnographic present reach-ing back into the ancient formative period of Chinese medical texts. Yet even those classic texts are not what Farquhar's ethnographic si-nology is about. While this rigorous pursuit of a single object of en-quiry is courageous and highly productive, it is also disconcerting. The sinology dominates the study so completely that ethnography may be the wrong word to describe either the research methodology or the book. Although Farquhar worked in a *danwei* (work unit), we learn very little about it. There is no local world in much of the book. Ob-servations about local prescriptions take up much more space than descriptions of clinical transactions. The lived experience of patients is absent, but so is the lived experience of practitioners—their uncer-tainty, their stake in particular cases (or treatments).

Nor do we have what Michael Herzfeld (1987:x) calls "an anthro-pology that makes an ethnographic problem of itself [that] offers pragmatic insight into the social worlds that it examines and to which it belongs." Still less are we presented with the usual materials and techniques of cultural analysis that are present in the burgeoning field of cultural studies of science and technology (compare the review be-low of Margaret Lock's contribution). What we do have is nonetheless important: a powerful evocation of practical epistemology in the sino-logical tradition that makes a serious, if oddly self-constrained, con-tribution to the study of East Asian medicine and that suggests new uses for at least certain aspects of ethnography in the philosophy and history of science.

Music and Medicine

One of the more interesting directions that ethnogra-phies of healing have taken is to explore the place of music in healing rituals and in the healing process. Work in this tradition builds upon useful contributions of ethnomusicologists (e.g., Feld 1982) and in fact overlaps with their subdiscipline. Because rhythm is an "ordered and recurrent alternation of strong/weak elements" that occurs in "breathing, walking, running, dancing, speaking, drumming, and other vital and expressive processes" and because it is also "the periodicity of molecular activities, of geophysical, business, sleep-wake or metabolic cycles, of mood swings, of oscillations in the electrical activity of the cells of the cerebral cortex or of variable qualitative changes in other biological and physiological processes," the idea that rhythm, and other musical processes too, may mediate changes between the social world and the inner, psychobiological world of the person has intrigued medical anthropologists (You 1994a). Social processes such as relationality and reciprocity might even be modeled in terms of rhythms that are actualized in phases of time as synchronized or resonating changes that jump from social networks to neural networks. Because there are so few other candidates for even drawing rough analogies with society-mind-body mediation, music suggests itself, along with absorption and the attentional processes of trance states, as a leading candidate. That music is a ubiquitous component of indigenous healing rituals, and of many activities in which trance is induced for other purposes as well, adds significance to this interest. In the Chinese tradition, for example, sinologists have long connected ideas of order, yin/yang, and rhythmicity to a network of cosmological, sociomoral, and physiological connections emphasized in various texts of traditional Chinese medicine (Granet 1968; Needham 1954; Sivin 1987; You 1994b); music has often been used as the source of metaphors to illustrate this connection: for example, harmony.

Recent ethnographies by Carol Laderman (1991) and Marina Roseman (1991) explore the relationship between music and medicine in the Malaysian peninsula among Malay and Temiar, respectively. Both volumes are broadly concerned with the aesthetics of healing performances in local rituals. After reviewing both books, I will turn to a third ethnography, by Robert Desjarlais, *Body and Emotion* (1992), which describes a study of Yolmo Sherpa shamans in Nepal, because Desjarlais presses even further the issue of the poetics and aesthetics of therapy. Then I will examine Thomas Csordas's *The Sacred Self: A Cultural Phenomenology of Charismatic Healing* (1994), which applies culture theory vis-à-vis a rapprochement of semiotics and phenomenology to the study of how symbols heal.

Laderman's *Taming the Winds of Desire: Psychology, Medicine, and Aesthetics in Malay Shamanistic Performance* (1991), her second volume in the University of California Press series "Comparative Studies of Health Systems and Medical Care," centers on the Malay construction of *angin* (inner winds) as a chief source of personality, desire, and health. "Everyone is born with angin, the traits, talents, and desires representing our ancestors' heritage, but some have more, or stronger, angin than the common run," reports one informant (p. 68). The inner winds accommodate a Malay ethnopsychological theory of temperament, vulnerability, and resilience. There is a typology of personality types based on the angin's types of desires. The inner winds are a source of capriciousness; the thwarting or blocking of the inner winds can result in sadness or sickness. Freely blowing or sublimated inner winds keep the person and society healthy. If ignored or repressed, angin will create *sakit berangin*—sickness due to blockage of the inner winds—with symptoms of backaches, headaches, digestive problems, dizziness, asthma, depression, or anxiety.

Treatment aims to free the inner winds so that they can express their desires. Treatment also relates to complementary ideas of hot-cold humoral balance, protection of the spirit or force of life, *semangat,* and a strong Malay emphasis on the individuality of the person.

Bomohs, the Malay shamans, counteract the "hot" breath of invading spirits that threaten the "fortress" of the individual self. In the Malay séance the shaman, rather than the patient, enters trance to incarnate spirits. The bomoh helps certain patients, however, to enter trance states through his influence on the vital force and inner winds intrinsic to their individuality. Trance, during which patients say they feel high winds blowing within their chests, a claim the ethnographer corroborates from her own trance experience, puts patients in touch with their inner world, their inner being. Whereas the shaman becomes possessed, the patient, under the shaman's control, acts out repressed parts of her inner personality. "Patients in trance feel the Inner Winds as experiential reality rather than merely metaphor" (p. 95). Thus, cultural norm is validated by personal experience, while personal desire is fulfilled through cultural expression.

Laderman specializes in the ethnographic account of the *main peteri,* the elaborate ritual that the bomoh conducts to heal the pain of patients who are suffering from problems of the inner winds, the vital force or invasion by external spirits. The shaman mobilizes, in Laderman's fetching phrase, the patient's spiritual immune system (p. 61).

The bomoh counteracts the hot breath of invading spirits with his own vital breath, made "cool" by incantation. Bomohs "are usually well acquainted with life circumstances of patients" (p. 44). They ask psychosocially telling questions and practice what Laderman characterizes as a kind of psychotherapy with similarities to Jungian analysis. Much of the book is made up of detailed descriptions of main peteri healing rituals. The book ends with an entire main peteri performance, including the Malay words, translation, and the musical score.

The shaman should possess a beautiful voice. The words he sings are powered by his breath. The shaman's inner wind emerges in the performance and transfers efficacy to the patients he treats. But the meaning of the words he sings is also part of the performative construction of efficacy. The audience, including most notably the patient's family, also has a stake in seeing that performative efficacy is achieved. The performance seeks to contribute to order in the human microcosm, in the social macrocosm, and in the cosmos. But it is constrained by a factor that Laderman identifies as the chief cultural constraint on symbolic order in the Malay community: folk practices like the main peteri are contested by Islamic religious commitments. They conflict with each other. Regrettably, Laderman does not examine in any depth the implications of this seemingly important instance of cultural contestation for healing.

Taking up the idea of Gilbert Rouget (1985) that trance universally involves music, with acceleration, stresses, and syncopation, Laderman points out that the main peteri's music does not display syncopation. She does indicate, however, ways in which the music of the ritual weaves a subtle harmony between patient and healer, a harmony that even if it can't be generalized on symbolic grounds to the community is seen by informants as necessary for healing to occur. Laderman analyzes three main peteri rituals in detail, of which the story of the "stifled talent" and the séance for a sick shaman are impressive examples of her theory of how indigenous therapy works. Paradoxically for the reviewer of ethnography, it is precisely this detailed working through of events, which gives the ethnography book its distinctive analytic power, that, because of its very length and detail, cannot be instated in the review.

Although Laderman's book is successful in many of the tasks it sets for itself, there are a few problems reminiscent of difficulties found in the volumes already reviewed. The analysis at times is too deterministic, too complete for the subtle personal and interpersonal problems described in the case vignettes. The ritual seems too multisided to try to interpret in full. Both cases and ritual performances expand beyond the frame of the analysis; the artistry of ethnography makes them come alive. They are too vitally human for encapsulation in a totalizing social theory.

Once again the ethnographer seems to search for the same control in the ethnography that the shaman seeks in the patient's trance and treatment. Curiously, while the angin of the patient is freed and refreshed as a result of the performance of the ritual, the performance of the ethnography fastens down the imaginings of the reader, forcing conclusions such as a fairly flat portrayal of personality and the distant analogy to Jungian therapy that seems strained. The discussion of placebo response is too narrowly organized around Thomas Scheff's (1979) idea of catharsis. This is an interesting notion to be sure—but it is one that is overly valued by the author at the expense of other perspectives on the placebo process that might have enriched her interpretation. This overmanagement of the interpretive process contrasts strikingly with the graceful depiction of the performances and the sensitive discussion of the ethnographer's own inner experiences during the rituals. It is also surprising that so little is made of performance theory—a rich vein in cultural analysis—to develop the theoretical implications of the analysis, which on the whole seem surprisingly thin when contrasted with the thick description of the performance. A final reaction: why is so little done in the analysis with all the musical materials that are presented? The reader is led to feel that there will be much more ethnomusicological method in the interpretation than actually occurs. It is as if the author is presenting a resource for others, who are better trained in ethnomusicological practices, to analyze. But the reader who works through the text and recorded performances will feel, as I did, disappointed that after so much effort so little is forthcoming in the way of demonstration of what technical analysis of musical performance can add to the interpretation. Laderman's fine descriptions make us feel much can be added, but we are never shown what that extra value is. This is especially noticeable in the gap between the standard assertion that symbolic performances heal and the absence of a convincing demonstration of what mediates that healing process.

Marina Roseman, an ethnomusicologically trained anthropologist, who apparently consulted on Laderman's research, possesses the methodological skills to conduct such a demonstration. Her book, *Healing Sounds from the Malaysian Rainforest: Temiar Music and Medicine* (1991), sets out to bridge the divide between theories of symbolic healing and ethnographic analysis. The setting is the deep interior, where there is an "intricate interpenetrability of settlement and forest" (p. 4), which is architecturally represented in stilt houses with spaces between bamboo slats in the floor and higher up on walls that allow an opening, fraught with local implication, between the community and the jungle. For these hunter-horticulturalists, the social system turns on generalized reciprocity; the cultural system invokes homology between detachable souls in plants, animals, landforms, and humans (head and heart souls). "Bounded souls can be liberated as unbounded spirit during dreams, trance, and illness . . . unbounded souls make interaction and the flow of information possible between human and non-human entities" (p. 6).

Spirits of the jungle and settlement can engage humans as helpful guides or as malevolent causes of illness. Spirit guides in dreams bestow a song on the dreamer: "singing that song during ceremonial performance, the person becomes imbued with the voice, vision, and knowledge of the spirit guide" (p. 6). Transformed by the spirit into a medium, the guided person can diagnose and treat illness.

In the local imagery, songs are paths. Choruses of singers follow the path as they sing contrapuntally with the mediums. Mediums sing of the route traversed by the spirit guide during its travels. Knowing the real path in the jungle, of course, can be the difference between life and death. Illness is said to result when the person's head soul gets lost. Treatment is the singing of a "way": finding the head soul and leading it back to the settlement. The key metaphor in song involves travel along paths between two different domains of knowledge: music and healing.

Roseman builds her analysis on performance theory, especially the conveying of symbols through "ritual frames; aesthetic distance; performance roles; audience participation and commitment to the performance reality" (p. 15). She also takes seriously Temiar performance theory, which holds, less abstractly and more to the point of society-mind-body transformations,

that pulsating sounds of the Malaysian rainforest, such as calls of particular birds and insects, move with the beat of the heart, and then move the listener to feel longing. The pulsing of the bamboo-tube percussion that accompanies

Temiar singing ceremonies is similarly structured, alternating high and low pitches in continuous rhythm. These socially structured sounds, sonic icons of the heartbeat, move the heart to longing. (p. 15)

Longing, attraction, enticement—all mediate between humans and spirits. Detachment and reattachment of bounded souls is an idea that underlies Temiar music and medicine. Bounded souls—tied to the conditions of everyday life, health, and safety—can be liberated as unbounded souls, the stuff of dreams and trance and singing and also of illness and other dangers.

Roseman places the performance theory in the context of a broader social theory that we have already encountered in certain of the other ethnographies. For the Temiar—a social group organized, like the Huli, Hutu, and Tutsi, around reciprocity—halting the flow of goods (not reciprocating) puts the affected person in a state of unfulfilled wanting that makes that person vulnerable to misfortune. Good exchange is good health. Connection is crucial; separation dangerous. The social dialectic is between "the cultural subscript of sociocentric interdependence" and "the continual reinstatement of an independent, bounded self" (p. 47).

The Temiar spirit medium-healer is the *Halaa*: a person with the capability to receive songs from spirit guides during dreams and later on with the ability to "manifest those spirit guides when singing the songs and trancing during ceremonial performance" (p. 53).

"Temiar mediums are singers of the landscape, translating the rainforest environment—jungle, field, and settlement—into culture as inhabitant spirits emerge, identify themselves, and begin to sing in dreams and ritual performances" (p. 58). The Halaa creates the cultural experience in the intersubjective space of the ritual as the flow of the spirit guide through the song in the symbolic form of a cool spiritual liquid. In this felt experience of the symbolic, cosmology, humoral theory, music, and healing merge. The dislocation of the illness experienced as loss of the soul is counterbalanced in healing by the song of landscapes that locate the spirits.

The Temiar healing ritual overlaps, and alternates, the singing of male medium and female chorus in keeping with the egalitarian social organization and system of generalized exchange. The interweaving in sound and movement announces, and undermines, differences: individual/community, male/female, jungle/settlement, human/nonhuman, bounded/unbounded. Through symbolic inversions and conjunctions in ritual performance, these differences are transcended. Tellingly the Temiar themselves refer to trancing as "transforming."

Roseman illustrates the dynamic process of symbolic transformation she has installed in the interpretation through an account of the Temiar's aesthetics of longing. "The duple rhythm of these beating tubes [male-female pairs of bamboo-tube stampers beaten by the chorus of women against a log in alternation] is linked in a web of local meanings that extends from pulsating sound of the rainforest to the beating of the human heart" (p. 151). The spirits are set in motion and the sentiment of longing—which pervades the spirit guide-medium relationship—is modulated through these fraught sounds and dance steps. Sound becomes remembrance; trance forgetfulness.

"In everyday life," writes Roseman, the calls of the cicada "are said to move one's heart to longing for a loved one" (p. 157). Pulsing at the frequency of the heartbeat, the cicada's song is said to make the heart whirl and thereby invokes the remembrance of deceased relations or of longing for a lover. "This aesthetic sensibility links longing and remembrance with the pulsating sounds of bird calls, insect sounds, and the bamboo-tube stompers of ceremonial trance-dancing sessions" (p. 158). The music-invoked longing has to do with absences and that which is "unobtainably distant."

Thus, the sentient metaphor of connecting and separating is found in the primary experience of the singing, in the representational form of the song, and in the invoked experience of illness/healing. Transformation in Temiar ethnomusicology and ethnomedicine is "a momentary intermingling of self and other" (p. 172). Thereby, concludes Roseman, "aesthetic configurations participate in a comprehensive pattern of reality and become therapeutically effective" (p. 184).

But just how does that mediation occur? Roseman's prose pulls us toward an acceptance of her conclusion: the style is resonant with the subject matter, the conclusion is prefigured, all the elements are assembled for understanding how social space and bodily space commingle. We are even told when it has happened. Yet, the analysis stays very much at the surface of things. What is missing is a deep study of the mediation itself. Neither the music nor the cases are described in enough detail to make the reader feel the conclusions are adequately supported. If a problem with Laderman's book is too much ethnographic material with too little close interpretation, a problem with Roseman's volume is too much interpretation with too thin an ethnography. Both are noble failures: noble failures in Ivan Morris's (1975:xiii–xv) use of the term to speak to the Japanese tradition's valuing of courageous acts that even their authors know cannot succeed, not only because they are fine attempts, but because nobody else has succeeded fully either. And each instructs by what it lacks: a convincing demonstration of the process of symbolic mediation.[1] Laderman provides all the materials but doesn't carry through the analysis; Roseman draws the conclusion and shows us each of the components in the analysis, but doesn't link them together. For all the remarkably resonant things she has to say about healing, Roseman is unable to open up the fine processes of healing because her ethnography is not rich enough in events, situations, or lives to sustain such an illumination of how intertextuality and polyphony actually transform persons through performance (see Feld and Fox 1994, for a discussion of what such an ethnomusicological ethnography of mediation might require). Both works, however, provide a firmer basis than has heretofore been available for finer-tuned, more broadly integrative studies.

While it is not a study of musical performance, Robert Desjarlais's *Body and Emotion* (1992) does wrestle with issues in the aesthetics of illness and healing similar to those Laderman and Roseman engage. Although his ambitious ethnographic account is also too limited in findings to fully succeed, he does carry the study of specifying how healing is mediated in therapeutic rituals deeper into the phenomenology of the sensuous experience of therapeutic change. That promising direction is taken by another study of the therapeutic process, Thomas Csordas's *The Sacred Self* (1994), which will complete our review of the mediation of healing.

Aesthetics, Performance, and the Experience of Healing

Desjarlais's intention is well captured by the quotation from George Eliot's *Middlemarch* that opens his account:

If we had a keen vision of all ordinary human life, it would be like hearing the grass grow or the squirrel's heart beat, and we should die of that roar which lies on the other side of silence.

The "ordinary human life" to which Desjarlais seeks to give voice is the world of Yolmo Sherpas, ethnic Tibetan people who live in north central Nepal. In this beautifully crafted volume, Desjarlais draws on his participation in healing ceremonies as an apprentice of a barefoot, illiterate shaman (*bombo*) called Meme. During the ceremonies, Desjarlais entered into a trance state that

paralleled the descent of Meme's gods into his body. . . . Tracked by the driving, insistent beat of the shaman's drum, my body would fill with energy. Music resonated within me, building to a crescendo, charging my body and the room with impacted meaning. Waves of tremors coursed through my limbs. Sparks flew, colors expanded, the room came alive with voices, fire, laughter, darkness. (p. 5)

Later on, Desjarlais reports, "I felt that my body developed a partial, experiential understanding of their world, from the ways in which they held their bodies to how they felt, hurt, and healed" (p. 13).

To explore the experiential world of Yolmo "soul loss" and the shaman's search for lost souls, Desjarlais uses his own liminal experiences to engage "the sensory, the visceral, the unspoken." For ethnographers in the tradition of cultural phenomenology, such as Michael Jackson and Paul Stoller, Desjarlais holds, the researcher needs to cultivate "negative capability"—Keats's appreciation of Shakespeare's genius of "being in uncertainties, mysteries, doubts, without any irritable reaching after fact or reason" (p. 34). This is the cultural sensibility that enjoins "a visceral engagement with symbolic forms" (p. 35); it is not an immediate empathy, but an understanding of the poetics and aesthetics of experience built up out of a prior understanding of the social order. Thus, Desjarlais's description of Yolmo bodies interweaves the somato-symbolic imagery of Tantric anatomy, the cultural architecture of the built environment, the structure of social relationships, and moral processes. Like Pierre Bourdieu's (1977) analysis of the homology between the physiology of the body and the structure of the Algerian house, Desjarlais shows a similar symbolic architectural principle that bridges the Yolmo house, bodily habitus, and moral meanings. Thus, "motifs" of inner/outer, depth/surface, openings/closures "pervade Yolmo understandings of psychology, knowledge, and medicine" (p. 45). Illness is penetration of spirits, ghosts, and other malignant forces into the body; healing works to "throw" demons out of the house of the body. In spite of separations, these boundaries are permeable and continuously crossed. They are the source of vulnerability and also of therapeutic efficacy.

For Desjarlais, the village he studied as well as particular families he came to know and the bodily processes of villagers involved in the shamanistic séances in which he participated, all contain a core structural tension between independence and interdependence that shapes the micropolitics—the political "physiology"—of each domain. Yolmo social organization derives from a historical conflict between kinship ties and temple-based inter-household alliances. This tension shapes relationships of exchange, hospitality, mutual support, and status. Status hierarchy is mapped onto household relations, where it conflicts with individual life trajectories. In the village as a whole, the "household's" place in the political hierarchy is more important today than the "family's" place in the lineage. In the family as in the village, individuals relate to each other through both hierarchical and egalitarian principles. Fission and fragmentation of the village and the family are a constant threat in Yolmo society. A household balances between autonomy and interdependence as does its members.

Desjarlais writes that Yolmo cultural sensibility extends this conflicted metaphor of social order deep within the body, where the *sems* (heart-mind) conflicts with the *klad pe* (brain). Emotions arise within the sems, and the emotionally laden sems travels outside of the body to the place and time envisioned in dreams. The klad pe is the inner, moral censor that sediments out of social hierarchy into interior space. This conflict deep within the person recreates the conflict in village and family. Fragmentation of villages and dispersal of villagers into multiethnic settings under the political forces of the present era ramify into division of families and the inner experience of dispersal and loss. The aesthetics of both illness and healing experiences—the tacit cultural forms, values, and sensibilities that lend styles and felt qualities to modes of being-in-the-world—take origin from this cultural system. For Desjarlais, then, ritual performance emerges out of the aesthetics of the everyday.

Thus, the Yolmo experience of the body as a fragile harmonium—unified and whole but liable to fragment because of the inherent tension between constituent parts—informs their way of being ill and undergoing treatment. In illness, the body is experienced as "incomplete, adulterated, off-balance, lacking" (p. 73). Soul loss is an omnipresent threat, in which the body declines and the life forces are diminished. Curing involves the experiences of restoration and homeostatic balance. Health involves self-resistance and control, the latter closely connected not only to the social interests already mentioned, but also to the kinesthetic attentiveness to surroundings that is salient for a mountain people.

Desjarlais's methodology is to examine common aspects of Yolmo experience—pain, sadness, the sensibility of loss—and then to interpret them through the interweaving of bodily experiences, poetry that casts such feelings into the intersubjective space of the collective, the Buddhist literary tradition, and ritual performances. Thus, Yolmo "heartache" is deconstructed as a special form of Buddhist *dukkha* (suffering). Its ritualization in the experiences of informants is used to animate the emotion and its role in pathology and healing. But at the same time, "heartache" is embedded in the Yolmo context of the social organizational instability of "companionship, intimacy . . . relationality" and also harmony, order, and homeostasis (p. 108). Making up a summary list like this in place of the fine-grained analysis of poetry and felt sensibility, especially the way Desjarlais elaborates their interconnection, seriously distorts a methodology that convinces the reader through the very process of aesthetic interpretation that it installs. Indeed, Desjarlais's skill as a writer of evocative prose is at the center of his methodology, which might be described as recreating the collective sensibility of therapeutic transformation.

With *tsher ka* [heartache], the difficulties in communicating distress are twofold, for an essential component of such pain is the inability to express one's plight to others precisely because the intimates with whom one is most able to share thoughts are absent. A vicious circle is thus created, and a sufferer of *tsher ka* is left without an open vehicle to express distress. Villagers told me that, within the karmic wheel of life, the greatest torment of animals—chickens, dogs, buffaloes—is that, deprived of a language, they cannot communicate the pains of their existence, particularly those burdens enacted on them by their human custodians. Yolmo, lacking an open vehicle to communicate distress, often resemble these creatures.

> If we stay our hearts will ache,
> if we go our little feet will hurt
> the sorrow of little feet hurting,
> to whom can we tell?
>
> (p. 117)

The song creates a collective sentiment of the commonality of loss and separation for those who are bereaved, for those who are ill, and for others such as young women who experience the homesickness of moving out of their natal family into the household of their husbands. The expression of emotion, which takes place in a shared idiom under the strong social constraint of an ethic of self-restraint that fosters support, strengthens bonds, and gives voice to pain, is the source of their efficacy. Until this point, the analysis, though impressively fine-grained, follows a course worked out by various theorists of the poetics of everyday experience; now it builds upon the ethnographic base in a more original direction.

The poetics of Yolmo songs, we are told, model the transformation of bereavement and healing. "Yolmo heartaches" entail a sense of loss, abandonment, and separation. These events are occasioned by pitfalls specific to Yolmo social life: the separation of family members, the patrilocal travels of women, the death of children and elders. Since the pitfalls are common ones, sentiments of tsher ka imply a core emotional pattern, a "plot" that narrates a loss, a separation, a sense of abandonment: the consequences of these events (weary bodies, pained hearts), and then a struggle to avoid, escape, or transcend those burdens. The pattern of experience accords with other sufferings. Earlier we learned that threats of loss, dispersal, and fragmentation disturb the physiology of Yolmo bodies, households, villages. Tsher ka is the visceral correlative of these images. Its dark presence speaks of broken bodies, lost birds, and downhill descents.

The funeral song works with *tsher ka*'s plotted sensibility to effect change. The lyrics retell a common story—a world of pain, a father remembered, a call to ignore the pain, and an attempt to "cut" it from the body. The singers, by giving image to grief, create a moment in which the bereaved realize some of the basic forms and tensions of their existence. . . . [T]he epiphany can be a powerful one for Yolmo, not only because the moment is revelatory but because the world revealed by it accords with basic bodily dispositions and so seems apt and valid and of the natural order of things. "What he encounters is his own story," Gadamer says of a spectator to a Greek tragedy. The same might be said of a villager dancing a song of separation. The singers move themselves and their audience through the successive stages of a burden that they usually do not wish to confront in their everyday lives. The song's ghostly rhythms, in telling a tale of grief, evoke the experiential contours of loss and, in so doing, summon the imaginative forces needed to soothe that grief. Toward that end, the messages hidden within the recesses and echoes of the poem are as significant as its discursive strategies.

Those messages often hold to the level of the body. Feet grow weary, hearts blossom, desire "sticks" to the body. The songs evoke and recall the most visceral of experiences, as if one of their key functions is to engage the body, to alter human sentience. The likelihood that Yolmo bodies are the true authors for, and audiences of, the songs implies a great deal. (p. 133)

Desjarlais, who laments the limits of symbolic analysis to get at the process of change, goes beyond the language of representation to use such terms as "incarnate," "animate," "resonance," "similitude" to evoke the aesthetic sensibilities of illness as a cultural mode of being; the same terms are crucial to his approach to healing. These "assume common structures, like disparate musical notes come to form distinct and well-known melodies" (p. 156). Healing for Yolmo is about arousing or rejuvenating the spirit and life force. The shaman "lends image to a felt sensibility," like an expert art critic evaluating a painting. Healing, we are told repeatedly, works through the felt experiences of the rites. "Shamanic rites of protection demarcate the geography of Yolmo forms, accenting what belongs within a body or household and what does not. The core experience pivots on an image that is instantaneous, mimetic, without narrative time" (p. 190). The body is reconstructed as closed, defended, protected, its boundaries maintained. This occurs through the symbolic analogy with the order of the house and the cosmos. It is the experience of the image, however, not the image as a representation, that produces the effect. That effect "incarnates" the experiences of sociopolitical tensions, interpersonal tensions (interdependence versus autonomy), and bodily distress. "Healing rites catalyze an ontology of experience patterned by a play of flow and stoppage, ingress and egress: ghosts are drawn, life forces relived, and body surfaces cleaned and protected" (p. 194). Thus exorcism is literally experienced as expulsion from the body. Healing is not so much about the meaning of transactional symbols as it is about the kinesthetic actions those symbols evoke. Mimesis allows the shaman's movement to move the patient to feel that movement, say, of pain leaving the body.

The shaman "changes how a body feels by altering what it feels. His cacophony of music, taste, sight, touch, and kinesthesia activate a patient's senses" (p. 206). For soul loss, he alters "the sensory grounds of a spiritless body" (p. 206).

The visceral sense of renewed health, which usually takes hold in the house after a rite and must last if the rite is to be considered successful, is the major criteria upon which villagers judge rites efficacious or not. In Helamba, a person does not feel better after being cured; she is cured after feeling better. (p. 209)

Desjarlais's model is a performative one. The healer's rites "lighten a heavy body" due to soul loss because "they activate the senses to spark sensibilities distinct from those of malaise" (p. 210). These sensibilities are part of Yolmo aesthetics of healthy experience: namely, the feelings of "presence, vitality, harmony, and repletion." The shamanic strategies of recovering lost vitality include: "selective attention to detail, an evocation of the senses, a mimetic presentation of a tangible reality, an invocation of the 'here,' and the use of wild images to induce attentiveness" (p. 218). Kinesthesia is used by the shaman to incorporate life, power, vitality in the body. And that is how patients experience healing, as an entering into the body of the vital and the powerful, felt "like a jolt of electricity" (p. 221).

An ethnography that dares so much, especially by installing a language of evocation and animation, assumes a weighty responsibility that the ethnographic narratives must support. If those narratives are limited, the ethnography is likely not to succeed completely. Nor does Desjarlais escape from this predicament. In spite of considerable repetition of the central themes, with a measure of cumulative success, the examples seem too trim and undeveloped to carry the argument. Rather, the incandescent language and fluid interpretations seem to outdistance the findings. The idea of being healed because you are made to feel different or better also begins to seem less and less like a highly original reversal of the commonsensical and more and more like tautology. That is to say, the theoretical elaboration of the aesthetics of everyday life, unlike their brilliantly effective evocation, leaves something central that is unfinished.[2] To his credit as an ethnographer, Desjarlais makes no attempt to disguise this limitation. Indeed he ends his impressive postmodernist account with a sensitive reflection on uncertainty and the limits of interpretation that is just what readers would expect of a writer who is so remarkably attuned to the inner tone of social experience.

In *The Sacred Self: A Cultural Phenomenology of Charismatic Healing*, Thomas Csordas reports on nearly twenty years of study of healing in the Catholic Charismatic Renewal movement. His thesis is that Charismatic Renewal, like religious healing systems generally, involves "an experiential specificity of effect": "that transformative meaning dwells, to borrow a phrase from the poet William Blake, in the 'minute particulars' of human existence taken up in the healing process. To approach that specificity, we must identify the locus of efficacy" (p. 3). For Csordas, "the locus of efficacy is not symptoms, psychiatric disorders, symbolic meanings, or social relationships, but the self in which all of these are encompassed." Thus, the problem of efficacy turns on the development of "a theory of self that will allow for the experience of the sacred as . . . an element that constitutes one kind of the specificity we seek" (p. 4). That theory of the self, argues Csordas, should begin with an understanding of the self as "indeterminate capacity to engage or become oriented in the world, characterized by effort and reflexivity" (p. 5). The self is a "conjunction" of the experience of the body, the culturally created world, and situational specificity. The self is an embodied orientation to the world, a locus for perception, says Csordas following Merleau-Ponty, the French phenomenological psychologist. This is the existential, preobjective grounds of experience, prior to cultural construction of the "person," yet based in the social formation of the habitus, argues Csordas, who melds the views of Merleau-Ponty with those of Bourdieu. The habitus—the socially informed body—is the locus of mediation of human practices, potentialities, and actions that are always and everywhere indeterminate. And it is this very indeterminacy that is the source of transformation and transcendence, in everyday life, in religion, and in healing. Csordas's ambitious theoretical aim is to unite the languages of phenomenology and semiotics—the conceptual frames of Merleau-Ponty and Bourdieu—around the intersubjective worlds within which healing is actualized. "To be healed is to inhabit the Charismatic world as a sacred self" (p. 24).

They [Charismatics] participate in the late-twentieth-century shift away from embracing suffering and self-mortification as an imitation of Christ's passion, and toward the relief of suffering through divine healing as practiced by Jesus in the gospels (Favazza 1987). Yet healing is not only the relief of illness and distress, and not only a "sign to unbelievers" of divine power, but an instrument for molding the sacred self *for both healers and patients.* This ideal self is inherently healthy, both for its own sake and for its capacity to contribute to the divinely appointed collective mission of bringing about the "Kingdom of God." (pp. 25–26)

For Charismatics, the self can be "wounded" or "broken" and healed by divine power, and it can achieve spiritual growth.

Csordas presents findings from his study of Charismatic healers and patients in the late 1980s in New England who engage in three types of healing that parallel the same tripartite structure of the self: "physical healing" for illnesses of the body, "inner healing" for emotional distress, and "deliverance" from the negative effects of evil spirits. He interprets the repertoire of Charismatic healing techniques under six general headings: empowerment (e.g., annointing, laying on of hands, glossolalia), protection (e.g., calling on the Virgin Mary), revelation (e.g., prophecy and visions), deliverance (e.g., casting out spirits, cutting ancestral bonds), sacramental grace (e.g., Eucharist and confession), and emotional release (forgiveness). But Csordas's chief concern is to develop a theory of how healing works through the transformation of the experiences of patients. Pointing to experiences such as changing habitual posture and altering bodily modes of attention, Csordas proposes that religious healing realizes "incremental efficacy" at the "margin of disability" through four specific therapeutic processes: the disposition of supplicants, experience of the sacred, elaboration of alternative possibilities, and actualization of change.

Csordas explicates this theory in the study of religious images. These he interprets not as representations or things, but as acts in the embodied consciousness that contribute to the actualization of performative efficacy. Thus, revelatory images engage sensory modalities. They are "a sense of" or "infused knowledge" in the modalities of vision, olfaction, hearing, proprioception, and also emotion. Csordas presents quantitative data from his interviews as well as detailed reports to support his argument for the performative force of therapeutic images. These images act in the body through the mediation of sensory, intersubjective, and cultural "force" to change habitual experience, including the experience of the self. In the late-twentieth-century North American cultural context, that alteration "incarnates" spontaneity, control, and intimacy in the social experience of the self as the locus of therapeutic efficacy.

There is a remarkable rigor in the effort Csordas makes to build an elaborate set of theoretical models out of the interweaving of ethnographic findings and densely detailed summaries of relevant theoretical literature. But that very strategy of writing, which yields highly original formulations, also creates problems. The writing is dense, which is as much the problem of the phenomenological tradition as it is Csordas's own predilection for long, complex sentences; the ethnographic descriptions appear in dribs and drabs; and the reader can watch the theory set up the presentation of the data, which then are made to stand for what they have already been prefigured to mean. At its best, the last gives an exhilarating sense of cumulative development and completion; at its worst, it seems forced and comes perilously close to tautology. Csordas is at his best when he stays close to his ethnography, as in his discussion of Charismatic "healing of memories," where he finally does present fuller accounts of the experiences of patients undergoing the process of therapy that are rich enough to support the elaboration of a theory of the "specificity" of efficacy with ethnographic exactness. This clearly is the case with the three ethnographic features that Csordas isolates in the description of the healing of memories: (1) the emergence of memories that hold autobiographical import but that are attributed to revelation; (2) the construal of those memories as traumas and the forgiving of the trauma perpetrators; and (3) the privileging of imagined performance of the trauma or enactment of some other troubled scenario with Jesus in the role of healer. Less coherent is Csordas's application of object-relations theory from psychoanalysis to understand alterity in the self as basis for the construction of the sacred self. Csordas is on sturdier grounds when he applies Edward Casey's (1987) phenomenological analyses of imagining and remembering to his materials.

In one of the most satisfactory meshes of theory and description, Csordas deploys Merleau-Ponty's idea of the presubjective to understand how patients who are experiencing demons switch the codes of experience from being in control to giving up control to another, often alienated, part of the self. Out of that code switch, culture, working through collective meanings, is what objectifies self into demon. Here Csordas has opened up a usable space to relate cultural, intersubjective, and psychological processes in understanding the experience of affliction, the experience of transformation when demons are cast out, and the instauration thereby of the experience of grace. Another impressive ethnographic success, with assistance from the writings of the phenomenological psychologist Erwin Strauss, is the application of the theory to the cultural phenomenology of "falling" in a Charismatic healing practice called "resting in the Spirit."

At his very best, Csordas can demonstrate that efficacy can only be understood through cultural ontologies that enjoin the anthropologist to work out changes in individual experiences in an epoch's context of changing collective experiences. Thus, healing for Charismatic Catholics in late-twentieth-century North America must be different not only from healing in other religious traditions but, more to the point, from healing in other Catholic communities in other historical contexts, because of the shift in cultural experience. It is one thing to say this, which other researchers do; it is quite another to demonstrate it, which is Csordas's chief accomplishment, a key achievement.

What Csordas does not succeed in doing is proving to the reader that the theory of self is essential for the framework required to understand healing. His most convincing ethnographic examples of healing, tellingly, are ones where the analysis of bodily practices and intersubjective interactions does not seem to require an ontology of the self. In developing a usable cultural psychology for medical anthropology, Csordas indirectly, and counter to his stated intention, suggests that it may be feasible to bypass a theory of the self altogether, since his model replaces self-awareness not only with somatic modes of experiencing, but with "processes of orientation and engagement." These processes are so thoroughly interpersonal they suggest that what is needed is a more serviceable social psychology and a brand new social physiology (p. 278).

At the Margin of Medical Anthropology

The margins of medical anthropology, with psychological anthropology, feminist studies, and the wider array of ethnographic concern with other forms of social suffering, contain works that hold different sorts of relevance. In her provocative ethnography *The Last Word: Women, Death, and Divination in Inner Mani,* Nadia Seremetakis (1991) looks at death rituals through "the optic of death": "death rites as an arena of social contestation, a space where heterogeneous and antagonistic cultural codes and social interests meet and tangle" (pp. 14–15). Death is the domain of women in Mani, a remote, inhospitable, violent territory in Greece where women, she claims, have been dominated by men, the church, the state, and, most recently, "medical rationalities." The women of Mani sing *moiroloi* (laments) that connote the crying of their fate. Their performances of grieving validate their *ponos* (pain). "Pain is crucial for truth-claiming strategies of Maniat women" (p. 4): it is a form of sociopolitical resistance, Seremetakis avers, through which women come to speak the last word on the culture of Mani.

Women were traditionally caught up in the clan warfare, alliances, and blood feuds of the region. They embody the kinship ethic of caring and tending the living, the dying, and the dead. Women mediate birth—the passage from outside to inside the local world—and death: the passage from inside to outside. Mourning obligations and personal grieving lasts for years, and includes participation in exhumation, where women divine the moral condition of the dead. The symbolism associated with the feminine in Mani includes pollution and destructive contact. And yet in screaming for the dead, the women themselves have the image in mind of a bent woman who stands up and stretches out to express her gendered personhood through a death lament, a lament that for the author mediates between worlds, contests the forms of this-worldly dominance, and offers an alternative commentary on suffering and much of the rest of social experience as well.

For the women of Mani, their experience of pain is of a burning fire that "liquifies" the self into tears. Pain is a "holocaust" (p. 115). Women's fate is to endure pain and labor for others. "Through pain Maniat women link kinship, the division of labor, agricultural and domestic economies—all male-dominated institutions—into an experiential continuum" (p. 115). Their pain authorizes the truth claims of their ritual laments to reveal fate, the forced entrance of the outside into the inside world. This passage of fate through the mediation of the female body into the social order is not only a form of social memory, but a teleological critique of male-dominated ideologies of modernization and urbanization.

The crucial event for the playing out of this socio-logic is the funeral, where death is rationalized by medical, social welfare, state, and even church rationalities, and that rationalization is resisted and ultimately undone by the female mourners (pp. 163–166). Those mourners transform *soma* (their body and the body of the dead) into *sema* (a key cultural sign). Seremetakis's analysis of ritual laments at the exhumation of the bones of the dead discloses that women are cynical because of their understanding of fate. By offering the last word, they use irony to authorize an alternative form of social memory that claims the male-dominated social order is "false" (p. 218).

Up to this point, Seremetakis's symbolic analysis seems so well founded in ethnographic description that, despite its flamboyant rhetoric, the view she offers of the morality and politics of women's experiences appears reasonable. But the book ends with a provocation so extreme that it vitiates the strong program of feminist analysis. Seremetakis's ending moves her from scholar to partisan of divination as holistic knowledge for women in their resistance to men.

Women and men are treated as pawns in a binary opposition that is so fundamental they never seem to interact. Divination becomes the antithesis of rational technical practice: the former is always good, the latter always bad. This extreme ideological separation raises serious questions about the validity of the ethnography. Seremetakis is to be complimented on another count, however, because, unlike most ethnographers of death and social mourning, she deals, at least partially, with the experience of grieving. It is a telling comment on the interests of anthropologists that the huge corpus of ethnographies of social mourning practices has so little to say about the social experience of bereavement. Seremetakis is interested in that symbolizing experience. Yet, since her interpretation rejects any psychological (or existential) orientation, she ends up unable to examine the emotional response of real people to real losses. The quite marvelous case descriptions are only deployed to authorize her symbolic analysis of collective experience; the personal experiences of the arresting tragedies she describes go largely unexamined (p. 156). Grief, for all its deeply resonant subjectivity, is handled largely as a source of powerful cultural symbols. Because she has provided effective and affecting descriptions, however, the reader feels he has the evidence he needs to argue with the author that these cases are about lived tragedies in everyday experience— including states of "endurance" and "martyrdom" as local forms of suffering—that require an examination of the cultural ontology of social experience as a complement to the symbolic analysis (pp. 144, 156, 201). Nonetheless, the Seremetakis ethnography is a good example, at least prior to its concluding pages, of the power that feminist readings of the contestation, fragmentation, and multiplicity of social life can bring to subjects that are of high salience to medical anthropology.

In passing from Seremetakis to Nancy Scheper-Hughes (1992), we may be going from the frying pan of provocation to the fire of accusation, yet the ethnography—*Death without Weeping: The Violence of Everyday Life in Brazil*—is one no medical anthropologist can (or should) avoid encountering. Scheper-Hughes traces the lineaments of her ethnography back to her early experience as a Peace Corps volunteer in the 1960s in a terribly poor *favela*, Bom Jesus, in northeastern Brazil where she lived as well as carried out community organization. "What, I wondered, were the effects of chronic hunger, sickness, death, and loss on the ability to love, trust, have faith, and keep it in the broadest senses of these terms?" (p. 15). For Scheper-Hughes: "The horror was the routinization of human suffering in so much of impoverished Northeast Brazil and the 'normal' violence of everyday life" (p. 16). She returned to conduct anthropological field research and to continue her community development work at various periods over the next several decades.

Bom Jesus is dry and dirty; there is very little water, and what water is available is polluted. She describes both personal and collective thirst, as well as deep anxiety over water and hunger. The average *favela* family with eight members uses ten gallons of water a day; the average Marin County household used four hundred gallons per day during the water restrictions brought on by the Northern California drought of the late 1980s. The historic backdrop to this local world of thirst and hunger is by now an all-too-well-known one of colonial "greed, exploitation, and retaliation," followed by the dominance of sugar plantation monoculture, destruction of peasant cultivators, rural-urban migration, and the development of a social system of middle-class bosses, working-class poor, and two groups at the very margin of social class dynamics: *pobrezinhos,* the "truly poor," "struggling souls" who are seasonal workers in the fields without security; and *pobritoes,* the "truly wretched," who literally have nothing and are occupied day and night with the most basic requirements of survival. This last group includes the physically disabled, the chronically mentally ill, and the "walking corpses" of the chronically sick poor.

Scheper-Hughes describes the local world as the outcome of a dynamic social process in which an older sugar plantation economy and a newer industrializing economy interpenetrate in such a way that tension between hierarchy and democratic trends becomes intense enough to create a divided, chaotic, anarchic society. In this fragmented local world, her research subjects are the *Matutos:* "They are the little people, the no-account people, those whose features, clothing, gait, and posture mark them as anachronisms in modern Bom Jesus." Darker, smaller (stunted owing to inadequate nutrition), the Matutos maintain a self-image of being weak, wasted, worn out. The descendants of slave, runaway slave, and Indian populations, they are under the pressure of racism and "operate in a world of gifts and favors, barter and cunning, loyalties and dependence, rumor and reputation" (p. 91). Rejecting the idea of a culture of poverty, Scheper-Hughes comes very close to describing just such a local ethos, which she represents as predicated on cynicism, pessimism, desperation, anomie, promiscuity, exploitation, predation, and abandonment. Patron-client interaction, which is the chief model of relations outside of the community, linking it to the wider city, "locks the social classes into a ruse, a travesty of interaction in which exploitation parades as benevolence and passive aggression masquerades as fawning dependency" (p. 125).

At times, Scheper-Hughes's view of the community becomes unsympathetic and accusatory. It is a bad-faith economy—financial and moral, she claims (p. 126). It is out of this bleak view that the central theme of the ethnography emerges: "where the threat of hunger, scarcity, and unmet needs is constant and chronic, traditional patterns of triage may determine the allocation of scarce resources within the household" (p. 135). As a result, the male head of the household may abscond, teenage children may run off via sexual unions or just disappear, and young, sickly infants and small children may undergo a kind of desperate neglect in the context of the slow starvation of the family. The upshot is a routinization of child death with a frighteningly high infant mortality rate of 116 per 1,000 live births, to which the rest of society has become indifferent. Even the mothers of dying children participate in a (necessary?) misrecognition, an anankastic misrepresentation that keeps them from seeing that hunger and starvation are at the root of child sickness and death.

Babies who are viewed as doomed because of their fraility are allowed to die of "mortal neglect" (p. 342). Mothers are placed in a situation where no mother should ever be placed. They are led to accept a "holy indifference" (p. 363). "Failed" babies are stigmatized. There are negotiations over terminality which in the local moral world can mean the option of withdrawing support. The doomed child, like Christ, is said to need to die to redeem the lives of others. The social construction of household triage leads to a terrible pragmatism in which salvage, neglect, and uncertainty are worked out. Mothers show pity, not grief, and resignation or indifference, not effective resistance. For Scheper-Hughes the misrecognition and indifference place a veil over the state, which is the ultimate source of responsibility for this terrible violence of everyday life.

Scheper-Hughes first seems to accept an earlier criticism by Marilyn Nations and L. A. Rebhun (1988) that she is blaming the victims by presenting them as unfeeling and negligent/incompetent in mothering, but later on she disagrees with them, specifically when she suggests that the mothers do not (cannot allow themselves to?) experience deep emotion. Clearly, Scheper-Hughes's own response is ambivalent, as how could it not be? At times she seems to indict the mothers and the community as broken, predatory, and dangerously failing in the tasks of everyday life; at other times she sees the denizens of Bom Jesus in a more sympathetic light as engaging in the tactics of survival under almost impossible odds; then again, at other places in this very long book, they become heroes and heroines in a cultural melodrama of capitalist oppression.

About the only hopeful event is the possibility *carnaval* offers of a space of forgetting, being subversive, and offering resistance. "If the everyday world is structured by the metaphor of the *luta* in which suffering (*sofrimento*), pain (*dor*), and sickness (*doenca*) mask one's passage through time and space along the path that leads inevitably to death, then once a year *carnaval* ruptures the linear and tragic trajec-tory" (p. 481). But in fact little in the way of effective criticism or resistance erupts into public space. The poor of Bom Jesus are not reb-els, they are skeptical of radical solutions, though the author seems to want to maintain the hope that they might revolt. Rather, by keeping the peace and enduring, they tell us about an even more terrible turn in the ontology of suffering that Scheper-Hughes does not explore: namely, that men and women can endure, survive, and even adapt to the most inhuman of conditions. Though Scheper-Hughes mentions transcendence and transformation, we don't see much of it in her de-scription, and the thrust of the ethnography makes the reader doubt that these terms could be anything but a romantic reaction to the mundane horror of it all. There are no heroes here.

Scheper-Hughes's considerable artistry helps her to conclude some-thing valuable about the place of social and personal meaning and action in the desperate world she has so impressively recreated for her readers: "in granting power, agency, choice, and efficacy to the oppressed subject, one must begin to hold the oppressed morally accountable for their collusions, collaborations, rationalizations, 'false consciousness,' and more than occasional paralysis of will" (p. 533). The ambiguity of her summary seems right to this reader for a subject in which the humanity of the victims is at war with the social reality of their participation in the victimization.

Scheper-Hughes's ethnography, despite many strengths, also has a number of problems. At times the voice of the author is shrill and polemical. Her use of "bad faith" as a criticism hints at a tendency to be extreme and one-sided that is generally controlled, yet occasionally bursts through the scholarly constraints. Calling the *favela* a bad-faith economy is not only one-sided but contrary to the generosity that the author otherwise extends to its members (pp. 126–127). Calling most physicians and anthropologists exemplars of bad faith because they fail to recognize the secret indignation of the poor and the hunger pains of starving communities is so extreme a claim as to render this part of the ethnography suspect of exaggeration and name-calling (pp. 167–177, 209). Whereas the section on the lived experience of hunger is an effective description of the everyday reality of chronic starvation and its effects (pp. 135–140), the equally important section on hun-ger and sex (pp. 163–166) is uncharacteristically superficial, as if this was one area of collective and personal life into which she felt con-strained not to trespass. Why? The view of *nervoso* (nerves) as an idiom of hunger is original and important, but surely *nervoso* is a social idiom for other kinds of distress as well. Scheper-Hughes's account of the experienced meaning of nerves as hunger alone is an example of anthropological reductionism to a single source.

In the course of this one-sided argument about "somatization," Scheper-Hughes discounts much of medical anthropology, for which this topic has been an important issue over several decades. Many of the conclusions she draws about the social sources and consequences of bodily forms of distress are presented as if they were original; in fact they represent long-standing conclusions in the field. For example, she accuses me of writing too narrow a medical and cognitive account of somatization, based upon the idea of defense mechanisms, which she dismisses with a wave of the hand; yet most of the conclusions she draws about somatization in 1992 (pp. 186, 195) are in fact conclusions I drew in my major publication on the subject in 1986, *Social Origins of Distress and Disease,* a work she fails to cite. The idea of defense mechanisms is not the main point Joan Kleinman and I make in the 1985 paper Scheper-Hughes does cite (p. 185). At the least, this self-serving lapse is a matter of poor scholarship.

Other problems include a tendency at times for a "good guys, bad guys" analysis that, precisely because the ethnographic descriptions are so thickly human and morally complex, seems simplistic and out of place (p. 244). The rhetoric heats up to revolutionary levels at these times, but given the atrocities she witnesses and the author's openness about her two-sided role as ethnographer and community organizer, this is readily understandable. The analysis properly accuses the state for its not so invisible hand in creating human misery. Yet the author would do well to push the political analysis further. Inasmuch as we live in a time of failed states—the former Yugoslavia, Liberia, Somalia, Rwanda, Cambodia, Afghanistan—where violence, which seems nearly uncontrollable, emerges out of anarchic ethnic and class and factional conflict, one might well wonder whether the inhabitants of Bom Jesus suffer only from the brutalities of state repression and the routinization of poverty, or perhaps also from an absence of social control because the state is unwilling to be present or incapable of exerting responsible local authority. If so, and sometimes the author seems to suggest that one of these alternatives may be the case, the analysis needs to go more originally beyond the conventions of the critique of the abuses of state power, to more fully interpret the failure of the state as a source of security and protector of well-being where the problem is the absence of appropriate state power. In a volume that in other ways is so ambitious and important, there is surprisingly little done to build original social theory about the violence of everyday life.

The author, in an act of courage and moral engagement, takes a child away from a mother who is neglectful, almost mortally neglectful (p. 343). Yet elsewhere in the book she criticizes middle-class Brazilians for doing the same thing. This would seem to be a double standard that calls for self-reflective enquiry. What we get instead is a description of a melodrama in which the author has become a chief actor with lines that are often hyperbolic, and therefore a missed opportunity for some deeper critical reflection (see p. 436). This problem probably explains why the analysis of women and grieving is less convincing than in Seremetakis's ethnography. It also keeps the author from probing into the complexities of person and actions on the part of her friend Biu. The photo of Biu (p. 466) is hauntingly complex; the biographical description is richly suggestive and highly germane; but there is little analysis of how Biu is to be understood. That Scheper-Hughes shies away from too intricate a description of a good friend whose behavior is personally troubling to her is understandable. But because Biu is such a larger-than-life protagonist in the book Scheper-Hughes's reticence leaves the reader ultimately disappointed.

Here, then, is an ethnography of considerable importance and deft artistry that works hard to be a serious contribution to the study of human misery as well. That it is marred by the problems I have noted also needs to be taken into account in summing up the value of the work. In his introduction to Emile Zola's *Germinal,* Leonard Tancock, the masterly translator, defends Zola against those critics who contend that the author exaggerates the suffering of the immiserated mid-nineteenth-century French miners who are the subject of his narrative. "It is," says Tancock, "a grandiose epic poem of human misery and the revolt of the oppressed, but in no sense a true account of affairs as they could ever have existed at a given time." That is to say, to produce the effect he wanted the tale to have on readers, Zola took liberty with details, dates, and occurrences. Scheper-Hughes's narrative also carries telltale signs of exaggeration, including a powerful narrative line stuffed with all the classical tropes of desperation and squalor, compression of events, selective presentation of detail, illiterate women whose voices are almost too fluidly eloquent, and a very thin line between the author's incandescent sense of injustice and her disciplined ethnographic description of "the facts" of everyday life. The reader wonders if this is tragedy masquerading as ethnography—an epic of wretchedness, not a social scientific treatise. Whatever it is, it is memorable, a major achievement, and will be, as the author intended, a provocation to other researchers of human suffering.

At about the same time that *Death without Weeping* appeared, Pierre Bourdieu published *La Misère du Monde* (1993), a volume of studies under his direction by his students and coworkers. This book, too, has to do with the violence of everyday life, in this instance among the poor in France and North America. A huge (900 pages), unwieldy, and fragmented collection, the "testimonies" of misery that its authors present are stitched together by Bourdieu with a running commentary that is complex and not always coherent. Yet Bourdieu's remarks occasionally flash with brilliant originality as he too grapples with the frustrating crosscurrents in everyday worlds of brutality and wretchedness. These are ideas that ethnographers of social suffering will find helpful in formulating theory for their difficult subject.

For example, in his introductory "Lecteur," Bourdieu writes about the "misery of position," the social tragedy that comes from being placed in a more or less fixed position in the social order, which he contrasts with the "great misery" of the worst of social worlds and circumstances.[3] Bourdieu theorizes that because of the hierarchy of positioning, there is a "characteristic suffering of the social order." This is due especially to placement in localities where there are no functioning institutions, where people are survivors of "an immense collective disaster" like the closing of factories, for which he has in mind American inner-city ghettos and impoverished, immigrant Parisian *banlieues* (suburbs). The social tragedy of its occupants also results from the collision of social interests. He describes one such *banlieue* where a factory had closed, leaving behind an urban desert, a big avenue without trees, without houses, walling in discrimination, despair, and fatalism among the survivors. Here the state is absent—there are no schools, no health institutions, not even police. Commenting as well on essays in the volume by Loïc Wacquant about the south side of Chicago and Philippe Bourgois on Manhattan's Spanish Harlem, Bourdieu writes about the *lieu*, the point of space where an agent is situated, a locality for memory and emotion, a social site characterized by its relative position vis-à-vis other social localities, so that the lieu can be characterized by what is not in it. Writing of how the lieu also materializes hierarchy, social distance, and political appropriations, Bourdieu argues for the theorizing of social space as the relationship between the distribution of agents and goods that defines the value of different socially reified fields. Later on in his comments on "The Struggle for the Appropriation of Space," Bourdieu brings habitus and the habitual into juxtaposition with habitat in order to suggest how his theory of symbolic, cultural, and linguistic capital can be applied to understand how social space and bodily space intersect. While never entirely convincing, and at times it is characteristically elliptical, Bourdieu's prose is a crucial struggle to develop social theory that will support comparative ethnographies of social suffering, so that ethnographers can go beyond personification to understand social misery as social experience. In this respect, *La Misère du Monde,* for all its wordiness, points to a telling absence in Scheper-Hughes's account. *Death without Weeping* does not offer a social theoretical interpretation to match its extraordinary intensity of descriptive prose. Yet, without social theory, it is uncertain how different ethnographies of the violence of everyday living can construct an ethnographic subject that differs from that of psychologists or novelists. I would hazard the suggestion, therefore, that the search for social theories of the human misery of violence, poverty, and oppression will preoccupy the next generation of ethnographers.

The Ethnography of Medical Education and Biomedical Science

Two of medical anthropology's senior members, who are among the most theoretically oriented in the field—Byron Good and Allan Young—have published many influential articles since the late 1970s. Curiously, both are publishing their first single-author book in the mid-1990s. Not surprisingly, then, both books are extraordinarily rich combinations of social theory and ethnography. Both Good and Young began their careers with studies of illness and healing in the non-Western world: a Turkish community in Iran and an ethnic region of Ethiopia, respectively. Both later turned to biomedicine in their own society: Good to the study of how medical students are initiated into the biomedical gaze, and Young to an ethnography of a clinical center for the treatment of posttraumatic stress disorder (PTSD) which is the basis for an exploration of psychiatric science. Taken together, these contributions substantially extend our understanding of the cultural grounds of biomedicine and of science generally. It is not accidental that two senior practitioners of medical anthropology have settled on the anthropology of science and technology. This is becoming a central topic in the discipline, even if the number of ethnographies of biomedical science is still quite limited. Reviewing both contributions will enable me to return to several themes developed in the essays in part 1 of this book.

Byron Good's (1994) *Medicine, Rationality, and Experience: An Anthropological Perspective,* hot off the press at the time I am writing this chapter, is a serious contribution to theory in medical anthropology and in anthropology more generally. Based upon the Lewis Henry Morgan Lectures that he gave at the University of Rochester in 1990, one of anthropology's most prestigious lecture series, Good's book packs together a variety of things including theoretical explorations across virtually the entire field of medical anthropology, several ethnographic chapters, and reexamination of anthropology's longstanding debate on rationality. His ideas will be discussed and debated over the years to come because they offer seminal observations on so many different themes in medical anthropology. It is not my purpose here to review the entire book; instead I focus narrowly on the book's main ethnographic contribution, a study of the education of medical students at Harvard Medical School. Although presented in only a single chapter, in fact the ethnographic materials in this chapter are the grounds for much of Good's analysis of medicine, science, and rationality, and they in turn are effective precisely because Good has prepared the way in his earlier chapters.

Good's orienting concern is well summarized by the chapter's title, "How Medicine Constructs Its Objects." He observes that "*medicine formulates the human body and disease in a culturally distinctive fashion*" (p. 65; italics are in the original). Medical students are taught in this distinctive manner an approach to the reality of diagnosis and the nature of treatment that seems "natural" and outside of culture. To the contrary, insists Good, "*biology is not external to but very much within culture*" (p. 66; italics are in the original). This large claim Good identifies as a continuation of Foucault's (1972) examination of the changing objects of medicine historically. But it is not the French historian and philosopher of science but rather Ernst Cassirer (1955) of the *Philosophy of Symbolic Forms* who provides Good with a *modus operandi:* namely, Cassirer's idea of "formative processes." In the long-term European debate between empiricism and idealism, Cassirer, a Kantian up to a point, proposed that symbolic forms (culture) organize reality distinctively. Cassirer was interested in the "formative principles" in language, myth, religion, art, and science that give to life its particular cultural shape. The formative principles create their own symbolic forms, which in turn constitute reality. The objects of religion, mythology, aesthetics, and science are those crucial symbolic forms. "The 'objects' of medicine are similar kind" (p. 68). Foucault's (1972) notion of the discursive practices subsumed under a particular discourse and the contemporary social anthropological concern with "practice" (Ortner 1994) are viewed by Good as ways of approaching this study of the symbolic mediation of reality, including medical reality. For Good, the materialist and moral components of medicine's symbolic forms are exemplified in "the role of medicine in mediating physiology and soteriology" (p. 70).

Medical students learn to construct medical reality through the practices of "seeing," "writing," and "speaking," which they undertake from day one in the medical school. For Good, medical education commences with anatomy: "entry into the human body" (p. 72). In anatomy laboratories the body as they have known and lived it is made over into a medical object. Reflecting on his own participant observation, Good observes: "One of the most shocking moments in anatomy lab was the day we entered to find the body prepared for dissecting the genitalia, the body sawn in half above the waist, then bisected between the legs. Students described their shock not at close examination of the genitalia, nor simply at the body being taken apart, but rather at the dismemberment, and at dismemberment that crossed natural boundaries."

Students are self-reflexive about learning a new way of seeing: along tissue planes, through gross dissection, under the microscope in finer and finer detail. Learning medicine is learning to reconstruct the world anew, medically. "Modern imaging techniques give a powerful sense of authority to biological reality. Look in the microscope, you can see it. Electron microscopy reveals histological concepts as literal. Look for yourself—there it is!" (p. 74).

In learning to see medically salient objects, students learn a hierarchical order of biological reality. The patient with the symptoms of a pathological entity like arthritis is compared to the pathological anatomical specimen. The gross specimen is compared to the microscopic picture; the latter is further reduced to derangement in biochemical processes at the molecular level. Thus, a student tells Good how he first learned about schizophrenia as behavior, then about genetics, and thereby came to see it as a disordered protein, still unknown, but lurking in nature as the "concrete" locus of the affliction. The strategy of teaching is to deconstruct a health problem by projecting a hierarchy of images from epidemiological slides of population-based data, through slides of individual patients, to slides at ever lower levels of the biological order of pathology. Like "the great chain of being" in an earlier epoch of Western civilization in which the ontological order is presented from animals to God, the late twentieth century's biological order instates a central hierarchy, but one in which "lower" rather than "higher" forms of reality are more fundamental. Thus, Good describes the cultural practices through which biological reductionism becomes the central vision of the medical student. Reductionism for the student is not epistemological commitment; rather, it is an active process of ontological genesis (objectification) of medical objects out of human problems.

From medical seeing, Good turns to learning medical writing and speaking. He demonstrates with examples from the experiences of Harvard medical students that the write-up of a medical case "is not a mere record of a verbal exchange. It is itself a formative practice, a practice that shapes talk as much as it reflects it, a means of constructing a person as a patient, a document, and a project" (p. 77). Writing authorizes the neophyte physician as an expert with a certain methodological expertise. It also organizes the interactions with the patient. Interviewing, writing, and speaking before a clinical audience instruct students on how to edit the person and the context out of the account of the disease and its treatment, the key elision in converting pathos into pathology.

One student described his early clinical experience: "I think the main thing . . . you learn [is] kind of the daily rhythm, which is rounds in the morning, work rounds, what are work rounds, what are attending rounds, what are visit rounds. . . . [A] big part of rounds is presenting cases, and in some ways that's probably the biggest thing medical students learn. . . . Doing case presentations is probably the main thing you concentrate on. . . . [For] the medical student, their one chance to be in the limelight is when they present, and it's also probably the area where you're most likely to either gain the respect or . . . the annoyance of your colleagues, and especially your superiors." (p. 79)

Good dissects student presentations as a genre of storytelling. "Virtually every student remembers the pain of telling a story poorly and enraging a resident or attending" (p. 79). The clinical presentation uses rhetorical strategies to "persuade your audience," as one of Good's medical students aptly puts it. "Students," observes Good, "become quickly aware of the performance dimension. They rehearse presentations, learn to give them without notes, even to make up details if they do not remember exactly, and are very aware of the response" (p. 80).

Clinical stories, for Good,

are one means of organizing and interpreting experience, of projecting idealized and anticipated experiences, a distinctive way of formulating reality and ideological ways of interacting with it. . . . [P]resenting cases is not merely a way of depicting reality but a way of constructing it. It is one of a set of closely linked formative practices through which disease is organized and responded to in contemporary American teaching hospitals. Case presentations represent disease as the object of medical practice . . . localized spatially in tissue lesions . . . and temporally in abstract, medicalized time. . . . The patient is formulated as a medical project. (p. 80)

Seeing, writing, and talking "medically," the student is authorized to be a participant in a Wittgensteinian "language game" that in turn creates a "way of life"—an ontology of being medical. And that ontology has "tremendous consequences in the real world" (p. 81). As one of the protagonists in his striking excerpts from interviews with informants troublingly puts it:

It often seems like as medical students we kind of slide into doing these kinds of things which can have just unimaginably great consequences for patients and we just sort of do it because we've incrementally learned about the biology and the science and the pathology and the pharmacology and we kind of inch into it and suddenly then we are saying, I'll write the orders that such and such be done to this patient. (p. 81)

Good demonstrates how the experiences of students in the totalizing environs of the hospital socialize them into a hierarchy whose control is exerted through the transformation of the arbitrary into the logical, the symbolic into the real, and that also teaches them to misrecognize what is "cultural" for what is "natural." In conducting this demonstration, Good is at pains to avoid posing the conventional criticisms of medicine that would seem to flow from his accounts. His cultural deconstruction has a more original and fundamental purpose. To understand "medicine as a symbolic formation," Good avers, it must be seen to contain not only the rational-technical organization of physiology, but also an existential, or as he puts it, soteriological dimension (p. 84). The medical student is part of a "moral drama" of human fear and suffering, and of a confrontation with death. When the moral erupts into the domain of the technical-rational, however, it is misrecognized as yet another technical-rational object. Thereby the life world is colonized by an instrumental rationality that cannot possibly engage moral questions. And yet, Good observes, based upon a long experience in medical settings, "Medical practice can never fully contain the moral and the soteriological" (p. 85). Students—not all but still many—want a passionate engagement with this human side of sickness. And this desire to be a healer of persons persists, in spite of all the technical training, in clinical practice. This is what makes medicine the particular form of experience that it is. But Good has even another turn of the screw in store for the reader.

"What I am suggesting is that medicine is deeply implicated in our contemporary image of what constitutes the suffering from which we and others hope to be delivered and our culture's vision of the means of redemption" (p. 86). In an epoch with a commitment to the cultural prisms of materialism and individualism, health replaces salvation. Thus, salvation becomes a hidden part of medicine's powerful technology and also contributes to popular outrage about the practice of medicine.

Regrettably, Good's discussion of this crucial question is barely long enough to set it firmly on the table. How do medical students and practitioners experience the soteriological? What is the ontology of redemption in medical work? What are its forms cross-culturally, especially when biomedicine is practiced outside the Judeo-Christian tradition, where redemption's lineaments are culturally authorized? Good deploys his formidable analytic structure to address many important aspects of illness, care, and medical science, aspects that will make his book influential, yet the theme of salvation, so resonant and so original, is not unpacked much further. A rapprochement between medical anthropology, the anthropology of religion, and anthropological approaches to ethics would seem a next step in the conversation on the culture of medicine that Good's impressive mix of social theory and ethnography so usefully facilitates.

That medical science and practice is a domain in which the moral, the existential, and the scientific traffic is a conclusion that Allan Young's (in press) account of posttraumatic stress disorder does not find inappropriate. Young's *The Harmony of Illusions*[4] examines the emergence of PTSD as a collective representation and as a new object in psychiatric science in order to understand "Western rationality" as consisting of a culturally specific way of narrating certain events and of asserting epistemological privilege. Leaning on the work of Ludwik Fleck (1979), Young takes the title of his ethnography from the idea that "rational inference is a way of narrating the production of facts, rather than a technique used for producing them." Fleck, himself a biological scientist, held that "scientific facts" are products of "thought collectives," networks of scientists with particular "thought styles." For Fleck, the "thought collective" is engaged in knowledge production and communication. The peculiar "thought style" of a collective, in Young's reformulation, is an assemblage that includes technologies, rhetorics, and paradigms. The stability of a network of scientists' agreements on concepts, methods, and outcome is not based in their rationality but is what Fleck, referring to the achievement of the collective's social process of knowledge production, calls "the harmony of illusions." It is this harmony of illusions based on the entire social apparatus of science as a form of social production that gives the scientist the sense of something in the real world that resists his studies and constrains his thinking. In actuality, every scientific object is a "technophenomenon" created out of the socially constructed process of rational-technical production. Only in after-the-fact accounts do scientists narrate a different story about the scientific process that separates it from the "reality" of its objects, the phenomena it studies *and* produces.

Young proceeds from a theoretical grounding in the anthropology of science to explore the gap between scientists' (and philosophers') formulations of the rationality of science as rule-guided by ideas of inference, contradiction, and falsifiability and the anthropological interpretation of the process of scientific work. The latter is closer to a view of science as the stuff of analogical thinking—metaphors, models, narration—working through instances and applications in local settings from which the particular is elaborated into the general. Much of Young's book is an effort—almost wholly convincing to my mind—to interpret PTSD as an example of these (and other) social processes.

Thus, Young shows how the community of researchers comes together, creates its object (traumatic memory), establishes its preformed template for generating knowledge, advocates official diagnostic status, creates consensus on instruments of measurement, authorizes the "validity" of *findings/facts* and diffuses and promotes the official narrative of what PTSD is and how it should be treated. Were Young's account an airtight blow-by-blow description of the forging of "entity" through community out of "meanings," it would be much less arresting than it is. What gives this volume its exhilarating effect are its extraordinary digressions. For in telling his story, Young tells many side and sub and supra stories, all part of the major account, yet several of which take on a life of their own, much to the fascination of the reader.

For example, Young dilates on constructions of probability in a section that starts off as an argument about testability, reliability, and validity, yet ends up with a surprising detour through the writings of statisticians and others whose work bears upon the much wider issue of the scientific meaning of "facts." Similarly, an arresting discussion of the social organization of time in scientific discourse is spun out of Young's interest in fallibility. But to my mind, the most intriguing discussion is Young's account of W. H. R. Rivers's contribution to the "discovery" of "traumatic memories."

Rivers initially appears in the ethnography near the beginning of the manuscript during Young's historical survey of the problem of war-related trauma in the Great War and the way such traumas were handled by military psychiatry. This is a much more detailed account than is needed if Young's point is to show how the psychiatric formulation of war neuroses is constrained by the experience of war, the work of psychiatrists, and the lineaments of psychiatric discourse. Indeed, this almost certainly is Young's purpose, but once he has gotten into the scholarship, it is as if Young does not want to let go. And thank goodness he doesn't. Because what is astonishing about the chapter is what Young tells us about Rivers. To my knowledge, no one else makes the claim that from the beginning (in his classical ethnographies) through the middle years of neurological experiments and development of psychological constructs, right through to the final phase of clinical work, Rivers's greatly diverse contributions carry a unity, a coherence of framework that links such seemingly disparate domains as his ideas about suggestion, pathogenic and therapeutic; protopathic and epicritic neurological sensitivity; mimesis, sympathy, and intuition; the simple and dynamic unconscious; and the treatment of "shell shock," hysteria, and neurasthenia. Usually, Rivers is portrayed in medical anthropology as something of a romantic failure. Brilliant contributor to at least four separate fields—social anthropology as ethnography, experimental neuropathology, comparative psychology, and psychotherapy—Rivers's failure, it is assumed (and I, too, held the assumption), is that he does not leave behind him a legacy of an integrated field.

That is to say, while Rivers certainly *did* medical anthropology in one phase of his distinguished career, he did not build a program for medical anthropology as a field. If Young's reading is correct, then Rivers's contribution must be rethought as having succeeded in bridging ethnography, social theory, psychosomatics, and psychotherapy with a set of principles that laced together theory, methods, and practice in an exemplary, if heretofore unappreciated, manner. That this is not the received version has more to do with the great flood tide of psychoanalysis which Pierre Janet, like so many others, saw burying alternative programs, including, Young suggests, Rivers's, in the sand of oblivion.

Young's contagious affection for Rivers leads him to question as well the dichotomous portrayal of the electrical treatment practiced by Lewis Yealland and the talk therapy practiced by Rivers as the classical materialization in treatment of Britain's fundamental divide between silent working-class soldiers, who are punished for suffering hysterical paralysis in the face of battle, and upper-class officers afflicted with neurasthenia, who are talked out of their remorse-laden dilemmas. Young gives us a sense of how cultural historians like Eric Leed and Elaine Showalter and novelists like Pat Barker have overcoded a divide that is more and more porous, fuzzy, and complexly human. Young's reconstruction of the case is a tour de force that could stand entirely on its own as an independent essay. Yet when woven into the book-length account it is not at all an unnecessary digression, but rather a highly instructive parenthesis that evokes the larger moral questions of how we understand warfare's traumatic effects at the same time that it develops the historical background for the military and psychiatric emergence of PTSD.

That same plethora of space encourages Young to include entire transcripts of group psychotherapy sessions in a Veterans Administration Hospital's "Center" for the treatment of Vietnam veterans suffering from PTSD as rich primary materials for understanding the discursive practices by which a psychoanalytic approach to trauma is used to construct the problem, to control the process, and to create the outcome of treatment—the social experience of efficacy—and its evaluation. Young's sensitivity in limiting his interpretation of these sessions makes the ethnographic materials all the more powerful as a demonstration of the social production of cure/treatment failure.

The limitations of this work are few, yet important. The description of the treatment unit is thin, as is discussion of the specific persons and groups engaged in PTSD as a collective project. Young is much more comfortable at interrogating or deconstructing the historical record and philosophical texts than he is in pursuing the interpretation of how the treatment sessions change the participants. Much of this story implicates American culture, yet the engagement with questions of power in American history and ethnography is limited. Surprisingly, Young has written himself largely out of the account. Yet, as a participant in the Vietnam War era, we need to learn more about how he is positioned. None of these problems seriously limits the significance of Young's accomplishment. At the end, we are led back to the moral and political abuses that American politicians, military leaders, and policy planners perpetrated on American soldiers, who quite obviously themselves became perpetrators as well as victims. Traumatic memories are more than objects of professional practice and scientific inquiry; they are a particular instance of the human atrocity of war for combatants and noncombatants alike. PTSD is part of this nasty legacy. For here medicine, politics, and morality are inescapably connected in cultural processes that construct the experience of trauma as well as the experience of diagnosing and treating its sources. (See chap. 8 above.) And here, too, science is implicated in the politics of history. As the Vietnam War recedes as memory of a distant past, the *DSM-IV* widens the criteria so that traumatic memory can encompass the fashionable human problems of the new world disorder.

Margaret Lock (1993a), Allan Young's colleague at McGill, has also written a book that contributes to the anthropology of biomedical science, although this is only one of its sides. *Encounters with Aging: Mythologies of Menopause in Japan and North America* is a curious, yet powerful, ethnography. It is curious from the perspective of ethnography because the research framework is a large survey of Japanese women regarding their experiences and ideas of menopause. Thus, there is no community or even network that grounds the study. Rather Lock and her associates traveled to many different settings in Japan to interview the survey's respondents, few of whom they knew well and many of whom lived and worked in locales that they did not study. What organizes the respondents' narratives is a focus on the social experience of aging in Japan and the place of menopause in that large cultural, moral, and political context. Playing off quantitative data against personal stories, Lock succeeds in creating an ethnographic focus that includes the cultural forms of Japanese society and their multifarious, contradictory, and changing contours. Against that huge ethnographic landscape, she contrasts materials from studies of menopause in Canada and the United States by sociologist colleagues— Patricia Kaufert and Sonja McKinley—with whom she has collaborated. The outcome is a success at comparative research that is even more impressive precisely because this style of work is becoming uncommon in anthropology.

Lock draws on the many studies she has conducted in Japan and her comprehensive knowledge of Japanese history and society to create a richly textured backdrop for her narratives and numbers. What starts out as research on menopause quickly takes on a much larger theme, as it becomes clear that the subject matter—as the book's title insists—is really aging, particularly the aging of women. Japanese women across the social spectrum do not seem fixated on the end of menstruation as a time of disruption or decrepitude. Nor are symptoms like hot flashes and drenching night sweats, which are commonplace in North America, either widely experienced by menopausal Japanese women or disturbing. The symptoms they focus upon, when they focus on complaints (and many don't), are different ones—shoulder stiffness, for instance. *Konenki,* the relevant Japanese term, "means something more encompassing than the end of menstruation . . . part of a general aging process in which greying hair, changing eyesight, and an aching and tired body appears to have more significance than does the end of the menstrual cycle" (p. 6). *Konenki* conveys the idea of "change of life," but even that is contradicted and contested by respondents. Konenki "is not a subject that generates a great deal of anxiety or concern" (pp. 10, 14). There is "no deep sense of loss at this time of life" (p. 45).

What regret there is, for some but by no means all Japanese respondents, is "about the way in which choices made by their parents when the women were very young imposed major limitations on what they can realistically expect to do in middle age" (p. 50). Many were simply not educated for jobs in the workforce, but were prepared only for marriage and family life. The burden of taking care of sick elderly relatives comes across in the narratives as a constraint on midlife options. But criticism of this or any other part of their life of service in the family is balanced by many positive aspects of that role which is seen as "natural" to the social experience of women. The narratives of aging informants provide Lock with a prism to refract the light of anthropological critique on the moral order of Japanese society. She canvasses, *inter alia,* the "natural" subjugation of women (p. 83), the domestic "cult of productivity" (p. 89), the image of the "good wife and wise mother" (p. 89), and the priority of interpersonal good over subjective desire in order to understand how cultural themes organize the life course of Japanese women. Yet within the norms she discloses the paradoxes: "society values hard work, perseverance, and self-discipline; but running a small modern household for a husband absent most of the time requires few of these virtues" (p. 101). Women work hard within the family and in a variety of positions outside, yet critics castigate them for boredom, a life of luxury and selfishness: "a moral disease accompanies the physical symptoms of *konenki*" (p. 103).

It is to Lock's credit as an ethnographic analyst sensitive to the complexity of ethnographic contexts that she evokes and then deconstructs this and other myths not because she wishes to expose a "different" reality, but because she wishes to show that social reality itself is plural and heterogeneous; it is formed, she avers, by a dynamic dialect between culture and psychobiology that sponsors multiple and differing outcomes. The narratives she recounts are filled with the peculiar details of distinctive lives and life worlds. Reading them, we feel we are brought into the midst of the multiplicity of experiences of aging Japanese women as fully as if we had read the relevant sections of highly condensed novels. Contrasting survey data with narratives empowers Lock to go back and forth between particular and shared themes.

Of the latter, the ones that impress themselves most insistently on the book are "fatigue from misery" (p. 123), the sacrifices of daughters-in-law in the generation born in the prewar era, who do not expect the care they have devoted to their elderly in-laws to be devoted to them, the "illusion of indolence," and the changing modes of social experience which make the feel of life as well as its meanings transitory. Lock shows the role of mythologies of aging as ideology in Japanese society, where that ideology supports the interests of a conservative order that has produced economic success and social harmony at the expense of personal flourishing. She provides many illustrations, enough to show us the atypical as well as the normative. The marvels of narrative are the intricacies of detail which color experience and enable us to appreciate the fine grain of improvisation, novelty, and difference that make life so much more than a model or statistic can convey. Lock lets the transcripts of her recordings proceed. She plays them at length so that we feel we get to know her respondents. And those respondents, it turns out, have a lot to say, much more than is coded into their numerical answers on the questionnaire. Yet there is also ample interpretive commentary so that the book is hers, not theirs.

At times, Lock seems frustrated with her subjects' passivity in the face of systematic pressure to be restrained and accepting of the naturalness of the ideology of male-dominated families. Lock clearly wants these Japanese women to fight back. Yet, though most of her informants seem resigned, they are not altogether unhappy. They find meaning and satisfaction as wives and mothers. The very process of naturalization gives them important status and even identity. And they are not terribly bothered by menopause, even though some, and perhaps many, regret the constraint on the self. Maturation within the Japanese social order is not "a search for a 'true,' autonomous self but rather a lifelong process . . . in which individuals come to understand themselves first and foremost as social beings, as products of units and forces larger than themselves and without which they could not exist" (p. 202). There is also self-cultivation, albeit in this decidedly social idiom, and Lock lets us see that, including its resonance with the "theme of self-discipline culminating in eventual escape from the toil of this world" that has cachet in the religious contour of Japanese history (p. 206).

The large body of materials on child development in Japanese society are put to excellent use in support of the overall argument. Hence, we learn how habitus is formed out of the cultural phenomenology of sensibility to the *interpersonal* as the bodily grounds of social life. Of the emotions, Lock suggests that loss and depression are not nearly as salient in the social experience of middle-aged Japanese women as they are in the West. Rather anger (more often irritability) and its control are central to the Japanese experience. Thus, the Japanese comparison undercuts leading Western perspectives on the life cycle.

"Reflecting on the entire female life span, we would say that middle age in Japan is relatively inviting, a transition from which individuals can both look back over the previous fifty years and forward to the next thirty and, given financial security, usually report good fortune and happiness. Nonetheless, a closer look at some of the narratives of middle-aged women reveals that beneath the surface of apparently unruffled lives a good deal of 'low-profile' resistance (Scott 1990, p. 198) takes place much of the time" (p. 240). This is the part of Lock's analysis which is least successful; probably because we would need ethnographic description of families and work settings over time in order to reveal the subtleties and longer-term effects of such techniques of resistance as "retreatism," "ritualism," and divorce.

Lock's success as an analyst comes in no small measure from her honesty about the kinds of data she doesn't possess and therefore the limits on her interpretation. How many researchers working with so much information and with so much at stake in the analysis would conclude as she does that no single pattern or cluster of relationships emerges from the study? There is no simple mapping of konenki onto distressing personal or family situations. The same sensibility to the refractory heterogeneity of social experience characterizes Lock's portrait of the diversity of medical responses. There is no doctor bashing, but neither is there any camouflaging of the confusion in the changing patterns of medical practice. Danger looms less from medicalization from the medical profession than from the building pressure of the drug industry. Nor does Lock fail to see the potential political danger of an essentializing, indigenous culture-biology discourse that picks up on racialist sentiment about "being Japanese."

There is another side to this book. Lock is effective at contrasting the sensitivity of the Japanese discourse on konenki to cultural peculiarity with the concern of North American and European discourses to sustain the universal nature of menopause. The making of menopause in the West is a story so substantial that it almost escapes from the limits of the book as Lock leads us through two centuries of Western medical writings. Yet, again her history as much as her anthropology is scrupulous about not caricaturing traditions. As she states, "there was (and is) no simple unveiling of scientific knowledge and no ready consensus in the medical world on an accurate representation of the menopausal transition; on the contrary, argument and speculation were (and remain) rife" (p. 317).

Lock's passion is clearly aroused when she describes the tendentious arguments of medical researchers in the West to the effect that menopause is a hormone-deficiency disease requiring endocrine replacement therapy, and when she attacks a misogynist psychoanalytic portrayal of the menopause that reads in the 1990s like an indictment of an entire discipline.

Menopause, Lock concludes, "is neither fact nor universal event but an experience that we must interpret in context" (p. 370). Her ethnography, like others featured in this review, is concerned with *lived experience* as the key to unlocking the mysteries of the social world. That understanding, she observes frequently, should be of "an intimate exchange between biology and culture" (p. 372) that shows that both are malleable and mutually constructive. Both are forms of local knowledge, of local experience.

Lock is also serious about theory. The prologue and epilogue frame the research and the review of the literature with a discussion of the way ideology enters into scientific discourse as well as into embodiment and subjectivity, with a reflection on the relationship of subjectivity and objectivity, and with an argument about the making of women as agents of social reproduction and as scientific facts. Particularly appealing is her discussion of the politics of knowledge, about which she gives so many telling examples in the book's 387 pages of text.

Any good book, and this is a good book, shows its limitations in building its strengths. Lock's combination of survey and ethnography points toward the culture-biology dialectic, yet doesn't say much about how it may be mediated. Perhaps this is because she tends to focus on the absence of hot flashes among Japanese women rather than on their own key symptoms. The reader suspects much more could be made of the social experiences of shoulder stiffness and fatigue among Lock's respondents as the interpenetration of memory, meaning, and moral physiology. But to do so would mean grounding them in interpersonal worlds. And so effective is Lock's description that we easily forget that this is not a study of any particular community. Also, for all the emphasis on the wider compass of aging, Lock's review of historical and ethnographic works does not engage the literatures in the history and anthropology of aging as much as one would expect. Although Lock makes excellent use of the work of Ian Hacking on the normal as norm and ideal, she doesn't choose to interrogate her own statistical data from this perspective.

Finally, the concluding interlude on hegemony seems stretched because the cultural account she has written is so sensitive to the multiplicity of social life. It is as if at the very end of her important volume, Lock felt the need to reassure herself that she was encompassing power sufficiently; hence the last few paragraphs on medicalization seem forced. Clearly, the hegemony she must deal with is much more diffused in family, work, and community. And what kind of hegemony can it be anyway if she can so convince us of pluralism, diversity, and change. One suspects that the nemesis is not medical but bodily. Japanese women do not routinely experience menopause as distress but neither do they experience life-cycle constraints and patriarchal oppression as distress. The hegemony perhaps is in the cultural illusion of bodily harmony, to put Fleck's attractive term to a different use, as social and personal well-being. And here perhaps Lock's aging Japanese women do get the last word, for by outliving men and crafting lives of significance, they suggest that the very idea of a burden or crisis of aging Japanese women is not their problem (strictly speaking it is a problem of their mothers and mothers-in-law) any more than menopause is, and it may not be their society's either. I take that to be one of the surprises that Margaret Lock wants her readers to consider.

There are other important ethnographies in this gathering wave besides those I have reviewed. The ethnography books written by Martha Balsham (1993), René Devisch (1993), Faye Ginsburg (1989), John Janzen (1992), Roland Littlewood (1993), Mark Nichter (1989), Lorna Rhodes (1991), Carolyn Sargent (1989), Unni Wikan (1990), and Francis Zimmermann (1987), to mention only a few, are serious and innovative contributions to the broad field of medical anthropology. They deserve to be reviewed too, but it is simply infeasible to describe them all. Although this review is restricted, I have tried to *illustrate* at least certain of the contributions that are remaking medical anthropology today. Their success means that there is no single agenda that dominates the field; instead, there are multiple styles, plural subjects, different methodologies, distinctive visions. In each ethnography, the working through of anthropology's cultural program and current concerns in social analysis takes a special turn. What is shared among the books derives as much from the recalcitrance of medical subjects as from the project of cultural analysis. After two decades in medical anthropology, I feel heartened by the quality of the ethnography, and by the promise it holds for scholarship. I do not doubt that ethnography is medical anthropology's most important contribution. Yet, as Charles Leslie[5] has reminded the practitioners of this interdisciplinary field, the measure of its success must also include evidence that it matters for people in the world outside the academy. That will require additional steps that bring medical ethnographies into the domain of policies, programs, and practices.[6]

Appendix:
Works by Arthur Kleinman

Books Authored

Kleinman, A. *Patients and Healers in the Context of Culture: An Exploration of the Borderland between Anthropology, Medicine, and Psychiatry.* Berkeley, Los Angeles, London: University of California Press, 1980. (427 pp.) Translated into Japanese: Kobundo, Tokyo.

Kleinman, A. *Social Origins of Distress and Disease: Neurasthenia, Depression, and Pain in Modern China.* New Haven, Conn.: Yale University Press, 1986 (264 pp.).

Kleinman, A. *The Illness Narratives: Suffering, Healing, and the Human Condition.* New York: Basic Books, 1988. (284 pp.) Translated into Japanese: Seishin Shobo Ltd., Tokyo; and French: Presses Universitaires de France, Paris; and Chinese: Laureate Book Co., Taipei, Taiwan.

Kleinman, A. *Rethinking Psychiatry: From Cultural Category to Personal Experience.* New York: Free Press, 1988. (237 pp.)

Edited Books

Kleinman, A., P. Kunstadter, E. R. Alexander, and J. L. Gale, eds. *Medicine in Chinese Cultures: Comparative Perspectives.* Washington, D.C.: U.S. Government Printing Office for Fogarty International Center, N.I.H., 1975. (803 pp.)

Manschreck, T. C., and A. Kleinman, eds. *Renewal in Psychiatry.* Washington, D.C.: Hemisphere Publishers, Halsted Press, 1977. (346 pp.)

Kleinman, A., P. Kunstadter, E. R. Alexander, and J. L. Gale, eds. *Culture and*

257

Healing in Asian Societies: Anthropological, Psychiatric, and Public Health Studies. Cambridge, Mass.: Schenkman Publishing Co., 1978. (462 pp.)

Eisdorfer, C., D. Cohen, A. Kleinman, and P. Maxim, eds. *Conceptual Models for Psychopathology.* New York: Spectrum, 1981. (276 pp.)

Eisenberg, L., and A. Kleinman, eds. *The Relevance of Social Science for Medicine.* Dordrecht, Holland: D. Reidel Publishing Co., 1981. (422 pp.)

Kleinman, A., and T. Y. Lin, eds. *Normal and Abnormal Behavior in Chinese Culture.* Dordrecht, Holland: D. Reidel Publishing Co., 1981. (436 pp.) Translated into Chinese: Chinese University of Hong Kong Press.

Kleinman, A., and B. Good, eds. *Culture and Depression.* Berkeley, Los Angeles, London: University of California Press, 1985. (535 pp.) Translated into Japanese: Sogensha, Osaka.

Osterweis, M., A. Kleinman, and D. Mechanic, eds. *Pain and Disability: Clinical, Behavioral, and Public Policy Perspectives.* Washington, D.C.: National Academy Press, 1987. (306 pp.)

Becker, J., and A. Kleinman, eds. *Psychosocial Aspects of Depression.* Hillsdale, N.J.: Lawrence Erlbaum, 1991. (254 pp.)

Chen, L., A. Kleinman, and N. Ware, eds. *Advancing Health in Developing Countries: The Role of Social Research.* Boston: Auburn House Publishers, 1992. (228 pp.)

Good, M.-J., P. Brodwin, B. Good, and A. Kleinman, eds. *Pain as Human Experience: An Anthropological Perspective.* Berkeley, Los Angeles, London: University of California Press, 1992. (214 pp.)

Chen, L., A. Kleinman, and N. Ware, eds. *Health and Social Change: An International Perspective.* Cambridge, Mass.: Harvard University Press, 1994. (508 pp.)

Desjarlais, R., L. Eisenberg, B. Good, and A. Kleinman, eds. *World Mental Health: Problems and Priorities in Low-Income Countries.* New York: Oxford University Press, 1995. (382 pp.)

Articles in Journals and Books

1973

Kleinman, A. "The Background and Development of Public Health in China: An Exploratory Essay." In *Public Health in the People's Republic of China,* ed. M. E. Wegman, T. Y. Lin, and E. F. Purcell, 1–23. New York: Josiah Macy, Jr., Foundation.

Kleinman, A. "Medicine's Symbolic Reality: A Central Problem in the Philosophy of Medicine." *Inquiry* 16:206–213.

Kleinman, A. "Some Issues for a Comparative Study of Medical Healing." *International Journal of Social Psychiatry* 19:159–165.

Kleinman, A. "Toward a Comparative Study of Medical Systems." *Science, Medicine, and Man* 1:55–65.

1974

Kleinman, A. "Cognitive Structures of Traditional Medical Systems: Ordering, Explaining, and Interpreting the Human Experience of Illness." *Ethnomedicine* 3:27–49.

Kleinman, A. "A Comparative Cross-Cultural Model for Studying Health Care in China." *Studies in Comparative Communism* 7:414–419.

Kleinman, A. "Cross-Cultural Studies of Illness and Health Care: A Preliminary Report." *Bulletin of the Chinese Society of Neurology and Psychiatry* 1(2): 1–5.

Kleinman, A. "Medical and Psychiatric Anthropology and the Study of Traditional Medicine in Modern Chinese Culture." *Journal of the Institute of Ethnology, Academica Sinica* 39:107–123.

Kleinman, A. "Social, Cultural, and Historical Themes in the Study of Medicine and Psychiatry in Chinese Societies: Problems and Prospects for the Comparative Study of Medical Systems." In *Medicine in Chinese Culture,* ed. A. Kleinman, P. Kunstadter, E. R. Alexander, and J. L. Gale, 589–644. Washington, D.C.: U.S. Government Printing Office for Fogarty International Center, N.I.H.

1977

Kleinman, A. "Depression, Somatization, and the New Cross-Cultural Psychiatry." *Social Science and Medicine* 11:3–10.

Kleinman, A. "Lessons from a Clinical Approach to Medical Anthropology." *M.A.N. (Medical Anthropology Newsletter)* 8(4): 11–15.

Kleinman, A. "Rethinking the Social and Cultural Context of Psychopathology and Psychiatric Care." In *Renewal in Psychiatry,* ed. T. C. Manschreck and A. Kleinman, 97–138. Washington, D.C.: Hemisphere Publishers, 1977.

1978

Kleinman, A. "Comparison of Traditional and Modern Practitioner-Patient Interactions in Taiwan: The Cultural Construction of Clinical Reality." In *Culture and Healing in Asian Societies,* ed. A. Kleinman, P. Kunstadter, E. R. Alexander, and J. L. Gale, 329–337. Cambridge, Mass.: Schenkman Publishing Co.

Kleinman, A. "Concepts and a Model for the Comparison of Medical Systems as Cultural Systems." *Social Science and Medicine* 12:85–93. Reprinted in *The Nation's Health,* ed. P. R. Lee (New York: Boyd and Frazer, 1981). Reprinted in *The Canadian Health Care System,* ed. C. Crichton, vol. 1 (Ottawa: Canadian Hospital Association, 1983). Reprinted in *Concepts of Health, Illness, and Disease: A Comparative Perspective,* ed. M. Stacey and C. Currer (Warwickshire, U.K.: Berg Publishing, 1986).

Kleinman, A. "International Health Care Planning from an Ethnomedical Perspective: Critique and Recommendations for Change." *Medical Anthropology* 2(2): 71–96.

Kleinman, A. "Native Healers." *Human Nature* 1(11): 63–69. Reprinted in *Emerging China*, ed. T. Draper, 186–194 (New York: H. W. Wilson Co., 1980), under the title "Taiwanese Folk Medicine." Reprinted in *Anthropology: Contemporary Perspectives*, 3d ed., ed. D. E. K. Hunter and P. Whitten, 266–269. Boston: Little, Brown and Co., 1982, under the title "The Failure of Western Medicine."

Kleinman, A. "Relevance for Clinical Psychiatry of Anthropological and Cross-Cultural Research: Concepts and Applied Strategies." *American Journal of Psychiatry* 135(4): 427–431.

Kleinman, A., and E. Mendelsohn. "Systems of Medical Knowledge: A Comparative Approach." *The Journal of Medicine and Philosophy* 3(4): 314–330.

Kleinman, A. "What Kind of Model for the Anthropology of Medical Systems?" *American Anthropologist* 80:662–665.

Kleinman, A., L. Eisenberg, and B. Good. "Culture, Illness, and Care: Clinical Lessons from Anthropological and Cross-Cultural Research." *Annals of Internal Medicine* 88:251–258.

1979

Kleinman, A. "Sickness as Cultural Semantics: Issues for an Anthropological Medicine and Psychiatry." In *Toward New Definitions of Health Psychosocial Dimension*, ed. P. Ahmed and G. Coelho, 53–66. New York: Plenum Press.

Kleinman, A., and D. Mechanic. "Some Observations of Mental Illness and Its Treatment in the People's Republic of China." *The Journal of Nervous and Mental Disease* 167:267–274.

Kleinman, A., and L. H. Sung. "Why Do Indigenous Practitioners Successfully Heal: A Follow-up Study of Indigenous Practice in Taiwan." *Social Science and Medicine* 13B:7–26.

1980

Kleinman, A. "Indigenous and Traditional Systems of Healing." In *Health for the Whole Person*, ed. Arthur C. Hastings, J. Fadiman, and J. S. Gordon, 427–442. Boulder, Colo.: Westview Press.

Kleinman, A. "Traditional Medicine in China." In *Committee on Scholarly Communication with the People's Republic of China: Rural Health in the People's Republic of China: Report of a Visit by the Rural Health Systems Delegation, June 1978*, 63–74. Washington, D.C.: U.S. Government Printing Office, Fogarty International Center, N.I.H. Publication No. 80-2124.

Chrisman, N., and A. Kleinman. "Health Beliefs of American Ethnic Groups." In *Harvard Encyclopedia of American Ethnic Groups*, 452–462. Cambridge, Mass.: Harvard University Press.

Eisenberg, L., and A. Kleinman. "Clinical Social Science." In *The Relevance of Social Science for Medicine,* ed. L. Eisenberg and A. Kleinman, 1–23. Dordrecht, Holland: D. Reidel Publishing Co.

Kleinman, A., and D. Mechanic. "Mental Illness and Psychosocial Aspects of Medical Problems in China." In *Normal and Abnormal Behavior in Chinese Culture,* ed. A. Kleinman and T. Y. Lin, 331–355. Dordrecht, Holland: D. Reidel Publishing Co.

Mechanic, D., and A. Kleinman. "Ambulatory Medical Care in the People's Republic of China: An Exploratory Survey." *American Journal of Public Health* 70(1): 62–66.

Mechanic, D., and A. Kleinman. "The Organization, Delivery, and Financing of Rural Medical Care in the People's Republic of China." In *Committee on the Scholarly Communication with the People's Republic of China: Report of a Visit by the Rural Health Systems Delegation, June 1978,* 17–22. Washington, D.C.: U.S. Government Printing Office for Fogarty International Center, N.I.H. Publication No. 80-2124.

1981

Katon, W., and A. Kleinman. "Clinical Social Science Interventions in Primary Care: A Review of Doctor-Patient Negotiation and Other Relevant Social Science Concepts and Strategies." In *The Relevance of Social Science for Medicine,* ed. L. Eisenberg and A. Kleinman, 253–278. Dordrecht, Holland: D. Reidel Publishing Co.

Kleinman, A. "The Meaning Context of Illness and Care: Reflections on a Central Theme in the Anthropology of Medicine." In *Science and Cultures, Sociology of the Sciences,* vol. 5, ed. E. Mendelsohn and Y. Elkana, 161–176. Dordrecht, Holland: D. Reidel Publishing Co.

Lin, K. M., and A. Kleinman. "Recent Development of Psychiatric Epidemiology in China." *Culture, Medicine and Psychiatry* 5(1): 135–144.

Lin, K. M., A. Kleinman, and T. Y. Lin. "Psychiatric Epidemiology in Chinese Cultures: An Overview." In *Normal and Abnormal Behavior in Chinese Culture,* ed. A. Kleinman and T. Y. Lin, 237–271. Dordrecht, Holland: D. Reidel Publishing Co.

Smilkstein, G., A. Kleinman, N. Chrisman, G. Rosen, and W. Katon. "Clinical Social Science Conference: A Biopsychosocial Teaching Instrument." *Journal of Family Practice* 12(2): 347–353.

1982

Kleinman, A. "Cultural Issues Affecting Clinical Investigation in Developing Societies." In *Cahiers de Bioethique,* vol. 4: *Medecine et Experimentation.* Quebec: Les Presses de L'Universite Laval.

Kleinman, A. "Medicalization and the Clinical Praxis of Medical Systems." In *The Use and Abuse of Medicine,* ed. Martin de Vries, R. L. Berg, and M. Lipkin, Jr., 42–49. New York: Praeger Scientific.

Kleinman, A. "Neurasthenia and Depression: A Study of Somatization and Culture in China." *Culture, Medicine and Psychiatry* 6(2): 117–189.

Kleinman, A. "The Teaching of Clinically Applied Medical Anthropology on a Psychiatric Consultation-Liaison Service." In *Clinically Applied Anthropology,* ed. N. Chrisman and T. Maretzki, 83–115. Dordrecht, Holland: D. Reidel Publishing Co.

Katon, W., A. Kleinman, and G. Rosen. "Depression and Somatization: A Review," part 1 and part 2. *American Journal of Medicine* 72(1): 127–135 and 72(2): 241–247.

Kleinman, A., and J. Gale. "Patients Treated by Physicians and Folk Healers: A Comparative Outcome Study in Taiwan." *Culture, Medicine and Psychiatry* 6(4): 405–423.

1983

Kleinman, A. "The Cultural Meanings and Social Uses of Illness Behavior: A Role for Medical Anthropology and Clinically Oriented Social Science in the Development of Primary Care Theory and Research." *Journal of Family Practice* 16(3): 539–545.

Chrisman, N., and A. Kleinman. "Popular Health Care and Lay Referral Networks." In *Handbook of Health, Health Care, and Health Professions,* ed. D. Mechanic. New York: Free Press.

Hahn, R., and A. Kleinman. "Belief as Pathogen, Belief as Medicine: 'Voodoo Death' and the 'Placebo Phenomenon' in Anthropological Perspective." *Medical Anthropology Quarterly* 14(4): 3, 16–19.

Hahn, R., and A. Kleinman. "Biomedical Practice and Anthropological Theory: Frameworks and Directions." In *Annual Review of Anthropology* 12: 305–333. Palo Alto, Calif.: Annual Reviews.

Rosen, G., and A. Kleinman. "Social Science in the Clinic: Applied Contributions from Anthropology to Medical Teaching and Patient Care." In *Behavioral Sciences in the Practice of Medicine,* ed. J. Carr and H. Dengerink, 85–104. New York: Elsevier Science Publishing Co.

1984

Kleinman, A. "Clinically Applied Medical Anthropology: The View from the Clinic." In *Advances in Medical Social Science,* vol. 2, ed. J. Ruffini, 269–288. New York: Gordon and Breach Science Publishers.

Kleinman, A. "Indigenous Systems of Healing: Questions for Professional, Popular, and Folk Care." In *Alternative Medicines: Popular and Policy Perspectives,* ed. J. W. Salmon, 138–164. London: Tavistock.

Kleinman, A. "Medical Anthropology." In *The Social Science Encyclopedia,* ed. Adam Kuper and Jessica Kuper. London: Routledge and Kegan Paul.

Kleinman, A. "Somatization." *Referential Journal of Psychiatry* (People's Republic of China, in Chinese) 11(2): 65–68.

Johnson, T., and A. Kleinman. "Cultural Concerns in Psychiatric Consultation." In *Manual of Psychiatric Consultation and Emergency Care,* ed. F. Guggenheim and M. Weiner, 275–284. New York: Jason Aronson.

1985

Kleinman, A. "Interpreting Illness Experience and Clinical Meanings: How I See Clinically Applied Anthropology." *Medical Anthropology Quarterly* 16(3): 69–71.

Good, B., and A. Kleinman. "Culture and Anxiety: Cross-Cultural Evidence for the Patterning of Anxiety Disorders." In *Anxiety and the Anxiety Disorders,* ed. A. H. Tuma and J. P. Maser, 297–324. Hillsdale, N.J.: Lawrence Erlbaum.

Kleinman, A., and Kleinman, J. "Somatization: Interconnections among Chinese Culture, Depressive Meanings, and the Experience of Pain." In *Culture and Depression,* ed. A. Kleinman and B. Good, 429–490. Berkeley, Los Angeles, London: University of California Press.

1986

Kleinman, A. "Anthropology and Psychiatry: The Role of Culture in Cross-Cultural Research in Illness." In *Psychiatry and Its Related Disciplines: The Next Twenty-Five Years,* ed. R. Rosenberg, Copenhagen: World Psychiatric Association.

Kleinman, A. "Illness Meanings and Illness Behavior." In *Illness Behavior: A Multi-Disciplinary Model,* ed. S. McHugh and T. M. Vallis, 149–160. New York: Plenum.

Kleinman, A. "Social Origins of Distress and Disease." *Current Anthropology* 27(5): 499–509.

Kleinman, A. "Some Uses and Misuses of Social Science in Medicine." In *Metatheory in Social Science,* ed. D. Fiske and R. Shweder, 222–245. Chicago: University of Chicago Press.

1987

Kleinman, A. "Anthropology and Psychiatry: The Role of Culture in Cross-Cultural Research on Illness." *British Journal of Psychiatry* 151:447–454.

Kleinman, A. "Culture and Clinical Reality." *Culture, Medicine and Psychiatry* 11:49–52.

Kleinman, A. "Symptoms of Relevance, Signs of Suffering: The Search for a Theory of Illness Meanings." *Semiotica* 65-1/2 (June): 163–174.

Brodwin, P., and A. Kleinman. "The Social Aspects of Chronic Pain." In *Handbook of Chronic Pain Management,* ed. G. Burrows, 109–120. Amsterdam: Elsevier.

Weiss, M., and A. Kleinman. "Psychosocial and Cross-Cultural Issues in Depression: A Prolegomenon for Culturally Informed Research." In *Psychology, Culture and Health: Toward Applications,* ed. P. Dassen and N. Sartorius. Beverly Hills, Calif.: Sage.

1988

Kleinman, A. "Medical Anthropology at Harvard: From Culture to Experience." *Symbols,* December 1988: 2–4.
Kleinman, A. "A Window on Mental Health in China." *American Scientist* 76(1): 22–27.
Lin, K. M., and A. Kleinman. "Psychotherapy and Clinical Course of Schizophrenia: A Cross-Cultural Perspective." *Schizophrenia Bulletin* 14(4): 555–567.

1989

Kleinman, A. "The Sources of Pain, Distress, and Misery: A Medical Anthropological Perspective on the Symbolic Bridge between Social Structure and Physiology." *Kroeber Anthropological Society Papers* 69–70:14–22.
Farmer, P., and A. Kleinman. "AIDS as Human Suffering." *Daedalus,* Spring 1989, 118(2): 135. Reprinted in *Living With AIDS,* ed. Stephen Graubard (Cambridge: MIT Press), 1990.
Jou, S. Y., J. K. Wen, A. Kleinman, J. Kleinman, Y. Wu, C. C. Chin, and M. Schiller. "A Pilot Study of Expressed Emotion of Relatives of Patients with Schizophrenia in Taiwan." *Chinese Psychiatry,* Supplement 1, 3:124–137.

1990

Csordas, T., and A. Kleinman. "The Therapeutic Process." In *Medical Anthropology: Contemporary Theory and Method,* ed. T. Johnson and C. Sargent, 11–25. New York: Praeger.
Guarnaccia, P. J., B. Good, and A. Kleinman. "A Critical Review of Epidemiological Studies of Puerto Rican Mental Health." *American Journal of Psychiatry* 147:11.

1991

Jenkins, J., A. Kleinman, and B. Good. "Cross-Cultural Studies of Depression." In *Psychosocial Aspects of Depression,* ed. J. Becker and A. Kleinman, 67–69. New York: Lawrence Erlbaum.
Kleinman, A. "Suffering, Healing, and the Human Condition." In *Encyclopedia of Human Biology,* vol. 7, 323–325. New York: Academic Press.
Kleinman, A., and J. Sugar. "Whither Culture in a Biological Era in Psychiatry?" *Anthropology UCLA,* Special Issue: "Essays in Honor of Harry Hoijer," Medical Anthropology Lecture Series, 20–43.
Sugar, J., A. Kleinman, and K. Heggenhougen. "Development's 'Downside': Social and Psychological Pathology in Countries Undergoing Social Change." *Health Transition Review* 1(2): 211–220.

1992

Kleinman, A. "Local Worlds of Suffering: An Interpersonal Focus for Ethnographies of Illness Experience." *Qualitative Health Research* 2(2) (May): 127–134.

Christakis, N., A. Kleinman, and N. Ware. "An Anthropological Approach to Social Science Research on the Health Transition." In *Advancing Health in Developing Countries: The Role of Social Science Research,* ed. L. Chen, N. Ware and A. Kleinman, 23–38. Westport, Conn.: Auburn House Publishing Co.

Sugar, J., A. Kleinman, and L. Eisenberg. "Psychiatric Morbidity in Developing Countries and American Psychiatry's Role in International Health." *Hospital and Community Psychiatry* 43(4): 355–361.

Ware, N., and A. Kleinman. "Culture and Somatic Experience: The Social Course of Illness in Neurasthenia and Chronic Fatigue Syndrome." *Psychosomatic Medicine* 54:546–560.

Ware, N., and A. Kleinman. "Depression in Neurasthenia and Chronic Fatigue Syndrome." *Psychiatric Annals* 22(4): 202–208.

1993

Hinton, W. L., IV, and A. Kleinman. "Cultural Issues and International Diagnosis." In *International Review of Psychiatry,* ed. J. A. Costa e Silva and C. C. Nadelson. Washington, D.C.: APA Press.

1994

Kleinman, A., and J. Kleinman. "How Bodies Remember: Social Memory and Bodily Experience of Criticism, Resistance, and Delegitimation Following China's Cultural Revolution." *New Literary History* 25(1): 707–723.

Xiong, W., M. Phillips, X. Hu, R. W. Wang, Q. Q. Dai, J. Kleinman, and A. Kleinman. "Family-Based Intervention for Schizophrenic Patients in China: A Randomized Controlled Trial." *British Journal of Psychiatry* 165: 239–247.

1995

Kleinman, A. "How Culture Is Important for *DSM-IV.*" In *Culture and Psychiatric Diagnosis,* eds. J. Mezzick, D. Parron, H. Fabrega, and A. Kleinman. Washington, D.C.: American Psychiatric Press. In press.

Kleinman, A., and J. Kleinman. "The Appeal of Experience, the Dismay of Images: Cultural Appropriations of Suffering in Our Time." *Daedalus.* In press.

Desjarlais, R., and A. Kleinman. "Violence and Demoralization in the New World Disorder." *Anthropology Today* 10(5): 9–12.

Notes

Chapter 1. Introduction

1. See the list of relevant publications in the Appendix.

Chapter 2. What Is Specific to Biomedicine?

1. A much more sophisticated misappropriation of holism occurred among those professional philosophers in Germany who became enthusiastic supporters of the Nazi Party after it gained control of the German state. Post-Nietzschean critiques of individualism, mechanism, and hegemonic Christian moral categories consorted with virulent anti-Semitism and aggressive nationalism in the philosophical support for the political program of National Socialism (Sluga 1993).

2. Carlo Ginzburg (1982), the celebrated Italian intellectual historian of Early Modern Europe, provides an illustration in the form of the inquisition of a sixteenth-century Northern Italian miller, Menocchio, whose alternative cosmology was treated as heresy and led to his eventual burning at the stake. It is instructive to read Menocchio's interchange with the inquisitors. They go to great pains to assist him to present his radical cosmology accurately and fully. Their terrible purpose, of course, is not to engage his ideas, but rather to specify with chilling exactness the degree of difference from orthodoxy so that the magnitude of his heresy can be measured in order to provide the right amount of punishment. For Menocchio, unfortunately, that meant death.

3. The relatively limited role that the medical profession has played in the Clinton administration's development of health care reform in America, even as a locus of resistance to change, is an example.

Chapter 3. Anthropology of Bioethics

1. Isaiah Berlin (1979:22–81), in a justly famous essay, deployed Archilochus's antique distinction between the hedgehog and the fox to characterize two types of intellectuals: the former who, concerning human experience, knows one big thing (e.g., the moral philosopher or the psychoanalyst) and the latter who knows many small things (e.g., the social historian or anthropologist).

2. Charles Taylor (1992) has gone on to point up the limitations of the cultural program of autonomy and authenticity even within moral philosophy. Yet, he still defends this program's basic thrust.

3. As with all cross-cultural generalizations about human experience, there are important exceptions. Malays have been described by Carol Laderman (1991) as having an individualized, inner-directed health philosophy in which one's obstructed "inner winds" (temperament) are held responsible for one's problems, and shamanistic therapy is oriented to assist the person to express the latent creative talents and energies that are blocked. Laderman does not comment on ethical decision making in rural Malay villages, but, if James Scott (1985), working in the same society, is correct, then a collective orientation inflected by class and factional conflict is crucial. Stephen Frankel (1986) and Fred Myers (1986) describe strong individualistic orientations among members of small-scale preliterate groups in the New Guinea highlands and the Australian desert.

Furthermore, ethical deliberation as a process and ethics as a discipline are at least in principle more open to the social sides of experience than economics, for example, seems to be. B. J. Reilly and M. J. Kyj (1994) recommend ethical models in economics for this reason. Thus, in relation to other fields, such as cognitive psychology and economics, for which the individual orientation is absolutely paramount, ethics would seem more vulnerable. That is one reason for this essay.

4. After creating the version of this essay that was published in the *Encyclopedia of Bioethics,* I read for the first time Patricia Marshall's (1992) useful contribution on the two-way relationship between anthropology and bioethics. I am impressed by the tone of Marshall's writing, which seems to be as interested in balancing the differences between each discipline as in searching out theoretical and programmatic *modi operandi* that would facilitate anthropologists' contributions to medical ethics questions. Among her recommendations is that anthropology play a role in registering and reformulating the unequal influence of doctor and patient on medical decision making in the clinical setting.

5. Hans Sluga (1993:5) makes this point about the debate over how to relate Heidegger's deeply troubling politics and his philosophy. The appropriate enquiry, Sluga avers, is to avoid factionalism and to leave questions open.

Sluga's idea of what characterizes genuine philosophizing is also worth quoting because it can be extended to the role of critical enquiry in the process of cultural formulation that I have sketched out. Philosophical thinking, says Sluga, is always at odds with itself. Even within a single mind or within a single philosophical text, thoughts run in different directions. There is always the battle that thinking must carry out for itself in order to restrain, to rope in, to hamper, or to let go of certain ideas. Even within philosophical periods that seem single-minded and unified in doctrine, there are divisions, forces that pull thoughts in different and opposing directions. Philosophy is essentially a discourse of dissent, of battling voices. (p. 11)

6. Cultural relativism, though characteristic of social anthropology, is by no means universally accepted within the discipline. Robert Edgerton (1992), speaking on behalf of an increasingly vocal minority, offers a telling, if overdrawn, critique of the limits of relativism as they relate to cross-cultural descriptions of human behavior. One need not agree with his adaptationist approach—and I do not—to feel the need to reconstruct relativism in response to the troubling critique he lodges.

7. See Daniel Gordon (1991) and the response to his article on female circumcision in Egypt and the Sudan for illustration of just how difficult the issue of ethical relativism is in medical anthropology. Yet, following even the most sensitive and detailed description of the historical and cultural basis of a practice that produces mortality and morbidity on the one side and culturally valued (and self-valued) women on the other, the dilemma remains of how to proceed (cf. Boddy 1989). Here bioethical concerns offer something valuable to anthropology. These troubling questions require that the medical anthropologist work through the clash of distinctive discourses—local (lay and biomedical) and international (biomedical and ethical)—in order to come to an engaged point of view with recommendations for action.

8. I am obliged to Debbora Battaglia for this point.

9. The current intellectual trends in social anthropology, especially postmodernism, which has had a number of positive effects, have undermined the profession's long-term commitment to comparison. Many anthropologists today speak as if they regard comparison as ordinarily invalid and perhaps even impossible. The project of cross-cultural comparison, ethnology, is to my way of thinking the logical consequence of ethnography. Without it, there is no possibility of conducting anthropology as a social science. Nor would it be possible, in the absence of comparison, to adequately address the moral issues canvassed in this essay. The implication of medical ethics for medical anthropology is that comparison across local worlds is possible and even ethically necessary.

Chapter 4. A Critique of Objectivity in International Health

1. The last decade and a half has been one of intense, perhaps excessive, anthropological preoccupation with problems that limit ethnographic description and interpretation. Great emphasis has been placed on detecting cultural bias, distortion in the dialogically constructed data of interviewing, the effect of trope and style in shaping informants' narratives, the role of professional

authority and dominant discourse in the writing of the ethnographic text, and on self-reflexive analysis of the influence of the ethnographer's personal experience on the ethnography. (See Clifford and Marcus 1986; Crapanzano 1980; Marcus and Fischer 1986.)

2. Crandon-Malamud (1991) goes so far as to suggest that when informants are telling stories of sickness to the ethnographer (or family and friends), they are principally involved in negotiating social status and ethnic identity in order to gain access to resources. The veracity of the story is less important, therefore, than its strategic uses, which leads to creative distortions. In this view, all illness narratives—whether told to or reported by the ethnographer— are tendentious. The Israeli novelist A. B. Yehoshua (1993) deepens the narrative puzzle when he observes that each story has another, even earlier story behind it, so that when to begin a story is itself problematic.

3. That ethnographies are not replicable is the result of changes in the communities studied as well as in the professional community of ethnographers and in intellectual discourse more generally. Control of a sort is provided by the critical evaluation of ethnographers who work in the same culture area.

4. If ethnographers forgo serious attempt at translation of their findings into a professional discourse, the ethnographies they write will lack comparative cross-cultural significance. In fact such forbearance is an impossibility. Yet, the fact that the ethnographer's translation comes as a final, not initial, step is what distinguishes the ethnographer's quest for local cultural validity from the economist's and international health expert's precommitment to a universal discourse, which makes local cultural validity difficult if not impossible to achieve.

5. Because ethnography, like history, is most effectively conveyed in a monograph, or a lengthy article in a collection, and is not easily given to the extremely short article format in which most international health research appears in print, it is not often found in international health journals, and when it is, it is much less convincing than in monograph form. The work ethnographers write up in the anthropological literature, moreover, is only infrequently consulted by international health researchers. This genre gap is as serious a problem as is the conceptual and methodological question of objectivity; in fact, the questions of objectivity, validity, and the relative dearth of ethnographic writing in international health publications and in the list of references of articles written by international health researchers are inseparable.

6. Self-reports by Puerto Ricans and their responses to questionnaires assessing mental health problems have repeatedly been found to overestimate the degree of psychopathology and underestimate their health. In part this may be due to the popular use of a normative idiom of *nervios* (nerves) to talk about various kinds of life problems, which is easily misinterpreted by mental health professionals and researchers as pathology (Guarnaccia et al. 1990).

7. Ironically, there are ethnographic descriptions of societies undergoing historical change which themselves offer ideas about their own experience of change that are utterly antithetical to the Western idea of progress applied to them by health planners. Stephen Frankel's (1986) description of the worldview of the Huli of the Southern Highlands of Papua New Guinea is such an example:

The Huli preoccupations with entropy, with decreasing yields, with a recent upsurge of human and porcine disease and with increasing strife are expressed . . . in terms of a predestined progression towards devastation that can only be averted by prescribed ritual acts. These afflictions that the Huli interpret as indicative of a fundamental deterioration in the ritual forces that maintain the natural and moral order can also be seen as the products of recent ecological changes that have affected horticulture and disease patterns. (p. 26)

8. I owe this analysis of Chinese society to Anne Kleinman's unpublished manuscript, "Across China: Regional Pluralism and Developmental Imbalance."

9. Peter Kunstadter (1990), Fred Dunn (1979), and Kris Heggenhougen (1988, 1990) are members of a small cadre of anthropologists who have made career-long contributions to international public health. Carol MacCormack (1992), Lenore Manderson (1987 [and Manderson and Aaby 1992]), Susan Scrimshaw (and Elena Hartado 1987), Dennis Willms (1983), and Carl Kendall (1988) also belong to this group. Members of this group, including Mary-Jo Good (1992b) and James Trostle (with John Simon 1992), have been particularly effective in training social scientists and physicians in Asia and Africa in an anthropological approach to international health problems.

Mark Nichter (1989) has developed international public health research that is grounded in anthropological theory. Judith Justice (1985) has done the same for international health policy. Stephen Frankel (1986) is one of a cohort of anthropologist-physicians and other anthropologists who are not also physicians who have worked to integrate epidemiological and anthropological studies around international health problems. (See also the work of Mitchell Weiss [1988], Marilyn Nations [1986], and Benedicte Ingstad [1992].)

I cite these works in order to indicate that there are varied anthropological contributions to international health, including a few that go beyond self-styled "critical" anthropology labels to organize empirical research on health within a framework generated by anthropological theory. Recently, the anthropological study of pharmaceutical use has added useful contributions as well (Whyte 1992). Indeed, so many useful contributions have been made in this branch of medical anthropology and international health that it is not feasible to list them all here. Yet attention needs to be drawn to the important work that Francophone authors have pioneered, among which Gilles Bibeau's many contributions stand out. That some of the more impressive works in recent years have been written by anthropologists from low-income societies is especially promising (see Das 1995; Madan 1980; Ramphele 1993; among others).

Chapter 5. Suffering and Its Professional Transformation

1. The idea that experience, whatever else it may be, is of overriding practical relevance to the persons engaged in transacting a lived world can be found in the writings of scholars from a wide range of orientations: John Dewey (1957), William James (1981), Alfred Schutz (1968), and Helmut Plessner (1970), the most important if the least well known of Continental

phenomenologists, and is echoed in Dan Sperber and Deidre Wilson's (1986) criticism of contemporary studies in psychology and anthropology, which they claim lack an appreciation of this central orientation. Calling "relevance" that which is at stake in living—that is, for survival, for coherence, for transcendence—has a long provenance in literature; it has become revivified for us as a resonant theoretical category in a dialogue with Unni Wikan (1987), with Veena Das (1994), with Vera Schwarcz (1991), and with the present and past members of the Harvard Seminar in Medical Anthropology: Byron J. Good, Mary-Jo DelVecchio Good, Thomas Csordas, Mitchell Weiss, Peter Guarnaccia, Pablo Farias, Norma Ware, Joyce Chung, Janis Jenkins, David Napier, John Sugar, Robert Desjarlais, and others, including our present and former graduate students: Paul Farmer, Paul Brodwin, Anne Becker, Jim Kim, Lawrence Cohen, Maya Dummermuth Todeschini, Richard Castillo, Scott Davis, Ana Ortiz, Tara AvRuskin, Karen Stephenson, Catherine Lager, Kate Hoshour, Eric Jacobson, Terry O'Neill, Linda Hunt, Liz Miller, Don Seeman, Matthew Kohrman, Cheungsatiansup Komatra, among others.

Michael Jackson (1989) develops a sophisticated argument for radical experientialism in ethnography whose focus is the personal experience of native informant and ethnographer. Writing earlier, in the same tradition, Renato Rosaldo (1984) draws upon his own experience of grief, following the death of his wife, to understand the "force" of emotion among the Ilongot. Paul Stoller (1989) is another contributor to this group. His focus on the sensory appreciation of cultural processes in taste, smell, sight, and sound suggests that ethnomusicologically informed ethnographies such as Steven Feld's (1982) as well as studies that focus on dance (Chernoff 1979) deserve to be included in this grouping. Francis Zimmermann's (1989) ethnomedical reconstruction of Ayurveda through metaphors of the terrain and taste of healing spices orients his work toward the experiential foundations of therapeutics. Marina Roseman's (1990) multichanneled sensory approach to Malaysian aboriginal healing rituals would also deserve to be categorized under the rubric of experience-near ethnography.

In this chapter we attempt to develop a somewhat different understanding of experience, though we do not mean to deny certain resonances with the works mentioned above. We define experience not as a subjective phenomenon—something that a single person "has"—but as an interpersonal medium shared by, engaged in, and also mediating between persons in a local world. Here we elaborate the Chinese paradigm into a position that claims cross-cultural validity.

Our intention is to dissolve the individual/collective dichotomy. Interpersonal experience is the grounds of sociosomatic mediation (in illness) and transformation (in healing). In the local field of experience, chunks of unified processes of memory, affect, and physiology can be described at a variety of levels: personal, familial, network, community. Yet it is the novel idea of experience as an interpersonal medium of mediation that we wish to emphasize, rather than its more usual categorization as a personal form. For this reason, we describe our approach as the ethnography of interpersonal experience, though perhaps we could equally well describe it as the sociodynamics of cultural experience, because we regard culture to be constitutive, through everyday processes and practices, of the interpersonal routines and rhythms of experience.

2. By *human conditions,* we mean to signify that there are only a limited number of ways of being human. We all must experience physical growth, personal transformations, hunger, injury, sickness (both minor and serious), fear, death, bereavement, and so on. We use the plural, however, because we wish to indicate that even human conditions may vary within and among groups. Not everyone will experience a grave childhood disorder or bereavement for an infant son or daughter, yet many will, and some groups will have more than their share of such experiences. That which is at stake for men and women is constrained by shared human conditions, and, at the same time, it is elaborated by the particularities of local life worlds and individuals. Thus, human conditions supersede the dichotomy between "universal" and "particular" forms of living.

3. Including, of course, what is at stake for the ethnographer—by which we mean to convey a much wider set of self "interests" than is captured by the postmodernist emphasis on intellectual paradigm and style of writing. Something akin to the ethnographer's countertransference of passions, abiding and momentary, is what we have in mind, but without the psychoanalytic specification of their allegedly universal content.

4. Here we argue that "cognition," "affect," "defense," and "behavior" not only are hegemonic Western psychological categories but are particularly inadequate as categories for the ethnography of experience. The separation of cognition from affect, in spite of all the words spilled to show the distortions produced by the residual dichotomies of the Western cultural tradition, is now taken for granted not just in psychology but in virtually all the human sciences. Yet even a moment's self-reflection is enough to illustrate amply that this dichotomy rends the unity of experience. Commitments to measurement make most researchers deaf to these objections. Defense, of course, carries the entire weight of the psychoanalytic paradigm, which converts the multiplicity and uncertainty and sheer originality of experience into "truths" whose validity and reliability have almost never been rigorously tested, while their use has infiltrated the everyday language of social scientists and physicians. The ethnography of experience would be better off if it were defenseless. "Behavior" reifies the narrowest possible vision of living, and is underpinned by theories that are the most vulnerable to dehumanizing applications. All of these terms reify an overly individualistic account of experience that obscures the intersubjectivity we wish to emphasize.

5. Max Scheler (1971:14, 52–53) defines the quality of resistance as the very essence of the person's experiencing of reality as real. "Representations and mediated thinking [inferences] can never give us anything but this or that quality in the world. Its reality as such is given only in an experience of resistance accompanied by anxiety" (pp. 52–53). Here Scheler's notion of what is the realness of our experience of the world is what we denote by its quality of

overriding relevance: namely, that which absorbs our attention. Social absorption, then, is the shared core of human conditions.

6. We are not saying there is no human nature. Rather, we insist that human nature is emergent in local worlds of experience; it is achieved and contains both universal and culturally specific elements. Ronald Melzack (1989) theorizes from considerable research in the neurosciences that the brain-self is a neuromatrix open to experience, yet largely preceding it, that gives rise to a particular neurosignature of the lived body. While we disagree with Melzack's biological reductionism, our vision of human nature encompasses a notion of the body-self that is the continuously achieved result of the interaction of social world and psychobiological processes (including the neuromatrix). In this dialectical model, human nature is emergent: constrained yet elaborated.

7. The concept of local moral worlds is developed further in Kleinman 1992. For our purposes here the idea is a kind of shorthand for the focus of ethnographic studies on microcontexts of experience in village, urban neighborhood, work setting, household networks, or communities of bounded relationships where everyday life is transacted.

8. This case is republished with a few alterations from *Social Origins of Distress and Disease: Neurasthenia, Depression and Pain in Modern China* (Kleinman 1986:127–131).

9. See the *Li Ji, Book of Ritual, Li yun* chapter: all people are born with these key emotions.

10. J. C. Scott (1985, 1990) refers to the "hidden transcript" as that set of ideas which subordinates, in a contested field of power relations, cannot express publicly because of the sanctions of their superordinates. The idea is close to the Chinese understanding save for the emphasis Scott places on class conflict. In the Chinese version, the hidden transcript is expressed only in the first and second compartments. The third compartment, even with members of the same social class or political stratum, still contains the public transcript.

11. Of course, the story of the victims and survivors of the Tiananmen Massacre and the present period of repression of the Democracy Movement would be another and more powerfully charged way to challenge Potter's argument that emotions in Chinese society are irrelevant to the legitimation of the social order. The grief and anger of overseas Chinese and students from the People's Republic in the West have been emphasized as a sign of moral revulsion with the current government, and with Communism more generally. In the Democracy Movement, emotion was central to the hunger strikes and to resisting the troops who were sent to Beijing. In both cases, its significance as moral authorization for resistance was widely understood.

12. This is one of the reasons why Mao Zedong, who came from the same region of China, the area of the ancient Kingdom of Chu, held Qu Yuan to be one of his cultural heroes.

13. Compare Liu Binyan's (1990) account of the life of an intellectual under Chinese Communism.

14. Compare Phillippe Aries's sardonic summary of the meaning of death in the modern Western world for professional thanatologists: "They [a small

elite of anthropologists, psychologists, and sociologists] propose to reconcile death with happiness. Death must simply become the discreet but dignified exit of a peaceful person from a helpful society that is not torn, not even overly upset by the idea of a biological transition without significance, without pain or suffering, and ultimately without fear" (1981:614).

15. Compare Dreuilhe (1988) or other personal accounts of persons with AIDS to see how Sontag's cultural analysis leaves out—purposefully, as she indicates in her introduction—precisely that lived experience of suffering that we take to be the focus of the ethnography of suffering.

16. Recent examples of such ethnographies include Ellen Oxfeld's (1992) study of the felt experience of conflicting commercial and familial modes of interaction in the life of a Chinese merchant in India; Michael Jackson's (1989) description of the intersubjective flow of experiencing everyday life activities in a Sierra Leone tribal society; and Steven Feld's (1982) attempt to render the sensibility of bereavement among the Kaluli of New Guinea across several sensory domains.

17. We have in mind Michael Taussig's tendentious interpretation of shamanism solely as political resistance of colonized Indians in Colombia, and his denigration of both the personal pains and distress that sick persons bring to shamans, which shamans try to cure, and the practical responses of the public health system to control diarrheal disease as a source of the high infant mortality rates afflicting Indian families. For critiques of the interpretations of suffering as resistance see Das (1994) and Kleinman (1992). Taussig's use of the fantasy and illusion of hallucinogen-derived montage makes for some extraordinary literary excursions, yet it obscures what is at stake in local worlds. His radically self-experiential experimentation, though innovative, distorts the authenticity of the worlds of others; it also inverts the legitimacy of their local accounts for the priority of a totalizing analysis of hegemonic ideology that is his own source of authority. That political inversion creates what Scott (1985: 346–350), following Barrington Moore (1978:459), rejects as a false sense of inevitability in the discourse on hegemony that "fail(s) completely to capture the texture of local experience." As Scott puts it,

To see the causes of distress instead as personal, as evil, as a failure of identifiable people in their own community to behave in a seemly way may well be a partial view, but it is not a wrong view. And not incidentally, it is quite possibly the only view that could, and does, serve as the basis for day-to-day resistance. (p. 348)

A not significant contribution, however, is Taussig's experiment with a form of writing aimed at challenging the authority of the author in describing the realities of other worlds. Genre and style of writing are clearly crucial to the ethnography of interpersonal experience, and either can clarify or obscure human conditions. Yet the vexed prose of postmodernism shows itself to be as corrosive for the voice of the subject as it is of the authorial voice, so that Taussig's extreme experiment eventually substitutes one abuse of language for another. Nonetheless by forcing attention to the language of ethnography, Taussig provokes a useful question about the words and style most suited to describe the flow of interpersonal worlds. Perhaps one of the benefits of the ethnography of experience is that it challenges the ethnographer to search for an authentic voice that can match both the scholarly and ethical requirements of its subject.

18. As for the magnitude of abuse, the professional transmogrification of experience via psychiatric or anthropological rhetoric is serious but certainly not nearly as dangerous as, say, the nineteenth-century idea of degeneracy and its twentieth-century revivification in the murderous eugenics of Nazism (Pick 1989). It would be a terrible scholarly error to exaggerate the former form of abuse. Even today the new eugenics strikes us as the most dangerous of discourses with respect to potential political abuse. Nonetheless the medicalization (or socialization) of suffering—what Bruno Latour (1988:116–129) might call the Pasteurization of suffering by biomedical (or social science) reductionism—is still a significant example of the dehumanizing consequences of contemporary professional discourse.

19. The chief problem with phenomenological theory is that it has over time become a special language whose conventions, accepted by initiates, are opaque to general readers. The neologisms invented by Edmund Husserl, Martin Heidegger, Maurice Merleau-Ponty, Arnold Gehlen, Helmut Plessner, and others obscure more than they illuminate about the felt quality of the flow of experience, and ultimately take on an essentialist tenor that is unacceptable for social analysis. Indeed, phenomenological theory often hides behind these abstruse terms. It has not taken on the responsibility of popularizing its conceptual advance through a rapprochement with broader intellectual currents. Nonetheless, as Jackson (1989) shows, the insights of the phenomenologists can be outstanding and breathtaking when effectively translated into ethnography.

20. The ethnographic and comparative historical analysis of suffering would provide something altogether different from a cross-cultural science of suffering. For example, suppose the Chinese materials canvassed in this essay were compared, say, with the moral meaning and political uses of suffering in the Polish tradition. Longina Jakubowska (1990:12) evokes the imagery of Jesus Christ on the cross as symbol of "despair, sacrifice and death, but also resurrection" and notes the popular association of "Jesus the Sorrowful," *Jesus Fasobliny*, with Poland itself. A historical and ethnographic comparison would contrast these quite distinctive religious and political images, but would also be enriched by taking into account how they contribute to the structuring of experience in local worlds in each society. We would also want to know what such an empirical comparison can tell us about the moral order and its significance for human conditions. The upshot would not be a new science (behavioral or otherwise) but an integrating focus for historical and anthropological and psychological/psychiatric studies.

21. Presented by Arthur Kleinman at the first conference of the Society for Psychological Anthropology: "On Current Thinking and Research in Psychological Anthropology," San Diego, 6–8 October 1989; the current chapter is a revision of a revision of the original draft.

Chapter 6. Pain and Resistance

1. A considerable body of writing touches on aspects of this anthropological focus on the grounding of meaning and experience in cultural worlds; see, for example, Abu-Lughod (1986); Geertz (1987); Hallowell (1967); Rosaldo (1980); Shweder and LeVine (1984); J. W. Stigler, R. Shweder, G. Herdt, eds., (1990).

2. E. Schieffelin (1976), writing on the same ceremony among Kaluli but from a different theoretical perspective, has also presented a sensitive ethnographic description of this particular cultural construction of bereavement.

3. In this paragraph, I follow Bourdieu's (1989) usage of the terms *structure* and *structural* and *structuring,* but I will hereafter freely substitute the words *construction, constructed* and *constructing,* and *constitutive,* within the same general conceptualization of the generative dialectic in social processes.

4. The latter usage of resistance is expanded in Kleinman and Kleinman (1991); the former usage builds on Scott (1976, 1985, 1990), who in turn appropriated the concept from an earlier, largely Marxist, generation of theoreticians, whom he also criticized; the idea of political resistance has been taken up in such ethnographic works in which suffering and healing figure as Comaroff (1985); Martin (1987); Ong (1987); Taussig (1980); among others. Scott (1985) emphasizes peasant resistance in class struggles with wealthy villagers; his focus is on the everyday routines and extraordinary actions of participants in rural communities, who, among other things, engage in the politics of reputation and the implicit threat of violence to defend their vulnerable positions. Particularly pertinent is his argument that political economic decisions that mandate planned development undermine the established routines in peasant communities, so that the very moral structure itself is threatened, including the established patterns of interaction across classes. This places the poor at great risk and also threatens their legitimated coping devices. The analogy can be transferred to the health field. There the structural vulnerability of subordinate groups to local social changes that result from political economic change in turn places greater pressure on the health status of the poor; it also is a means of highlighting, albeit provocatively, the increasing gap between the technological power and cognitive control of health professionals and the threat of increasing powerlessness felt by patients from the lowest socioeconomic stratum. Under these conditions, the patient-doctor relationship can become such an unequal engagement that poor patients find noncompliance one of their only ways of resisting paternalistic authority and asserting what little personal efficacy they believe to be available to them. The consequence, as Scott (1985, 1990) shows for the agricultural domain and political order generally, may be to worsen their material conditions, yet the intention is to resist authority and to struggle for more control, symbolic and pragmatic. The same processes of resistance, I contend, occur in the therapeutic relationship and affect the moral economy of health. The political imagery will seem exaggerated and even inappropriate to many health care providers and planners.

Yet I would suggest that for at least some patients of poverty and perhaps for many others with chronic illness, the feeling that they are deploying "weapons of the weak" in unequal engagements both with the practical realities of health care and with those symbolic apparatuses that support society's "tyranny of health," which holds them responsible for their misfortune, is neither irrational nor without its uses, particularly if the partisan language of class warfare is replaced by the experiential terminology of the ethnography of suffering.

5. For a useful discussion of embodiment of distress and disease from a phenomenological perspective, see Csordas (1990), which can be read as a complement to this operational description of suffering.

6. In the Jewish tradition, as A. Mintz (1984) discloses in his remarkable survey of responses to catastrophe in Hebrew language literature, writers have been torn by two questions that are highly relevant to the issues explored in this chapter. First, how should the suffering of the collective be portrayed? (Ever since Lamentations the device has been personification via the experience of particular individuals.) And second, how should unexplained and undeserved suffering be dealt with? The emphasis has been on cognitive disorientation and subsequent restoration of the paradigm of meaning (Mintz 1984: 21). This meaning-dominated concern with suffering, which has been so fateful for the Western tradition, periodically gave way, especially after the pogroms and the Holocaust, to a concern with resistance, as in Bialik's poem, "In the City of Slaughter," which rebukes passive acceptance of oppression by Russian Jews following a pogrom:

> For since they have met pain with resignation
> And have made peace with shame,
> What shall avail thy consolation?
> They are too wretched to evoke thy scorn.
>   (Mintz 1984:140)

The implication is that resistance is both authorized by undeserved suffering and the only morally justifiable response. Thus, the idea of resistance is charged with special moral significance in the Western tradition, a significance that echoes in Marx and in the writings of anthropologists who have picked up this question. This Western orientation toward suffering, especially as it has been refracted in the writings of existential authors, has clearly influenced my own contributions: first toward a meaning-centered medical anthropology, and more recently toward an anthropology of experience.

7. See Aaron Cicourel's tripartite model as described in Bourdieu (1989).

8. To protect the anonymity of the research subjects whose stories of pain I elicited, through five to ten hours of interviewing of each subject, I have changed identifying details and provided each subject with a pseudonym. The information contained in this chapter, though altered for this purpose, accurately conveys the essence of the research I conducted. When I have made changes to protect anonymity of patients and practitioners, I have drawn on findings from the entire group of the chronic pain patients I interviewed in order to insure that the changes held general validity.

9. A full treatment needs to consider each of these aspects of pain. By

focusing narrowly, I neither discount these other interpretations nor seek to contribute to a fallacy of misplaced concreteness. Resistance and delegitimation are components of a complex, contradictory, only incompletely understandable, positioned picture. I draw them out because others have paid insufficient attention to these moral sides of pain, and they support the larger conception of suffering I seek to develop.

10. I cannot here go further into the place of this religious implication of a fall from divine grace in the Hoff family's Huguenot tradition of Protestantism in Catholic France, but it is worth remembering that besides apostasy and forced uprooting, the spirit of resistance remained a strong component of the Huguenots' ethnic identity. Dr. Hoff's family took their religious tradition as serious business, and Hoff's building of her own career lends itself quite easily to the Weberian interpretation of the Calvinist roots of secular success. Hence, it would also seem appropriate to follow Weber further in his analysis of suffering as *resentment,* a critique of cultural authority from those below the established hierarchy or from those who, having fallen out of grace, take on a pariah status for which they seek retribution (Weber 1978:518–602). Furthermore, as shown in Philip Hallie's (1979) study of how the French Huguenot village of Le Chambon saved Jews from the Nazis and their Vichy collaborators, this tradition of Protestantism has supported political resistance of a remarkable quality, a tradition that Dr. Hoff's family prized.

11. In research with patients suffering from chronic fatigue syndrome in Boston, my colleague Norma Ware and I have noted that their exhaustion, once defined and sanctioned as a medical illness, though it frequently seems to be the result of exhausting lifestyles, can also authorize basic shifts in the pace and control over activities in their family and work. Some of these sick persons, most of whom are women, once they are diagnosed as chronic fatigue patients, make such fundamental decisions as changing or giving up jobs and intimate relationships, and end up transforming the very structure of their lives and even such daily social rhythms as when and how they sleep, eat, exercise, and spend their time (Ware and Kleinman 1992). Illness, then, relegitimates their flow of experience and reorganizes their engagements and transactions, authorizing greater control. Michel de Certeau (1984:43) avers that "everyday practices depend on a vast ensemble which is difficult to delimit but which we may originally designate as an ensemble-of-procedures." Our chronic fatigue patients, at least some of them, altered the "ensemble of procedures" and thereby everyday practices, too, through the experience of illness. I believe this can happen in chronic illness generally, including chronic pain.

12. The phases of this delegitimation crisis are several. During the Great Famine, from 1959 to 1961, when 30 million Chinese died of starvation, hunger reached most Chinese families, yet the press falsely reported bountiful harvests, thus removing the possibility for effective public criticism that might support a challenge to the moral legitimacy of Communist Party rule. The depredations of various Anti-Rightists campaigns and the chaos of the Cultural Revolution led to widespread private condemnation of Communist ideology and authority. This condemnation was such that in the period of economic

reforms, from 1979 onward, the party itself switched its ideological justification for Communist rule from the erstwhile class warfare to the new claim that Communism had improved and would continue to improve the lives of most people, though it was admitted that 10 percent of the population still lived in abject poverty. This ideological reform was an attempt to shift the grounds for moral legitimacy to rule—what the Chinese have traditionally called the Mandate of Heaven—at a stage when massive cynicism had seeped into virtually every corner of the state. The Tiananmen Massacre completed the delegitimation of the moral order. Mainland China today is ruled through military power alone without any vestige of cultural legitimacy. For the citizen in his family circle, delegitimation moved from passionate affirmation of Marxism to bitterly enervating disillusionment, and onward to involuntary compliance with discredited authority. Cynicism followed misplaced loyalty. Foot-dragging, false compliance, and passive hostility followed political fervor and revolutionary ardor. The embodied effects of this trauma are deep and pervasive. (See Thurston 1987; Liang and Shapiro 1983; Cheng 1986; Liu 1990, among others.)

13. The breakdown of the moral code in Chinese society is canvassed in Shu (1989), *The Spiral Road*; Liu (1990), *A Higher Kind of Loyalty*; Marsden (1984), *Morality and Power in a Chinese Village*; Siu (1989), *Agents and Victims in South China*; and Tu (1992:251–252), "The Exit from Communism." For ethnographic and clinical findings on the issue pertinent to this chapter see Kleinman (1986), *Social Origins of Distress and Disease*.

14. See, for example, Black and Munro (1993), *Black Hands of Beijing: Lives of Defiance in China's Democracy Movement*.

15. Perhaps the clearest North American example of pain as resistance to political authority that I came across in the chronic pain sample was a middle-aged lawyer from a suburban town who had arthritis in his hips and knees. Emile Sachar represented local working-class clients in negotiations with developers and the town authorities in a local dispute. Once his adversaries had recognized that Mr. Sachar's chronic condition worsened over the course of the day and required that he periodically get up, walk around, and even lie down, they pressed for meetings that lasted longer and longer, at which Mr. Sachar found himself sitting in chairs that lacked proper support. He felt certain that the behavior of his adversaries was aimed at worsening his complaints so that he would more readily agree to a compromise that favored their interests over that of his clients. Mr. Sachar responded by deliberately using his disability to authorize official delays in the negotiations. He also pointedly emphasized his pain and its effects on his posture and gait to gain a more sympathetic hearing for his clients' position and even to project the image that they were victims. The downside of this oppositional response, besides its limited tactical success, was the undermining effect the illness behavior had on Emile Sachar's personal life, including his marriage. Indeed, Mr. Sachar's demoralization seemed to arise as much from the social intensification of his disabled role as from his increasing despair over the possibilities for social justice in American society. Thus, like the Chinese patients whose neurasthenia had become the embodied scar of the Cultural Revolution, the bodily mode of

resistance seemed to deepen personal crisis while not succeeding as a form of political protest or change.

16. For an alternative analysis of the cultural mediation of experience, see Jackson (1989:1–18).

Chapter 7. The Social Course of Epilepsy

1. The authors wish to express their appreciation to the following colleagues for their assistance with the study: Professors Jia-ren Song and Fan-yuan Kong, Ningxia Medical College; Professor Run-min Yan and Dr. Yu-qing Yuan, Changzhi Medical College; and Dr. Lip Chai Seet, Ciba-Geigy, Singapore. This chapter was prepared while Arthur Kleinman was a Fellow at the Center for Advanced Study in the Behavioral Sciences. He is grateful for financial support provided by the John D. and Catherine T. MacArthur Foundation #8900678; the Foundations' Fund for Research in Psychiatry Fund at the Center; and the Guggenheim Foundation. The research project was funded by Ciba-Geigy.

2. See a longer version of Dwyer (1992) in *Framing Disease: Studies in Cultural History,* ed. Charles Rosenberg and Janet Golden (New Brunswick, N.J.: Rutgers University Press, 1992, 248–274). The full story of the effect of the theory of biological degeneracy on the chronically ill and the disabled among others can be found in Pick (1989), *Faces of Degeneration: A European Disorder, 1848–1918.* For the Nazi approach to the chronically ill as degenerates requiring an ultimate solution, see Proctor (1988), *Racial Hygiene: Medicine under the Nazis.*

3. Alvarado et al. (1992); Tekle-Haimanot et al. (1991); El-Hilu (1990); Nkwi and Ndonko (1989). Attitudes toward epilepsy patients have improved in the West as has the illness experience of epileptics: see Jensen and Dam (1992); Jacoby (1992).

4. See, for example, Farmer and Kleinman (1989); A. Kleinman and J. Kleinman (1991); Ware and Kleinman (1992); Desjarlais (1992); and Farmer (1992).

5. Epilepsy as a clinical syndrome was recognized in ancient Chinese society and has held a place in traditional Chinese medicine texts through the present. It was originally associated with wind, later with mucus or phlegm blocking the cardiac system. Other diseases associated with similar causes included mental disorders like manic psychosis. Thus, the stigma associated with epilepsy may possibly be related to the stigma of mental illness in Chinese society, which continues to be powerful. See Sivin (1987:246) and Hillier and Jewell (1983:384). On the thorny question of relating traditional Chinese medical and biomedical disease terminologies, see Paul Unschuld's "Terminological Problems," in Unschuld (1989:97–106).

6. On the idea of resistance as strategic action and cultural performance via concealment, foot-dragging, and so on, see Scott (1990:45–55).

7. See the chapter on epilepsy and the law in Wyllie (1993).

8. Compare with the similar situation of overprotection of the chronically mentally ill by their families in China; see Phillips (1993).

Chapter 8. Violence, Culture, and the Politics of Trauma

1. Portions of this section drew upon Arthur Kleinman and Joan Kleinman (in press-b).

2. The *DSM-IV* draft criteria of 1 March 1993 have six components: (1) exposure to a traumatic event—now no longer described in terms of what is presumed to be normative or normal—that involves "actual or threatened death or serious injury," which elicits "intense fear, helplessness, or horror"; (2) persistent reexperience of the traumatic event; (3) "persistent avoidance of stimuli associated with the trauma and numbing of general responsiveness"; (4) increased arousal; (5) the symptoms must last for more than one month; (6) a requirement that there is significant distress, social or occupational impairment, or other important impairments in functioning. Although this streamlined draft removes certain of the cultural and political assumptions criticized in this text, most of the criticisms raised still are pertinent.

3. For a discussion of how the most common diagnosis that is applied to patients like Mrs. Fang in China—namely, neurasthenia—patterns the experience of distress and thereby becomes part of the social experience of politically generated symptoms, see Kleinman (1986).

4. A further mistake in the analysis of involuntary abortion as part of China's single-child family is created when we examine the overall consequences of this policy, which have been to significantly reduce the rate of fertility in China from 2.5 percent in 1988 to 1.9 percent in 1992. Thus, practices that have trampled all over human rights have succeeded, as nothing else had, in reining in growth of China's immense population; uncontrolled growth had threatened to outstrip China's food supply and the possibility for raising the economic standards of most workers and peasants (Kristoff 1993). The response to China's abuse of human rights in population control by critics in the West has often been to indict China without understanding the resentment of Chinese for what they view as the imposition of Western standards aimed at unfairly criticizing China and placing its development once again under Western control. Thus, charge and countercharge fly about without attention to the historically derived political-moral controversy that is the horizon of interpretation for making sense of the uses and abuses of local cases like Mrs. Fang's. That is to say, crucial to the ethnographic emphasis on local worlds is a broad interpretive framework that allows large-scale forces to enter the picture.

5. On this point, useful things have been written by Pierre Bourdieu in *La Misère du Monde* (1993), and by his former student Luc Boltanski (1993) in his important volume *La Souffrance à Distance.*

6. Since this chapter was written, the appalling human plight of Hutu refugees in Zaire, some of whom themselves had perpetrated ethnocidal violence on Tutsi neighbors, and who were running away from the new Tutsi-dominated government, forced the international aid agencies and the press to begin to address the moral complexities and politics of trauma.

Chapter 9. The New Wave of Ethnographies in Medical Anthropology

1. My reading of Devisch's (1993) evocative account of Yaka healing in Zaire suggests the same problem as that found in the works of Laderman, Roseman, and Desjarlais (see below). Devisch uses the appealingly integrative metaphor of "weaving" to connect social context and bodily processes. Over the course of his argument, the metaphor of "weaving the threads of life" is itself treated as if it adequately conveys what happens in the process of healing; indeed, it is as if "weaving" not only represents but constitutes the cultural-somatic processes that actually mediate therapeutic change. That is to say, an illuminating analogy gets materialized as the embodied reality itself. Instead of pointing toward the qualities and activities in the interaction, the metaphor, understood on multiple levels, becomes the interaction between those levels. I find this *modus operandi* unfinished, because the nature of the mediation needs to be much more precisely specified so that we understand what "weaving" means in sociosomatic terms. That is unfinished business not only for Devisch but for all of us in medical anthropology who are concerned with how healing works.

2. See note 1.

3. Translation of Bourdieu's (1993) passages is by Anne Simone Kleinman.

4. I read Allan Young's book in a 1994 manuscript, and refer therefore to that manuscript version.

5. Remarks delivered by Charles Leslie at the close of the symposium that celebrated Harvard's Department of Social Medicine and its Medical Anthropology Program, May 1992.

6. There are a few early indications of at least small success in this effort to inform health affairs and medical practice with ethnography. Ethnographies are occasionally, though not often, taught in medical school courses in the humanities and ethics and in schools of public health which have programs in international health and community development, where ethnographic assessment has attracted interest. The *World Mental Health Report* that I collaborated on with colleagues in the Department of Social Medicine at Harvard Medical School used ethnographic materials. But this is decidedly unusual in the discourse of health policy. Finding a more effective means to project ethnography into that discourse remains a goal for the future.

References

Abu-Lughod, L.
  1986   *Veiled sentiments: Honor and poetry in a Bedouin society.* Berkeley,
          Los Angeles, London: University of California Press.
Ainlay, S. C., G. Becker, and L. M. Coleman, eds.
  1986   *The dilemma of difference: A multidisciplinary view of stigma.* New
          York: Plenum.
Alvarado, L., F. Ivanovic-Zuvic, X. Candia, M. Mendez, X. Ibarra, and
    J. Alarcon
  1992   Psychosocial evaluation of adults with epilepsy in Chile. *Epilepsia*
          33(4): 651–656.
American Psychiatric Association
  1987   *DSM-IIIR* (Diagnostic and Statistical Manual of Mental Disor-
          ders, 3d ed., revised version). Washington, D.C.: American Psy-
          chiatric Association.
Ames, R. T.
  1991   Introduction. In *Interpreting culture through translation,* a fest-
          schrift for D. C. Lau, ed. R. T. Ames, S. W. Chen, and K. M. S.
          Ng. Hong Kong: The Chinese University Press.
Annegers, J. F., W. F. Hauser, and L. R. Celoeback
  1979   Remission of seizures and relapse in patients with epilepsy. *Epi-
          lepsia* 20:729–737.
Aries, P.
  1981   *The hour of our death.* New York: Alfred A. Knopf.
Augé, M.
  1975   *Theorie des pouvoirs et ideologie. Etude Cas en Cote-d'Ivoire.* Paris:
          Hermann.
  1984   Ordre biologique, ordre social: La maladie forme elementaire, de
          l'evenement. In *Le sens du mal,* ed. M. Augé and C. Herzlich.
          Paris: Editions des Archives Contemporaries.
  1986   L'anthropologie de la maladie. *L'Homme* 261(1–2): 81–90.

Balsham, M.
    1993   *Cancer in the community: Class and medical authority.* Washington, D.C.: Smithsonian Institution Press.
Barker, D. C., A. I. Rabcenell, A. Pomphrey, E. Cox, V. D. Weisfeld, and J. K. Hollendonner, eds.
    1991   *Challenges in health care: A chartbook perspective.* Princeton, N.J.: Robert Wood Johnson Foundation.
Barker, Pat
    1992   *Regeneration.* New York: Dutton.
Battaglia, D.
    1990   *On the bones of the serpent: Person, memory, and mortality in Sabarl Island society.* Chicago: University of Chicago Press.
Becker, J., and A. Kleinman, eds.
    1991   *Psychosocial aspects of depression.* Hillsdale, N.J.: Lawrence Erlbaum.
Beiser, M.
    1977   Ethics in cross-cultural perspective. In *Current perspectives in cultural psychiatry,* ed. E. F. Foulks, R. M. Wintrob, J. Westermeyer, and A. R. Favazza. New York: Spectrum.
Berger, P., and T. Luckmann
    1967   *The social construction of reality.* New York: Doubleday.
Bergson, H.
    1889   *Les donnees immediates de la conscience.* Paris: Alcan.
Berlin, I.
    1979   The hedgehog and the fox. In *Russian thinkers.* Harmondsworth, Middlesex: Penguin.
Black, G., and R. Munro
    1993   *Black hands of Beijing: Lives of defiance in China's democracy movement.* New York: Wiley.
Boddy, J.
    1989   *Wombs and alien spirits: Women, men, and the Zar in Northern Sudan.* Madison: University of Wisconsin Press.
Boltanski, L.
    1993   *La souffrance à distance.* Paris: Metailie.
Bosk, C.
    1979   *Forgive and remember: Managing medical failure.* Chicago: University of Chicago Press.
Bottero, J.
    ND   Le magic et la medicine regnent a Babylone. *L'histoire* 74:12–23.
Bourdieu, P.
    1977   *Outline of a theory of practice.* New York: Cambridge University Press.
    1989   Social space and symbolic power. *Sociological Theory* 7(1): 14–24.
    1990   *The logic of practice.* Stanford, Calif.: Stanford University Press.
    1993   *La misère du monde.* Paris: Editions du Seuil.
Bowker, J.
    1970   *The problem of suffering for the religions of the world.* Cambridge: Cambridge University Press.

Brody, H.
    1977   *Placebos and the philosophy of medicine*. Chicago: University of Chicago Press.
Burrows, G., D. Elton, and G. V. Stanley, eds.
    1987   *Handbook for the management of chronic pain*. New York and Amsterdam: Elsevier.
Caldwell, J., S. Findley, P. Caldwell, G. Santon, W. Cosford, J. Braid, and
        D. Broers-Freeman, eds.
    1990   *Health transitions: The cultural, social, and behavioral determinants of health*. Canberra: Australian National University Press.
Callahan, D.
    1987   *Setting limits*. New York: Simon and Schuster.
    1990   *What kind of life*. New York: Simon and Schuster.
Canguilhem, G.
    1989   *The normal and the pathological*. New York: Zone Press.
    [1966]
Caputo, J. D.
    1993   *Against ethics*. Bloomington: Indiana University Press.
Casey, Edward S.
    1987   *Remembering: A phenomenological study*. Bloomington: Indiana University Press.
Cassell, E.
    1982   The nature of suffering and the goals of medicine. *New England Journal of Medicine* 306(11): 639–644.
    1991a   Recognizing suffering. *Hastings Center Report* 21(3): 24–31.
    1991b   *The nature of suffering and the goals of medicine*. New York: Oxford University Press.
Cassell, J.
    1991   *Expected Miracles: Surgeons at Work*. Philadelphia: Temple University Press.
Cassirer, E.
    1953–   *The philosophy of symbolic forms*. Vols. 1–3. Trans. Ralph Manheim.
    1957   New Haven, Conn.: Yale University Press.
    1962   *An essay on man*. New Haven, Conn.: Yale University Press.
Cavell, S.
    1994   *The pitch of philosophy*. Cambridge: Harvard University Press.
Chaplin, J. E., R. Yepez Lesso, S. D. Shorvan, and M. Floyd
    1992   National general practice study of epilepsy: The social and psychological effects of a recent diagnosis of epilepsy. *British Medical Journal* 304(6839): 1416–1419.
Chen, L. C., A. Kleinman, and N. Ware, eds.
    1994   *Health and social change: An international perspective*. Series on Population and International Health, Harvard School of Public Health. Cambridge, Mass.: Harvard University Press.
Cheng, N.
    1986   *Life and death in Shanghai*. New York: Grove Press.
Chernoff, J. M.
    1979   *African rhythm and African sensibility: Aesthetics and social action in African musical idioms*. Chicago: University of Chicago Press.

Christakis, N.
    1988   The ethical design of an AIDS vaccine trial in Africa. *Hastings Center Report* 18(3): 31–37.
Clifford, J., and G. Marcus, eds.
    1986   *Writing culture*. Berkeley, Los Angeles, London: University of California Press.
Cohen, L.
    1992   No aging in India: The uses of gerontology. *Culture, Medicine, and Psychiatry* 16(2): 123–161.
Comaroff, J.
    1985   *Body of power, spirit of resistance: The culture and history of a South African people*. Chicago: University of Chicago Press.
Commission on Epilepsy, Risks, and Insurance, International
    Bureau of Epilepsy
    1993   Workshop on epilepsy, risk, and insurance. *Epilepsia* 34(4): 590–591.
Connerton, P.
    1989   *How societies remember.* Cambridge: Cambridge University Press.
Connolly, W. E.
    1993a   *Political theory and modernity*. Ithaca, N.Y.: Cornell University Press.
    1993b   Beyond good and evil: The ethical sensibility of Michael Foucault. *Political Theory* 21(3): 365–389.
Corbett, K. K.
    1986   Adding insult to injury: Cultural dimensions of frustration in the management of chronic back pain. Ph.D. diss., joint doctoral program in medical anthropology, University of California, Berkeley and San Francisco.
Crandon-Malamud, L.
    1991   *From the fat of our souls: Social change, political process, and medical pluralism in Bolivia*. Berkeley, Los Angeles, Oxford: University of California Press.
Crapanzano, V.
    1980   *Tuhami: Portrait of a Moroccan*. Chicago: University of Chicago Press.
Csordas, T.
    1990   Embodiment as a paradigm for anthropology. *Ethos* 18(1): 5–47.
    1994   *The sacred self: A cultural phenomenology of charismatic healing*. Berkeley, Los Angeles, London: University of California Press.
Das, V.
    1994   Moral orientations to suffering: Legitimation, power, and healing. In *Health and social change: An international perspective*, ed. L. C. Chen, A. Kleinman, and N. Ware. Cambridge, Mass.: Harvard University Press.
    1995   *Critical events: An anthropological perspective on contemporary India*. New Delhi: Oxford University Press.

Dasgupta, P.
1993   *An inquiry into well-being and destitution.* New York: Oxford
        University Press.
Davis, D.
1991   Rich cases: The ethics of thick description. *Hastings Center Re-
        port* 21(4): 12–17.
Davis, L. S.
1992   On the eccentric position of shamanism in Taiwan. Ph.D. diss.,
        Department of Anthropology, Harvard University, Cambridge,
        Mass.
de Certeau, M.
1984   *The practice of everyday life.* Trans. Steven Rendall. Berkeley, Los
        Angeles, London: University of California Press.
Deleuze, G.
1988   *Foucault.* Minneapolis: University of Minnesota Press.
Desjarlais, R.
1992   *Body and emotion: The aesthetics of illness and healing in the Nepal
        Himalayas.* Philadelphia: University of Pennsylvania Press.
Desjarlais, R., L. Eisenberg, B. Good, and A. Kleinman, eds.
1995   *World mental health: Problems and priorities in low-income coun-
        tries.* New York: Oxford University Press.
Desjarlais, R., and A. Kleinman
1994   Violence and demoralization in the new world disorder. *Anthro-
        pology Today* 10(5): 9–12.
Devisch, R.
1993   *Weaving the threads of life: The Khita gyn-eco-logical healing cult
        among the Yaka.* Chicago: University of Chicago Press.
Dewey, J.
1957   *Human nature and conduct.* New York: Modern Library.
[1922]
Dressler, W.
1991   Stress and adaptation in the context of culture: Depression in a
        Southern black community. Albany, N.Y.: SUNY Press.
Dreuilhe, E.
1988   *Mortal embrace: Living with AIDS.* New York: Hill and Wang.
Dunn, F.
1979   Behavioral aspects of the control of parasitic diseases. *Bulletin of
        the World Health Organization* 57(4): 499–512.
Dwyer, Ellen
1992   Stories of epilepsy. *Hospital Practice,* Sept. 30:65–92.
Edgerton, R.
1992   *Sick societies: Challenging the myth of primitive harmony.* New York:
        Free Press.
Eisenberg, D., R. C. Kessler, C. Foster, F. E. Norlock, D. R. Calkins, and
        T. L. Delbanco
1993   Unconventional medicine in the United States. *New England Jour-
        nal of Medicine* 328(4): 246–252.

El-Hilu, S. M.
    1990   Social aspects of epilepsy in Kuwait. *International Journal of Social Psychiatry* 36(1): 68–73.
Eliot, George
    1986   *Middlemarch.* Ed. David Carroll. New York: Oxford University Press.
Elvin, M.
    1985   Between the earth and heaven: Conceptions of the self in China. In *The category of the person,* ed. M. Carrithers, S. Collins, and S. Lukes. Cambridge: Cambridge University Press.
Emanuel, E. J.
    1991   *The ends of human life: Medical ethics in a liberal polity.* Cambridge: Harvard University Press.
Fabrega, H.
    1974   *Disease and social behavior: An interdisciplinary perspective.* Cambridge: M.I.T. Press.
    1990   An ethnomedical perspective on medical ethics. *Journal of Medical Philosophy* 15:592–627.
Farmer, P.
    1992   *AIDS and accusation: Haiti and the geography of blame.* Berkeley, Los Angeles, Oxford: University of California Press.
Farmer, P., and A. Kleinman
    1989   AIDS as human suffering. *Daedalus* 118(2): 135–162.
Farquhar, J.
    1994   *Knowing practice: The clinical encounter of Chinese medicine.* Boulder, Colo.: Westview Press.
Favazza, A.
    1987   *Bodies under siege: Self-mutilation in culture and psychiatry.* Baltimore: Johns Hopkins University Press.
Fei X. T.
    1992   *From the soil: The foundations of Chinese society.* Trans. G. G. Hamilton and W. Zheng. Berkeley, Los Angeles, Oxford: University of California Press.
Feld, S.
    1982   *Sound and sentiment: Birds, weeping, poetics, and song in Kaluli expression.* Philadelphia: University of Pennsylvania Press.
Feld, S., and A. A. Fox
    1994   Music and language. *Annual Review of Anthropology* 23:25–54.
Fernandez, J. W.
    1990   Tolerance in a repugnant world and other dilemmas in the cultural relativism of Melville J. Herskovits. *Ethos* 18(2): 140–164.
Field, M. J.
    1960   *Search for security: An ethno-psychiatric study in rural Ghana.* London: Faber and Faber.
Fleck, L.
    1979   *Genesis and development of a scientific fact.* Chicago: University of Chicago Press.

Foucault, M.
   1972   *The archaeology of knowledge.* Trans. A. M. Sheridan Smith. New York: Pantheon.
   1973   *The birth of the clinic.* New York: Pantheon.
   1980   *Power/knowledge: Selected interviews and other writings, 1972–1977.* New York: Pantheon.
   1985   *The use of pleasure.* New York: Vintage.
Fox, R.
   1990   The evolution of American bioethics. In *Social science perspectives on medical ethics,* ed. G. Weisz. Hingham, Mass.: Kluwer.
Fox, R., and P. Swazey
   1984   Medical morality is not bioethics—Medical ethics in China and the United States. *Perspectives in Biology and Medicine* 27(3): 336–340.
Frank, J.
   1974   *Persuasion and healing.* New York: Schocken.
Frankel, S.
   1986   *Huli response to illness.* Cambridge: Cambridge University Press.
Frankl, V.
   1967   *The doctor and the soul.* New York: Bantam.
   [1946]
Freidson, G.
   1986   *Professional powers.* Chicago: University of Chicago Press.
Frenk, J., J. L. Bobadilla, J. Sepúlveda, and M. López Cervantes
   1989   Health transition in middle-income countries. *Health Policy Planning* 4(1): 29–39.
Freudenberg, W. R.
   1993   Risk and recreancy: Weber, the division of labor, and the rationality of risk perceptions. *Social Forces* 71(4): 909–932.
Frye, N.
   1982   *The great code: The bible and literature.* New York: Harcourt Brace Jovanovich.
Fussell, P.
   1975   *The great war and modern memory.* New York: Oxford University Press.
Garcia, J.
   ms.   Dimensions of cultural relativity in the moral realm. Unpublished.
Geertz, C.
   1987   *Local knowledge.* New York: Basic Books.
   1988   *Works and lives: The anthropologist as author.* Stanford, Calif.: Stanford University Press.
Giddens, A.
   1991   *Modernity and self-identity: Self and society in the late modern age.* Stanford, Calif.: Stanford University Press.
Gilbert, M.
   1989   *Second World War: A complete history.* New York: Henry Holt.
Ginsburg, F.
   1989   *Contested lives: The abortion debate in an American community.* Berkeley, Los Angeles, Oxford: University of California Press.

Ginzburg, C.
    1982   *The cheese and the worms: The cosmos of a sixteenth-century miller.*
            Trans. J. Tedeschi and A. Tedeschi. New York and London: Pen-
            guin Books.
Gladney, D.
    1993   The Muslim face of China. *Current History* 92(575): 275–280.
Goffman, E.
    1963   *Stigma.* New York: Simon and Schuster.
Good, B. J.
    1977   The heart of what's the matter: The semantics of illness in Iran.
            Culture, Medicine, and Psychiatry 1:25–28.
    1994   *Medicine, rationality, and experience.* Cambridge: Cambridge Uni-
            versity Press.
Good, B. J., and M.-J. Good
    1994   In the subjunctive mode: Epilepsy narratives in Turkey. *Social Sci-
            ence and Medicine* 38:855–862.
Good, M.-J.
    1992a   Local knowledge: Research capacity building in international health.
            Social Science and Medicine 35(11): 1359–1367.
    1992b   Research capacity building in international health: Definitions, eval-
            uations, and strategies for success. *Social Science and Medicine*
            35(11): 1321–1324.
Good, M.-J., P. Brodwin, B. Good, and A. Kleinman, eds.
    1992   *Pain as human experience: An anthropological perspective.* Berke-
            ley, Los Angeles, London: University of California Press.
Good, M.-J., Linda Hunt, T. Munakata, and Y. Kobayashi
    1992   A comparative analysis of the culture of biomedicine: Disclosure
            and consequence for treatment and the practice of oncology in
            the United States, Japan, and Mexico. In *Sociological perspectives
            on international health,* ed. Peter Conrad and Eugene Gallagher.
            Philadelphia: Temple University Press.
Gordon, D. R.
    1988   Tenacious assumptions in Western medicine. In *Biomedicine ex-
            amined,* ed. M. Lock and D. R. Gordon. Boston: Kluwer.
Gordon, D.
    1991   Female circumcision and genital operations in Egypt and the Su-
            dan: A dilemma for medical anthropology. *Medical Anthropology
            Quarterly* 5(1): 3–14.
Granet, M.
    1968   *La Pensée Chinoise.* Paris: Editions Albin Michel.
Gregory, C.
    1982   *Gifts and commodities.* London: Academic Press.
Grunebaum, G.
    1982   The movement against clitoridectory and infibulation in Sudan.
            Medical Anthropology Newsletter 13:4–12.
Guarnaccia, P., V. DeLaCancela, and E. Carrillo
    1989   The multiple meanings of ataques de nervios in the Latino com-
            munity. *Medical Anthropology* 11:47–62.

Guarnaccia, P., B. Good, and A. Kleinman
    1990   A critical review of epidemiological studies of Puerto Rican mental health. *American Journal of Psychiatry* 147(11): 1449–1456.
Gusfield, J. R.
    1981   *The culture of public problems: Drinking-driving and the symbolic order.* Chicago: University of Chicago Press.
Gussow, Z., and G. Tracy
    1970   Stigma and the leprosy phenomenon. *Bulletin of the History of Medicine* 44:425–449.
Gutmann, A.
    1993   The challenge of multiculturalism in political ethics. *Philosophy and Public Affairs* 22:171–206.
Hallie, P.
    1979   *Lest innocent blood be shed.* New York: Harper and Row.
Hallowell, A. I.
    1967   *Culture and experience.* Philadelphia: University of Pennsylvania
    [1955]   Press.
Harrington, A.
    In press   *Hunger for wholeness: Holistic science and German culture, 1890–1945.* Princeton, N.J.: Princeton University Press.
Hauser, W. A.
    1993   The natural history of seizures. In *The Treatment of Epilepsy,* ed. E. Wyllie. Philadelphia: Lea and Febiger.
Heggenhougen, K.
    1988   *Traditional medicine and primary health care.* London: London School of Hygiene and Tropical Medicine Publication.
    1990   *Medical anthropology and primary health care.* London: London School of Hygiene and Tropical Medicine Publication.
Helman, C.
    1992   *Culture, health, and society.* 2d ed. Boston: Wright.
Henderson, G.
    1990   Increased inequality in health care in China. In *China on the eve of Tiananmen,* ed. D. Davis and E. Vogel. Cambridge: Harvard University Press.
Heritier, F.
    1983   Sterilité, aridité, secheresse: Quelques invariants de la pensée symbolique. In *Le Sens du mal,* ed. M. Auge and C. Herzlich. Paris: Editions des Archives Contemporaries.
Herzfeld, M.
    1987   *Anthropology through the looking-glass: Critical ethnography in the margins of Europe.* Cambridge: Cambridge University Press.
Hilbert, R. A.
    1984   The acultural dimension of chronic pain: Flawed reality construction and the problem of measuring. *Social Problems* 31(4): 365–378.
Hillier, S. M., and J. A. Jewell
    1983   *Health care and traditional medicine in China, 1800–1982.* London and Boston: Routledge and Kegan Paul.

Hoffmaster, B.
    1992   Can ethnography save the life of medical ethics? *Social Science and Medicine* 35(12): 1421–1432.
Hsu, F.
    1985   Field work, cultural differences, and interpretations. In *The Chinese family and its ritual behavior,* ed. J. C. Hsieh and Y. C. Chuang. Taipei: Institute of Ethnology, Academic Sinica.
Huang, S. M.
    1989   *The spiral road.* Boulder: Westview.
Hunt, L.
    1992   Cancer in Oaxaca. Ph.D. diss., Department of Anthropology, Harvard University, Cambridge, Mass.
Hwang, K. K.
    1987   Face and favor: The Chinese power game. *American Journal of Sociology* 92(4): 944–974.
Idler, E.
    1992   Self-assessed health and morality: A review of studies. In *International Review of Health Psychology,* ed. S. Maes, H. Leventhal, and M. Johnston. New York: Wiley.
Idler, E., S. V. Kasl, and J. H. Lemke
    1990   Self-evaluated health and mortality among the elderly. *American Journal of Epidemiology* 131(1): 91–103.
Ingstad, B.
    1992   Care for the elderly, care by the elderly: The role of elderly women in a changing Tswana society. *Journal of Cross-Cultural Gerontology* 7:379–398.
Jackson, M.
    1989   *Paths toward a clearing: Radical empiricism and ethnographic inquiry.* Bloomington: Indiana University Press.
Jacoby, A.
    1992   Epilepsy and quality of everyday life. *Social Science and Medicine* 26:657–666.
Jakubowska, L.
    1990   Political drama in Poland: The use of national symbols. *Anthropology Today* 6(4): 10–13.
James, W.
    1981   The consciousness of self. In *The principles of psychology.* Cam-
    [1890]   bridge: Harvard University Press.
Janes, C. R., R. Stall, and S. Gifford
    1986   *Anthropology and epidemiology.* Hingham, Mass.: Kluwer.
Janzen, J.
    1978   *The quest for therapy in Lower Zaire.* Berkeley, Los Angeles, London: University of California Press.
    1992   *Ngoma: Discourses of healing in Central and Southern Africa.* Berkeley, Los Angeles, Oxford: University of California Press.
Jecker, N., J. Carrese, and R. A. Pearlman
    1995   Caring for patients in cross-cultural settings. *Hastings Center Reports* 25(1): 6–14.

Jennings, B.
  1990   Ethics and ethnography in neonatal intensive care. In *Social science perspectives on medical ethics*, ed. G. Weisz. Hingham, Mass.: Kluwer.
Jensen, R., and M. Dam
  1992   Public attitudes toward epilepsy in Denmark. *Epilepsia* 33(3): 459–463.
Jilek-Aall, L., and H. T. Rwiza
  1992   Prognosis of epilepsy in a rural African community. *Epilepsia* 33(4): 645–650.
Jones, E. E.
  1984   *Social stigma: The psychology of marked relationships.* New York: Freeman.
Justice, J.
  1985   *Policies, plans, and people.* Berkeley, Los Angeles, London: University of California Press.
Keegan, J.
  1976   *The face of battle.* New York: Viking Press.
Keen, D.
  1994   In Africa, planned suffering. *New York Times,* 15 August, p. A15.
Kekes, J.
  1993   *The morality of pluralism.* Princeton, N.J.: Princeton University Press.
Kendall, C.
  1988   The implementation of a diarrheal disease control program in Honduras. *Social Science and Medicine* 27(1): 17–23.
Keyes, C.
  1985   The interpretive basis of depression. In *Culture and depression,* ed. A. Kleinman and B. Good. Berkeley, Los Angeles, London: University of California Press.
King, A.
  1991   *Kuan-hsi* and network building. *Daedalus* 120(2): 63–84.
Kirk, S. A., and H. Kutchins
  1992   *The selling of DSM: The rhetoric of science in psychiatry.* New York: Aldine De Gruyter.
Kleinman, A.
  1977   Depression, somatization, and the new cross-cultural psychiatry. *Social Science and Medicine* 11:3–10.
  1980   *Patients and healers in the context of culture: An exploration of the borderland between anthropology, medicine, and psychiatry.* Berkeley, Los Angeles, London: University of California Press.
  1982   Problèmes culturels associes aux recherches cliniques dans les pays en voie de developpement. In *Cahiers de bioethique: Médecine et experimentation.* Quebec: Les Presses de l'Université Leval.
  1986   *Social origins of distress and disease: Neurasthenia, depression, and pain in modern China.* New Haven, Conn.: Yale University Press.
  1988a   *The illness narratives: Suffering, healing, and the human condition.* New York: Basic Books.

1988b   *Rethinking psychiatry: From cultural category to personal experience.* New York: Free Press.

1992   Pain and resistance: The delegitimation and relegitimation of local worlds. In *Pain as human experience: An anthropological perspective,* ed. M.-J. Good, P. Brodwin, B. Good, A. Kleinman. Berkeley, Los Angeles, Oxford: University of California Press.

Kleinman, A., and J. Kleinman

1985   Somatization. In *Culture and depression,* ed. A. Kleinman and B. Good. Berkeley, Los Angeles, London: University of California Press.

1991   Suffering and its professional transformations: Toward an ethnography of experience. *Culture, Medicine and Psychiatry* 15(3): 275–301.

1994   How bodies remember: Social memory and bodily experience of criticism, resistance, and delegitimation following China's Cultural Revolution. *New Literary History* 25:707–723.

in press-a   Morality and health in Chinese society. In *Morality and Health,* ed. A. Brandt and P. Rozin. New York: Routledge.

in press-b   The appeal of experience, the dismay of images: Cultural appropriations of suffering in our time. *Daedalus.*

Kleinman, A., and J. Gale

1982   Patients treated by physicians and folk healers: A comparative outcome study in Taiwan. *Culture, Medicine and Psychiatry* 6(4): 405–423.

Korbin, J., ed.

1981   *Child abuse and neglect: Crosscultural perspectives.* Berkeley, Los Angeles, London: University of California Press.

Kotarba, J.

1983   *Chronic pain: Its social dimensions.* Beverly Hills, Calif.: Sage Publications.

Kristoff, N.

1993   China's crackdown on births: A stunning and harsh success. *New York Times,* 25 April, pp. A1 and A12.

Kunstadter, P.

1980   Medical ethics in cross-cultural perspective. *Social Science and Medicine* 14B:289–296.

1990   Health transition in Thailand. In *Health transitions,* ed. J. Caldwell, S. Findley, P. Caldwell, G. Santow, W. Cosford, J. Braid, and D. Broers-Freeman. Canberra: Australian National University Press.

Laderman, C.

1991   *Taming the winds of desire: Psychology, medicine, and aesthetics in Malay shamanistic performance.* Berkeley, Los Angeles, Oxford: University of California Press.

Lai, C. W., X. S. Huang, Y. H. Lai, Z. Q. Zhang, G. S. Liu, and M. Z. Yang

1990   Survey of public awareness, understanding, and attitudes toward epilepsy in Hunan Province, China. *Epilepsia* 31(2): 182–187.

Latour, B.

1988   *The pasteurization of France.* Cambridge: Harvard University Press.

Lazarus, R., and R. Launier
  1978   Stress-related transitions between persons and environment. In
          Perspectives in international psychology, ed. L. Pervin and M. Lewis.
          New York: Plenum.
Lefebvre, H.
  1991   *The production of space*. Trans. D. Nicholson-Smith. Oxford: Basil
          Blackwell.
Legge, J., ed.
  1960   *The Chinese classics*. Vol. 4. Oxford: Oxford University Press.
  [1935]
Leslie, C., ed.
  1976   *Asian medical systems*. Berkeley: University of California Press.
Leslie, C., and A. Young, eds.
  1992   *Paths to Asian medical knowledge*. Berkeley, Los Angeles, Oxford:
          University of California Press.
Levi, P.
  1988   *The drowned and the saved*. Trans. from the Italian by Raymond
          Rosenthal. New York: Summit Books.
Levinas, E.
  1988   Useless suffering. In *The provocation of Levinas*, ed. R. Bernagconi
          and D. Wood. London: Routledge.
Lewis, G.
  1975   *Knowledge of illness in a Sepik society*. London: Athlone Press.
  1980   *Day of shining red: An essay on understanding ritual*. Cambridge:
          Cambridge University Press.
Li, S. C., B. S. Schoenberg, C. C. Wang, X. M. Cheng, S. S. Zhou, and C. L.
          Bolis
  1985   Epidemiology of epilepsy in urban areas of the People's Republic
          of China. *Epilepsia* 26(5): 391–394.
Li, S. X., and M. Phillips
  1990   Witchdoctors and mental illness in Mainland China. *American
          Journal of Psychiatry* 147:221–224.
Liang, H., and J. Shapiro
  1983   *Son of the revolution*. New York: Alfred A. Knopf.
Lieban, R.
  1990   Medical anthropology and the comparative study of medical ethics.
          In *Social science perspectives on medical ethics*, ed. G. Weisz. Hing-
          ham, Mass.: Kluwer.
Lin, N.
  1988   Chinese family structure and Chinese society. *Bulletin of Institute
          of Ethnology. Academica Sinica* (Taiwan) 65:59–129.
Lindholm, C.
  1990   *Charisma*. Cambridge, Mass.: Basil Blackwell.
Littlewood, R.
  1993   *Pathology and identity: The work of mother earth in Trinidad*.
          Cambridge: Cambridge University Press.
Liu, B. Y.
  1990   *A higher kind of loyalty*. New York: Pantheon.

Lock, M.
  1993a   *Encounters with aging: Mythologies of menopause in Japan and North America.* Berkeley, Los Angeles, Oxford: University of California Press.
  1993b   The politics of mid-life and menopause: Ideologies for the second sex in North America and Japan. In *Knowledge, power, and practice: The anthropology of medicine and everyday life,* ed. S. Lindenbaum and M. Lock. Berkeley, Los Angeles, Oxford: University of California Press.
  1995   Contesting the natural in Japan: Moral dilemmas and technologies of dying. *Culture, Medicine, and Psychiatry* 19(1): 1–38.

Lock, M., and C. Honda
  1990   Reaching consensus about death: Heart transplants and cultural identity in Japan. In *Social science perspectives on medical ethics,* ed. G. Weisz. Hingham, Mass.: Kluwer.

Lock, M., and D. Gordon, eds.
  1988   *Biomedicine reexamined.* Hingham, Mass.: Kluwer.

Loewy, E.
  1991   *Suffering and the beneficent community.* Albany, N.Y.: SUNY Press.

Lu H. [Lu X.]
  1963   *Selected stories.* Trans. H. Y. and Gladys Yang. Peking: Foreign Languages Press.

MacCormack, C.
  1992   Health care and the concept of legitimacy in Sierra Leone. In *The social basis of health and healing in Africa,* ed. S. Feierman and J. Janzen. Berkeley, Los Angeles, Oxford: University of California Press.

Madan, T. N.
  1980   *Doctors and society: Three Asian case studies.* Sahabadad and New York: Vikas.

Manderson, L., and P. Aaby
  1992   An epidemic in the field: Rapid assessment procedures and health. *Social Science and Medicine* 35(7): 839–850.

Manderson, L., ed.
  1987   Hot-cold food and medical theories. *Social Science and Medicine* 25(4): 329–417.

Manning, O.
  1981   *The Balkan trilogy.* New York: Penguin.
  [1960]

Marcus, G., and M. Fischer
  1986   *Anthropology as cultural critique.* Chicago: University of Chicago Press.

Marsden, R.
  1984   *Mortality and power in a Chinese village.* Berkeley, Los Angeles, London: University of California Press.

Marshall, P. A.
  1992   Anthropology and bioethics. *Medical Anthropology Quarterly* 6(1): 49–73.

Martin, E.
1987   *The woman in the body.* Boston: Beacon Press.
McGuire, M.
1988   *Ritual healing in suburban America.* New Brunswick, N.J.: Rutgers University Press.
Melzack, R.
1989   Phantom limbs, the self, and the brain. *Canadian Psychology* 30: 1–16.
Merleau-Ponty, M.
1962   *Phenomenology of perception.* London: Routledge and Kegan Paul.
Mintz, A.
1984   *Hurban: Response to catastrophe in Hebrew literature.* New York: Columbia University Press.
Mizrahi, T.
1986   *Getting rid of patients: Contradictions in the socialization of physicians.* New Brunswick, N.J.: Rutgers University Press.
Montaigne, M. de
1992   *The complete essays of Montaigne.* Trans. Donald M. Frame. Stan-
[1958] ford, Calif.: Stanford University Press.
Moore, B.
1978   *Injustice: The social basis of obedience and revolt.* London: Macmillan.
Morris, D.
1991   *Culture of pain.* Berkeley, Los Angeles, Oxford: University of California Press.
Morris, I.
1975   *The nobility of failure.* New York: Holt, Rinehart and Winston.
Murray, C. J. L., and L. C. Chen
1994a Understanding morbidity change. In *Health and social change,* ed. L. C. Chen, A. Kleinman, and N. Ware. Cambridge: Mass.: Harvard University Press.
1994b A conceptual approach to understanding transitions in morbidity. In *Health and social change,* ed. L. C. Chen, N. Ware, and A. Kleinman. Cambridge: Harvard University Press.
Myers, F.
1986   *Pintupi country, Pintupi self.* Washington, D.C.: Smithsonian Institution Press.
Nagel, T.
1986   *The view from nowhere.* New York: Oxford University Press.
Nakayama, S.
1984   *Academic and scientific traditions in China, Japan, and the West.* Trans. J. Dusenberg. Tokyo: Tokyo University Press.
Nations, M.
1986   Epidemiologic research of infectious diseases: Quantitative rigor or rigor mortis?—Insights from ethnomedicine. In *Anthropology and epidemiology,* ed. C. R. Janes, R. Stall, and S. Gifford. Hingham, Mass.: Kluwer.

Nations, M., and L. A. Rebhun
    1988   Angels with wet wings won't fly: Maternal sentiment in Brazil and the image of neglect. *Culture, Medicine and Psychiatry* 12(2): 141–200.

Needham, J.
    1954   *Science and civilization in China.* Vol. II. Cambridge: Cambridge University Press.

Newman, K.
    1989   *Falling from grace: Downward social mobility in the American middle class.* New York: Random House.

Nichter, M.
    1989   *Anthropology and international health: South Asian case studies.* Boston: Kluwer.

Nichter, M., and C. Kendall
    1991   Beyond child survival: Anthropology and international health in the 1990s. *Medical Anthropology Quarterly* 5(3): 195–203.

Nkwi, P. N., and F. T. Ndonko
    1989   The epileptic among the Bamileke of Maham in the NDe Division, West Province of Cameroon. *Culture, Medicine and Psychiatry* 13:437–448.

Nussbaum, M.
    1990   *Love's knowledge.* New York: Oxford University Press.

Oakeshott, M.
    1985   Experience and its modes. Cambridge: Cambridge University
    [1933] Press.

Ohnuki-Tierney, E.
    1994   Brain death and organ transplantation: Cultural bases of medical technology. *Current Anthropology* 35(3): 233–242.

Ong, A.
    1987   *Spirits of resistance and capitalist discipline: Factory women in Malaysia.* Albany, N.Y.: SUNY Press.

Osterweis, M., A. Kleinman, and D. Mechanic, eds.
    1987   *Pain and disability: Clinical, behavioral, and public policy perspectives.* Washington, D.C.: National Academy Press.

Ortner, S. B.
    1994   Theory in anthropology since the sixties. In *Culture/power/history,* ed. N. B. Dirks, G. Eley, and S. B. Ortner. Princeton, N.J.: Princeton University Press.

Oxfeld, E.
    1992   Individualism, holism, and the market mentality: Notes on the recollection of two Chinese entrepreneurs. *Cultural Anthropology* 7(3): 267–300.

Parry, J., and M. Bloch
    1989   Introduction. In *Money and the morality of exchange,* ed. J. Parry and M. Bloch. New York: Cambridge University Press.

Pellegrino, E. D.
    1993   The metamorphosis of medical ethics: A thirty-year retrospective. *Journal of the American Medical Association* 269(9): 1158–1162.

Phillips, M.
1993   Strategies used by Chinese families in coping with schizophrenia. In *Chinese families in the 1980s,* ed. D. Davis and S. Harrell. Berkeley, Los Angeles, Oxford: University of California Press.
Pick, D.
1989   *Faces of degeneration: A European disorder, 1848–1918.* Cambridge: Cambridge University Press.
Plessner, J.
1970   *Laughing and crying: A study of the limits of human behavior.* Evanston, Ill.: Northwestern University Press.
Plough, A. L.
1981   Medical technology and the crisis of experience. *Social Science and Medicine* 15F:89–101.
Polanyi, M., and H. Prosch
1975   *Meaning.* Chicago: University of Chicago Press.
Potter, S. H.
1988   The cultural construction of emotion in rural Chinese social life. *Ethos* 16(2): 181–208.
Proctor, R.
1988   *Racial hygiene: Medicine under the Nazis.* Cambridge: Harvard University Press.
Putnam, H.
1981   *Reason, truth, and history.* Cambridge: Cambridge University Press.
1987   *The many faces of realism.* La Salle, Ill.: Open Court.
1989   Model, theory, and the factuality of semantics. In *Reflections on Chomsky,* ed. A. George. Oxford: Basil Blackwell.
1993   Objectivity and the science-ethics distinction. In *The quality of life,* ed. M. Nussbaum and A. Sen. Oxford: Clarendon Press.
Ramphele, M.
1993   Adolescents and violence in South Africa. Working Papers, World Mental Health, Center for the Study of Culture and Medicine, Department of Social Medicine, Harvard Medical School.
Read, K.
1955   Morality and the concept of the person among the Gahuku-Gama. *Oceania* 25(4): 233–282.
Reid, J.
1983   *Sorcerers and healing spirits.* Canberra: Australian National University Press.
Reilly, B. J., and M. J. Kyj
1994   Meta-ethical reasoning: Applied to economics and business principles. *American Journal of Economics and Sociology* 53(2): 142–162.
Rhodes, L.
1991   *Emptying beds: The work of an emergency psychiatric unit.* Berkeley: University of California Press.

Rogler, L.
   1990   The meanings of culturally sensitive research in mental health. *American Journal of Psychiatry* 146: 296–303.
Rosaldo, M.
   1980   *Knowledge and power: Ilongot notions of self and social life*. Cambridge: Cambridge University Press.
Rosaldo, R.
   1984   Grief and a headhunter's rage: On the cultural force of emotions. In *Text, play, and story: The construction and reconstruction of self and society*, ed. S. Plattner and E. Bruner. Washington, D.C.: American Ethnological Society.
Roseman, M.
   1990   Head, heart, odor, and shadow: The structure of the self, the emotional world, and ritual performance among senior Temiar. *Ethos* 18(3): 227–250.
   1991   *Healing sounds from the Malaysian rainforest: Temiar music and medicine*. Berkeley, Los Angeles, Oxford: University of California Press.
Rosenberg, C.
   1985   The therapeutic revolution. In *Sickness and health in America*, 2d ed., ed. J. Leavitt and R. Numbers. Madison: University of Wisconsin Press.
   1987   *The care of strangers: The rise of America's hospital system*. New York: Basic Books.
Rothman, D. J.
   1990   Human experimentation and the origins of bioethics in the United States. In *Social science perspectives on medical ethics*, ed. G. Weisz. Hingham, Mass.: Kluwer.
   1991   *Strangers at the bedside: A history of how law and bioethics transformed medical decision making*. New York: Basic Books.
Rouget, G.
   1985   *Music and trance*. Trans. D. Coltman and B. Biebayck. Chicago: University of Chicago Press.
Rubel, A., C. W. O'Nell, and R. Collado-Ardón
   1984   *Susto, a folk illness*. Berkeley, Los Angeles, London: University of California Press.
Said, E.
   1978   *Orientalism*. New York: Pantheon.
Santiago, D.
   1990   The aesthetics of terror, the hermeneutics of death. *America* 162(11): 292–294.
Sargent, C.
   1989   *Maternity, medicine, and power: Reproductive decisions in urban Benin*. Berkeley, Los Angeles, London: University of California Press.
Sartre, J. P.
   1956   *Being and nothingness: An essay on phenomenological ontology*. Trans. H. E. Barnes. New York: Philosophical Library.

Scarry, E.
1985   *The body in pain.* New York: Oxford University Press.
Scheff, T.
1979   *Catharsis in healing, ritual, and drama.* Berkeley, Los Angeles, London: University of California Press.
Scheler, M.
1971   *Man's place in nature.* Trans. H. Meyerhoff. New York: Noonday
[1928] Press.
Scheper-Hughes, N.
1992   *Death without weeping: The violence of everyday life in Brazil.* Berkeley: University of California Press.
1987   *Child survival.* Hingham, Mass.: Reidel/Kluwer.
Schieffelin, E.
1976   *The sorrow of the lonely and the burning of the dancers.* New York: St. Martin's Press.
1985   The cultural analysis of depressive affect: An example from New Guinea. In *Culture and depression,* ed. A. Kleinman and B. Good. Berkeley, Los Angeles, London: University of California Press.
Schutz, A.
1968   *On phenomenology and social relations.* Chicago: University of Chicago Press.
Schwarcz, V.
1991   Mnemosyne abroad: Reflections on the Chinese and Jewish commitment to remembrance. *Points East* 6(3): 1–16.
Scott, J. C.
1976   *The moral economy of the peasant.* New Haven, Conn.: Yale University Press.
1985   *The weapons of the weak.* New Haven, Conn.: Yale University Press.
1990   *Domination and the arts of resistance: Hidden transcripts.* New Haven, Conn.: Yale University Press.
Scrimshaw, S., and E. Hartado
1987   *Rapid assessment procedures for nutrition and primary health care: Anthropological approaches to improving program effectiveness.* Los Angeles: UCLA Latin American Center Publications.
Sen, A.
1994   Objectivity and position: Assessment of health and well-being. In *Health and social changes,* ed. L. C. Chen, A. Kleinman, and N. Ware. Cambridge: Harvard University Press.
Seremetakis, N.
1991   *The last word: Women, death, and divination in inner Mani.* Chicago: University of Chicago Press.
Shore, B.
1990   Human ambivalence and the structuring of moral values. *Ethos* 18(2): 165–179.
Showalter, E.
1985   *The female malady: Women, madness, and English culture, 1830–1980.* New York: Pantheon.

Shweder, R.
    1985   Menstrual pollution, soul loss, and the comparative study of emotions. In *Culture and Depression,* ed. A. Kleinman and B. Good. Berkeley, Los Angeles, London: University of California Press.
    1990   Ethical relativism: Is there a defensible version? *Ethos* 18(2): 205–218.
    1991   *Thinking through culture.* Cambridge: Harvard University Press.
Shweder, R., and R. LeVine, eds.
    1984   *Culture theory.* New York: Cambridge University Press.
Siu, H.
    1989   *Agents and victims in South China.* New Haven, Conn.: Yale University Press.
Sivin, N.
    1987   *Traditional medicine in contemporary China.* Ann Arbor: Center for Chinese Studies, University of Michigan.
Sluga, H.
    1993   *Heidegger's crisis: Philosophy and politics in Nazi Germany.* Cambridge: Harvard University Press.
Sontag, S.
    1989   *AIDS and its metaphors.* New York: Farrar, Straus and Giroux.
Sperber, D., and D. Wilson
    1986   *Relevance: Communication and cognition.* Oxford: Basil Blackwell.
Stagna, S. J.
    1993   Psychiatric aspects of epilepsy. In *The treatment of epilepsy,* ed. E. Wyllie. Philadelphia: Lea and Febiger.
Starr, Paul
    1983   *The social transformation of American medicine.* New York: Basic Books.
Sternbach, R., ed.
    1978   *The psychology of pain.* New York: Raven Press.
Stigler, J. W., R. A. Shweder, and G. H. Herdt, eds.
    1990   *Cultural psychology.* Cambridge: Cambridge University Press.
Stoller, P.
    1989   *The taste of ethnographic things: The senses in anthropology.* Philadelphia: University of Pennsylvania Press.
Stouffer, S. A.
    1949   *The American soldier: Combat and its aftermath.* Vol. 2. Princeton, N.J.: Princeton University Press.
Strauss, A., ed.
    1970   *Where medicine fails.* New York: Transaction.
Tambiah, S.
    1990   *Magic, science, religion, and the scope of rationality.* New York: Cambridge University Press.
    1993   Friends, neighbors, enemies, strangers: Aggressor and victim in civilian ethnic riots. Working Paper, Center for the Study of Culture and Medicine, Department of Social Medicine, Harvard Medical School.

Taussig, M.
  1980   *The devil and commodity fetishism in South America.* Chapel Hill: University of North Carolina Press.
  1987   *Shamanism, colonialism, and the wild man.* Chicago: University of Chicago Press.
Taylor, Charles
  1990   *Sources of the self: The making of the modern identity.* Cambridge: Harvard University Press.
  1992a   *The ethics of authenticity.* Cambridge, Mass.: Harvard University Press.
  1992b   The politics of recognition. In *Multiculturalism and the politics of recognition,* ed. C. Taylor and A. Gutmann. Princeton, N.J.: Princeton University Press.
Taylor, Christopher
  1992   *Milk, honey, and money: Changing concepts in Rwandan healing.* Washington, D.C.: Smithsonian Institute Press.
Tekle-Haimanot, R., M. Abehe, L. Forsgren, A. Gebre-Mariam, J. Heubel, G. Holmgren, and J. Ekstedt
  1991   Attitudes of rural people in central Ethiopia toward epilepsy. *Social Science and Medicine* 32(2): 203–209.
Temkin, O.
  1945   *The falling sickness: A history of epilepsy from the Greeks to the beginnings of modern neurology.* Baltimore: Johns Hopkins University Press.
Thurston, A. F.
  1987   *Enemies of the people: The ordeal of the intellectuals in China's great cultural revolution.* New York: Alfred A. Knopf.
Trawick, M.
  1992   Death and nurturance in Indian systems of healing. In *Paths to Asian medical knowledge,* ed. C. Leslie and A. Young. Berkeley, Los Angeles, Oxford: University of California Press.
Tronto, J. A.
  1993   *Moral boundaries: A political argument for an ethics of care.* New York: Routledge.
Trostle, J. A.
  1988   Medical compliance as ideology. *Social Science and Medicine* 27 (12): 1299–1308.
Trostle, J. A., W. A. Hauser, and I. S. Susser
  1988   The logic of noncompliance: Management of epilepsy from the patient's point of view. *Culture, Medicine and Psychiatry* 7(1): 35–56.
Trostle, J., and J. Simon
  1992   Building applied health research capacity in less developed countries: Problems encountered by the ADDR Project. *Social Science and Medicine* 35(11): 1379–1387.
Tu, W. M.
  1992   Exit from communism. *Daedalus* 12(2): 251–292.

Turk, D. C., D. Meichenbaum, and M. Genest
    1983   *Pain and behavioral medicine: A cognitive-behavioral perspective.*
            New York: Guilford Press.
Turner, V.
    1967   *The forest of symbols.* Ithaca, N.Y.: Cornell University Press.
Unschuld, P.
    1975   Medico-cultural conflicts in Asian settings: An explanatory the-
            ory. *Social Science and Medicine* 9:303–312.
    1979   *Medical ethics in imperial China.* Berkeley, Los Angeles, London:
            University of California Press.
    1985   *Medicine in China: A history of ideas.* Berkeley, Los Angeles,
            London: University of California Press.
    1987   Traditional Chinese medicine: Some historical and epistemologi-
            cal reflections. *Social Science and Medicine* 24(12): 1023–1029.
    1988   Seminar presented to the Medical Anthropology Program, Har-
            vard University, Cambridge, Mass.
    1989   Terminological problems. In *Approaches to traditional Chinese med-
            ical literature.* Boston: Kluwer.
Wagner, R.
    1986   *Symbols that stand for themselves.* Chicago: University of Chicago
            Press.
Waley, A.
    1940   *Translations from the Chinese.* New York: Alfred A. Knopf.
    [1919]
Ware, N., and A. Kleinman
    1992   Culture and somatic experience: The social course of illness in
            neurasthenia and chronic fatigue syndrome. *Psychosomatic Med-
            icine* 54:546–560.
Waxler, N.
    1984   Behavioral convergence and institutional separation: An analysis
            of plural medicine in Sri Lanka. *Culture, Medicine and Psychiatry*
            8(2): 187–205.
Weaver, P.
    1994   Selling the story. *New York Times,* 29 July, p. A27.
Weber, M.
    1978   Theodicy, salvation, and rebirth. In *Economy and society,* vol. 1, ed.
    [1922] G. Roth and C. Wettich. Berkeley, Los Angeles, London: Univer-
            sity of California Press.
Weisberg, D. H., and S. O. Long, eds.
    1984   Biomedicine in Asia. *Culture, Medicine and Psychiatry* 8(2): 117–
            205.
Weiss, M.
    1988   Cultural models of diarrheal illness: Conceptual framework and
            review. *Social Science and Medicine* 27(1): 5–13.
Weisz, G., ed.
    1990   *Social science perspectives on medical ethics.* Hingham, Mass.: Klu-
            wer.

Westerbrook, L. E., L. J. Bauman, and S. Skinner
   1992   Applying stigma theory to epilepsy. *Journal of Pediatric Psychology* 17(5): 633–649.
Whyte, S. R.
   1992   Pharmaceuticals as folk medicine: Transformations in the social relations of health care in Uganda. *Culture, Medicine and Psychiatry* 16(2): 163–186.
Whyte, S. R.
   1995   Constructing epilepsy: Images and contexts in East Africa. In *Disability and culture,* ed. B. Ingstad and S. R. Whyte. Berkeley, Los Angeles, London: University of California Press.
Wikan, U.
   1980   *Life among the poor in Cairo.* London: Tavistock.
   1987   Public grace and private fears: Gaiety, offense, and sorcery in Northern Bali. *Ethos* 15:337–365.
   1989   Illness from fright or soul loss: A North Balinese culture-bound syndrome? *Culture, Medicine and Psychiatry* 13(1): 25–50.
   1990   *Managing turbulent hearts: A Balinese formula for living.* Chicago: University of Chicago Press.
Williams, B.
   1981   Introduction. In *Concepts and categories,* ed. I. Berlin. Harmondsworth, Middlesex: Penguin.
Willms, D.
   1983   Community-based health care programs in Kenya. In *Third World medicine and social change,* ed. J. H. Morgan. New York: University of America Press.
Wing, D. H.
   1976   *Skeptical sociology.* New York: Columbia University Press.
Wong, D. B.
   1984   *Moral relativity.* Berkeley, Los Angeles, London: University of California Press.
World Bank
   1992   *China: Long-term issues and options in the health transition.* Washington, D.C.: World Bank.
Wrong, D.
   1976   Oversocialized conceptions of man in modern sociology. In *Skeptical sociology.* New York: Columbia University Press.
Wyllie, E., ed.
   1993   *The treatment of epilepsy: Principles and practice.* Philadelphia: Lea and Febiger.
Xiong, W., M. Phillips, M. R. Hu, X. Wang, Q. Q. Dai, J. Kleinman, and A. Kleinman
   1994   Family-based intervention for schizophrenic patients in China. *British Journal of Psychiatry* 165(2): 239–247.
Yang, K. S.
   1987   *The Chinese people in change.* Vol. 3, *Collected works on the chinese people.* Taipei: Kuei Kuan Book Co. (In Chinese.)

Yang, L. C., and K. Y. Cao
   1989   Epidemiology of epilepsy in rural and minority areas of China.
           Chinese Journal of Neurosurgery (Supplement) 5:22–28.
Yehoshua, A. B.
   1993   *Mr. Mani*. New York: Harcourt Brace Jovanovich.
Yelin, E., M. Nevitt, and W. Epstein
   1980   Toward an epidemiology of work disability. *Milbank Memorial
           Fund Quarterly/Health and Society* 58(3): 386–415.
You, H. L.
   1994a   Defining rhythm: Aspects of an anthropology of rhythm. *Culture,
           Medicine and Psychiatry* 18(3): 361–384.
   1994b   Rhythm in Chinese thinking: A short question for a long tradi-
           tion. *Culture, Medicine and Psychiatry* 18(4): 463–482.
Young, A.
   1990   Moral conflicts in a psychiatric hospital treating combat-related
           posttraumatic stress disorder. In *Social science perspectives on med-
           ical ethics,* ed. G. Weisz. Hingham, Mass.: Kluwer.
   1993   A description of how ideology shapes knowledge of a mental dis-
           order (posttraumatic stress disorder). In *Knowledge, power, and
           practice: An anthropology of medicine and everyday life,* ed. S. Lin-
           denbaum and M. Lock. Berkeley, Los Angeles, London: Univer-
           sity of California Press.
   In press *The harmony of illusions: An ethnographic account of posttrau-
           matic stress disorder.* Princeton, N.J.: Princeton University Press.
Young, M.
   1990   *Justice and the politics of difference.* Princeton, N.J.: Princeton
           University Press.
Zhang J. B.
   1710   *Qing Yue quan shu* (Qing Yue's Complete Works). Guiji: Guiji
   [1624] Lushi Ranben.
Zhou, S. S.
   1989   Spontaneous remission of epilepsy. *Chinese Journal of Neurosur-
           gery* 5 (Supplement): 31–34.
Zimmermann, F.
   1987   *The jungle and the aroma of meats: An ecological theme in Hindu
           medicine.* Berkeley, Los Angeles, London: University of Califor-
           nia Press.
   1989   *Le discours des remèdes au pays des épices. Enquête sur la médecine
           Hindune.* Paris: Editions Payot.
Zola, Emile
   1969   *Germinal.* Trans. Leonard Tancock. Baltimore: Penguin.
Zussman, M.
   1992   *Intensive care: Medical ethics and the medical profession.* Chicago:
           University of Chicago Press.

Index

Abortion, forced, 183, 185
Aging, in Japan, 250–256
AIDS, 82, 90, 116, 211–218
Alvarado, Louis, 149
American Psychiatric Association, DSM-IIIR of, 177–182; DSM-IV of, 178, 180, 282 n.2
Ames, R. T., 28
Anthropology: and bioethics, 44, 53–67; British, 205, 206; on chronic pain, 121–122; dehumanizes subject, 96–97; delegitimates pain, 96; on doctor-patient relationship, 268 n.4; feminist, 60–61, 232–240; French, 201, 203; on institutions' role, 55–56; and international health, 90–91; on local world, 53–54; medical, 41, 42, 44–45, 149–150, 152, 193–256; and psychology overlap, 196; social, 58, 205, 206; on somatization, 117; on suffering, 100–101, 123
Archilochus, 268 n.1
Aries, Phillippe, 274–275 n.14
Augé, Marc, 201, 203
Augustinian imperative, 27, 28–29
Ayurveda, practice, 27, 28, 36

Balance, in health, 27, 106, 216, 224
Barker, Pat, 249
Becker, Joseph, 14–15
Beiser, Morton, 42
Berger, Peter, 78

Berlin, Isaiah, 268 n.1
Bioethics, 41–67; anthropology contributes to, 44, 53–67; on biomedical settings, 50–52; in Chinese medicine, 43; on chronic pain, 120–121; in Greek medicine, 43; and informed consent, 57; on local context of illness, 54–55; and organ transplants, 43; on patient's perspective, 54–55; suffering ignored by, 50, 51, 52; universalism in, 58; used to control access, 44
Biomedicine, 24; Asian medicine compared to, 29, 34–35; and bioethics, 50–52; on charismatic healing, 33; ethnography of, 241–256; as hard or soft science, 30; institutionalized, 37–38, 39; materialism in, 29–30, 31, 36; monotheism in, 27–28, 29–30; on placebos, 33; professionalized, 38; as progressive, 34–36; role of nature in, 29, 30; as social control, 38–39; suffering ignored in, 31–32; teleology rejected by, 50; on vitalism, 36; as Western, 25–26
Blake, William, 228
Bloch, Maurice, 144
Bloom, Harold, 4
Bolivia, medical pluralism in, 24, 197–201
Bourdieu, Pierre, 76, 97, 123, 223, 229, 240–241
Bourgois, Philippe, 240

Designer: UC Press Staff
Compositor: Prestige Typography
Text: 10/13 Galliard
Display: Galliard
Printer: Haddon Craftsmen, Inc.
Binder: Haddon Craftsmen, Inc.